Robotics in Otolaryngology

Editors

UMAMAHESWAR DUVVURI
ARUN SHARMA
ERICA R. THALER

OTOLARYNGOLOGIC CLINICS OF NORTH AMERICA

www.oto.theclinics.com

Consulting Editor
SUJANA S. CHANDRASEKHAR

December 2020 • Volume 53 • Number 6

ELSEVIER

1600 John F. Kennedy Boulevard • Suite 1800 • Philadelphia, Pennsylvania, 19103-2899

http://www.oto.theclinics.com

OTOLARYNGOLOGIC CLINICS OF NORTH AMERICA Volume 53, Number 6
December 2020 ISSN 0030-6665, ISBN-13: 978-0-323-77838-1

Editor: Stacy Eastman
Developmental Editor: Julia McKenzie

Otolaryngologic Clinics of North America (ISSN 0030-6665) is published bimonthly by Elsevier, Inc., 360 Park Avenue South, New York, NY 10010-1710. Months of issue are February, April, June, August, October, and December. Business and Editorial Offices: 1600 John F. Kennedy Blvd., Suite 1800, Philadelphia, PA 19103-2899. Customer Service Office: 6277 Sea Harbor Drive, Orlando, FL 32887-4800. Periodicals postage paid at New York, NY and additional mailing offices. Subscription prices are $424.00 per year (US individuals), $947.00 per year (US institutions), $100.00 per year (US & Canadian student/resident), $548.00 per year (Canadian individuals), $1200.00 per year (Canadian institutions), $592.00 per year (international individuals), $1200.00 per year (international institutions), $270.00 per year (international student/resident). Foreign air speed delivery is included in all *Clinics*' subscription prices. All prices are subject to change without notice. **POSTMASTER:** Send address changes to *Otolaryngologic Clinics of North America*, Elsevier Health Sciences Division, Subscription Customer Service, 3251 Riverport Lane, Maryland Heights, MO 63043. **Telephone: 1-800-654-2452 (U.S. and Canada); 314-447-8871 (outside U.S. and Canada). Fax: 314-447-8029. E-mail: journalscustomerservice-usa@elsevier.com (for print support); journalsonlinesupport-usa@elsevier.com (for online support).**

Reprints. For copies of 100 or more of articles in this publication, please contact the Commercial Reprints Department, Elsevier Inc., 360 Park Avenue South, New York, NY 10010-1710. Tel.: 212-633-3874; Fax: 212-633-3820; E-mail: reprints@elsevier.com.

Otolaryngologic Clinics of North America is also published in Spanish by McGraw-Hill Interamericana Editores S.A., P.O. Box 5-237, 06500 Mexico D.F., Mexico.

Otolaryngologic Clinics of North America is covered in *MEDLINE/PubMed (Index Medicus), Current Contents/Clinical Medicine, Excerpta Medica, BIOSIS, Science Citation Index,* and *ISI/BIOMED.*

Contributors

CONSULTING EDITOR

SUJANA S. CHANDRASEKHAR, MD, FACS, FAAOHNS
Past President, American Academy of Otolaryngology–Head and Neck Surgery,
Secretary-Treasurer, American Otological Society, Partner, ENT & Allergy Associates,
LLP, Clinical Professor, Department of Otolaryngology–Head and Neck Surgery, Zucker
School of Medicine at Hofstra-Northwell, Hempstead, New York, USA; Clinical Associate
Professor, Department of Otolaryngology–Head and Neck Surgery, Icahn School of
Medicine at Mount Sinai, New York, New York, USA

EDITORS

UMAMAHESWAR DUVVURI, MD, PhD, FACS
Associate Professor of Otolaryngology, University of Pittsburgh Medical Center,
University of Pittsburgh, VA Pittsburgh Health System, Pittsburgh, Pennsylvania,
USA

ARUN SHARMA, MD, MS, FACS
Associate Professor, Division Chief, Head and Neck Surgery, Director of Clinical
Research, Department of Otolaryngology–Head and Neck Surgery, SIU School of
Medicine, Springfield, Illinois, USA

ERICA R. THALER, MD, FACS
Professor and Vice Chair, Directory of General Otorhinolaryngology: Head and
Neck Surgery, Department of Otorhinolaryngology: Head and Neck Surgery, University of
Pennsylvania School of Medicine, Philadelphia, Pennsylvania, USA

ZARA M. PATEL, MD
Associate Professor, Director of Endoscopic Skull Base Surgery, Department of
Otolaryngology–Head and Neck Surgery, Stanford University School of Medicine, Palo
Alto, California, USA

AUTHORS

SYED AHMED ALI, MD
House Officer, Department of Otolaryngology–Head and Neck Surgery, Michigan
Medicine, Ann Arbor, Michigan, USA

ABDALLAH S. ATTIA, MD
Department of Surgery, Tulane University, School of Medicine, New Orleans, Louisiana,
USA

BRANDON J. BAIRD, MD
Department of Surgery, Section of Otolaryngology–Head and Neck Surgery, University of
Chicago, Chicago, Illinois, USA

RANDALL A. BLY, MD
Assistant Professor, Department of Otolaryngology–Head and Neck Surgery, Division of Pediatric Otolaryngology, University of Washington, Seattle Children's Hospital, Seattle, Washington, USA

GRAINNE BRADY, MRes, MRCSLT
Clinical Lead Speech and Language Therapist, Department of Speech, Language and Swallowing, The Royal Marsden NHS Foundation Trust, London, United Kingdom

ROBERT M. BRODY, MD
Assistant Professor, Department of Otorhinolaryngology–Head and Neck Surgery, University of Pennsylvania Health System, Philadelphia, Pennsylvania, USA

JAMES KENNETH BYRD, MD
Associate Professor, Otolaryngology–Head and Neck Surgery, Medical College of Georgia, Augusta University, Augusta, Georgia, USA

MICHELLE M. CHEN, MD, MHS
Clinical Lecturer, Department of Otolaryngology–Head and Neck Surgery, University of Michigan, Ann Arbor, Michigan, USA

DANA L. CROSBY, MD, MPH
Associate Professor, Department of Otolaryngology, SIU School of Medicine, Springfield, Illinois, USA

MORGAN E. DAVIS, MD
Department of Surgery, Division of Otolaryngology–Head and Neck Surgery, UC San Diego School of Medicine, San Diego, CA

JOHN R. DE ALMEIDA, MD, MSc, FRCSC
Departments of Otolaryngology–Head and Neck Surgery, and Surgical Oncology, Princess Margaret Cancer Centre/University Health Network, University of Toronto, Toronto General Hospital, Toronto, Ontario, Canada

JENNIFER E. DOUGLAS, MD
Department of Otorhinolaryngology–Head and Neck Surgery, University of Pennsylvania Health System, Philadelphia, Pennsylvania, USA

UMAMAHESWAR DUVVURI, MD, PhD, FACS
Associate Professor of Otolaryngology, University of Pittsburgh Medical Center, University of Pittsburgh, VA Pittsburgh Health System, Pittsburgh, Pennsylvania, USA

AHMAD ELNAHLA, MD
Department of Surgery, Tulane University, School of Medicine, New Orleans, Louisiana, USA

HUDSON FREY, MD
Resident Physician, Department of Otolaryngology–Head and Neck Surgery, University of Mississippi Medical Center, Jackson, Mississippi, USA

AJITH GEORGE, FRCS
Consultant Head and Neck Surgeon, University Hospitals North Midlands, North Staffordshire, England; Senior Lecturer, Keele University Medical School, Staffordshire, United Kingdom

NEAL RAJAN GODSE, MD
Resident Physician, Department of Otolaryngology, University of Pittsburgh, Pittsburgh, Pennsylvania, USA

DEENA HADEDEYA, MD, MHS
Department of Surgery, Tulane University, School of Medicine, New Orleans, Louisiana, USA

JOHN HARDMAN, BSc (Hons), MSc, MRCS
Head and Neck Unit, The Royal Marsden NHS Foundation Trust, London, United Kingdom; Specialty Registrar in ENT, North London, United Kingdom

MITCHELL HEUERMANN, MD
Resident, Department of Otolaryngology, SIU School of Medicine, Springfield, Illinois, USA

PAUL T. HOFF, MS, MD
Assistant Professor, Department of Otolaryngology–Head and Neck Surgery, Michigan Medicine, Ann Arbor, Michigan, USA

KATHERINE A. HUTCHESON, PhD
Associate Professor, Department of Head and Neck Surgery, Division of Radiation Oncology, The University of Texas at MD Anderson Cancer Center, Houston, Texas, USA

GINA D. JEFFERSON, MD, MPH, FACS
Professor, Department of Otolaryngology–Head and Neck Surgery, University of Mississippi Medical Center, Jackson, Mississippi, USA

EMAD KANDIL, MD, MBA, FACS
Department of Surgery, Tulane University, School of Medicine, New Orleans, Louisiana, USA

CYRUS KERAWALA, FDSRCS, FRCS
Consultant Head and Neck Surgeon, Head and Neck Unit, The Royal Marsden NHS Foundation Trust, London, United Kingdom; Visiting Professor, Faulty of Health and Wellbeing, University of Winchester, Winchester, United Kingdom

NEERAJA KONUTHULA, MD
Department of Otolaryngology–Head and Neck Surgery, Division of Pediatric Otolaryngology, University of Washington, Seattle Children's Hospital, Seattle, Washington, USA

KEVIN J. KOVATCH, MD
House Officer, Department of Otolaryngology–Head and Neck Surgery, Michigan Medicine, Ann Arbor, Michigan, USA

ROBERT F. LABADIE, MD, PhD
Department of Otolaryngology, Vanderbilt University Medical Center, Nashville, Tennessee, USA

KELLY M. MALLOY, MD, FACS
Associate Professor, Department of Otolaryngology–Head and Neck Surgery, University of Michigan, Ann Arbor, Michigan, USA

GUILLERMO MAZA, MD
Department of Otolaryngology–Head and Neck Surgery, SIU School of Medicine, Springfield, Illinois, USA

ALEX P. MICHAEL, MD
Resident, Division of Neurosurgery, Neuroscience Institute, SIU School of Medicine, Springfield, Illinois, USA

VINIDH PALERI, MS, FRCS
Consultant Head and Neck Surgeon, Head and Neck Unit, The Royal Marsden NHS Foundation Trust, Professor of Robotic and Endoscopic Head and Neck Surgery, The Institute of Cancer Research, London, United Kingdom

REBECCA PAQUIN, MD, DMD
Resident, Otolaryngology–Head and Neck Surgery, Medical College of Georgia, Augusta University, Augusta, Georgia, USA

HARMAN S. PARHAR, MD, MPH
Clinical Instructor, Department of Otorhinolaryngology–Head and Neck Surgery, University of Pennsylvania Health System, Philadelphia, Pennsylvania, USA

SANJAY R. PARIKH, MD
Professor, Department of Otolaryngology–Head and Neck Surgery, Division of Pediatric Otolaryngology, University of Washington, Seattle Children's Hospital, Seattle, Washington, USA

DIEGO PRECIADO, MD, PhD
Vice-Chief and Fellowship Program Director, Pediatric Otolaryngology, Children's National Health System, Professor of Surgery and Pediatrics, George Washington University School of Medicine, Washington, DC, USA

CHRISTOPHER H. RASSEKH, MD
Department of Otorhinolaryngology–Head and Neck Surgery, University of Pennsylvania Health System, Philadelphia, Pennsylvania, USA

SCOTT M. RICKERT, MD, FACS
Chief, Division of Pediatric Otolaryngology, Associate Professor, Department of Otolaryngology, Pediatrics, and Plastic Surgery, Hassenfeld Children's Hospital at NYU Langone, NYU Langone Health, New York, New York, USA

KATHERINE E. RIOJAS, BS
Department of Mechanical Engineering, Vanderbilt University, Nashville, Tennessee, USA

ROSH K.V. SETHI, MD, MPH
Associate Surgeon, Division of Otolaryngology–Head and Neck Surgery, Brigham and Women's Hospital, Boston, Massachusetts, USA

ARUN SHARMA, MD, MS, FACS
Associate Professor, Division Chief, Head and Neck Surgery, Director of Clinical Research, Department of Otolaryngology–Head and Neck Surgery, SIU School of Medicine, Springfield, Illinois, USA

AREEJ SHIHABI, MD
Department of Surgery, Tulane University, School of Medicine, New Orleans, Louisiana, USA

STEVEN E. SOBOL, MD, MSc, FRCS(C)
Fellowship Program Director, Division of Otolaryngology, Associate Professor, Department of Otorhinolaryngology–Head and Neck Surgery, Children's Hospital of

Philadelphia, Perelman School of Medicine, University of Pennsylvania, Philadelphia, Pennsylvania, USA

C. KWANG SUNG, MD, MS
Division of Laryngology, Department of Otolaryngology–Head and Neck Surgery, Stanford University, Stanford, California, USA

ERICA R. THALER, MD, FACS
Professor and Vice Chair, Directory of General Otorhinolaryngology–Head and Neck Surgery, Department of Otorhinolaryngology–Head and Neck Surgery, University of Pennsylvania School of Medicine, Philadelphia, Pennsylvania, USA

ESTHER X. VIVAS, MD
Associate Professor, Department of Otolaryngology–Head and Neck Surgery, Emory University School of Medicine, Atlanta, Georgia, USA

BENJAMIN WAHLE, MD
Resident Physician, Department of Otolaryngology–Head and Neck Surgery, Washington University School of Medicine, St Louis, Missouri, USA

CHRISTOPHER Z. WEN, BA
Perelman School of Medicine, University of Pennsylvania, Philadelphia, Pennsylvania, USA

CAROL H. YAN, MD
Assistant Professor of Rhinology and Skull Base Surgery, Department of Surgery, Division of Otolaryngology–Head and Neck Surgery, UC San Diego School of Medicine, San Diego, CA

CHRISTOPHER M.K.L. YAO, MD
Fellow, Advanced Head and Neck Surgical Oncology and Microvascular Reconstruction, Department of Head and Neck Surgery, The University of Texas at MD Anderson Cancer Center, Houston, Texas, USA

CHRISTINA M. YVER, MD
Resident Physician, Department of Otorhinolaryngology–Head and Neck Surgery, University of Pennsylvania Health System, Philadelphia, Pennsylvania, USA

JOSE ZEVALLOS, MD, MPH
Division Chief of Head and Neck Surgery, Joseph B. Kimbrough Professor, Department of Otolaryngology–Head and Neck Surgery, Washington University School of Medicine, St Louis, Missouri, USA

TOBY SHEN ZHU, BS
Medical Student, University of Pittsburgh, School of Medicine, Pittsburgh, Pennsylvania, USA

Contents

> Robotic-assisted surgery embodies the latest in technological advancement and is being applied to operative management of patients. The current concept of robotic surgery involves performance of surgical procedures by using small wristed instruments attached to a robotic arm. Its extension to otolaryngology is only natural, because it allows for precise surgery through anatomic orifices, often allowing for preservation of critical anatomic structures and functions. Transoral robotic surgery is an effective and safe tool for head and neck surgeons. Its speed of recent growth and the imminent addition of innovative technology could signal the advent of a new era in surgery.

> The development and acceptance of transoral robotic surgery from an experimental procedure to widespread acceptance in the management of head and neck cancers and other disease states occurred over the course of about a decade, from 2005 to 2015. Transoral robotic surgery has cemented its' place in the treatment of pharyngeal and laryngeal cancer. Education and training was key to broad use and acceptance. This article traces the history and evolution of transoral robotic surgery to its current practice. The process of surgical innovation in this arena is followed from early cadaveric studies to recent large systemic reviews of outcomes.

 Video content accompanies this article at http://www.oto.theclinics.com.

> The incidence of oropharyngeal squamous cell carcinoma (OPSCC) is increasing dramatically and is conclusively linked to increasing rates of human papillomavirus (HPV) infection. HPV-related oropharyngeal cancers have been shown to occur in a unique demographic group and show favorable oncologic outcomes compared with HPV-negative OPSCC. There has been a paradigm shift in the treatment of early-stage OPSCC, with most patients now undergoing primary surgery in

the United States. Transoral robotic surgery is associated with excellent oncologic and functional outcomes in the treatment of OPSCC and is increasingly being used for a broader range of oropharyngeal indications.

John R. de Almeida

Unknown primary squamous cell carcinoma metastatic to cervical lymph nodes is a relatively rare tumor presentation, although the incidence may be increasing along with the rising incidence of human papilloma virus–mediated oropharyngeal cancers. Traditional diagnostic methods with palatine tonsillectomy and panendoscopy may identify the minority of primary tumors. The addition of a transoral lingual tonsillectomy may improve the diagnostic yield of identifying a primary tumor. Incorporation of transoral robotic surgery may be used for diagnostic purposes to identify a primary site and also for therapeutic purposes, whereby a primary tumor may be completely resected and combined with a neck dissection.

Benjamin Wahle and Jose Zevallos

This article outlines the ways that transoral robotic surgery and transoral laser microsurgery relate to treatment de-escalation in the treatment of head and neck cancer. Treatment de-escalation has particular importance in context of human papillomavirus–related oropharynx squamous cell carcinoma, which responds well to therapy but leaves many survivors with decades of treatment-related sequelae. We compare these less invasive transoral approaches with previously used open approaches to the oropharynx. We discuss the topic of treatment de-escalation in human papillomavirus–related disease and outline completed and ongoing clinical trials investigating the choice of primary treatment modality and de-escalation of adjuvant therapy.

Gina D. Jefferson and Hudson Frey

Transoral robotic surgery is a useful minimally invasive technique in the treatment of oropharyngeal squamous cell carcinoma, both human papilloma virus (HPV)-positive and HPV-negative patients in certain instances. This treatment modality often has proven useful for certain tumor persistences or recurrences. Good outcomes are possible given appropriate patient selection, both oncologically and functionally.

Neeraja Konuthula, Sanjay R. Parikh, and Randall A. Bly

Robotic surgery has been shown to be feasible and successful in several areas of pediatric head and neck surgery. However, adoption has been limited. Robotic surgery may be better integrated into practice with advanced preoperative surgical planning and the design of new robotic platforms with instrumentation specific for the application. With continued investigations, computer-aided surgical planning techniques including three-dimensional printing, virtual reality, multiobjective cost function for optimization of approach, mirror image overlay, and flexible robotic instruments may demonstrate value and utility over current practice.

Introduced in 2010, transoral robotic surgery (TORS) is recognized as an effective treatment of moderate to severe obstructive sleep apnea (OSA) in the setting of lymphoid and muscular tongue base hypertrophy. Upper airway stimulation (UAS) or hypoglossal nerve stimulation has emerged as a promising treatment of patients with moderate to severe OSA who have failed continuous positive airway pressure. UAS has shown favorable success rates and low morbidity compared with traditional soft tissue and skeletal framework surgery. UAS is in its infancy as a surgical procedure and concerns exist regarding narrow candidacy criteria, postimplant device titration, and durability of treatment response.

Through the past decades, there was a tremendous revolution in the surgical approaches for thyroidectomy. Remote access approaches (RAA) use the axillary approach, the axillary-bilateral breast approach, the bilateral axilla-breast approach, the retroauricular approach, and the transoral approach. The installation of the robotic system in surgery overcomes many limitations of the RAA. Although there are various types of robotic thyroidectomy by far, transaxillary is the commonly used approach. Moreover, the transoral approach is the most novel approach. In this article, the authors demonstrate the benefits and the constraints of each method and future directions of robotic thyroidectomy.

Management of head and neck squamous cell carcinoma necessitates a multimodal approach. The neck dissection has evolved over many years but is well established as the key surgical intervention for management of nodal disease in the neck. The open neck dissection has many varieties based on location and degree of disease but is the gold standard surgical technique. Robot-assisted neck dissections have emerged in recent years as an alternative. More research is required to establish long-term oncologic outcomes achieved with robot-assisted surgery and to assess whether cost and operative times decrease with experience.

This article summarizes major and minor complications following transoral robotic surgery in the head and neck. Overall, transoral robotic surgery is extremely safe; however, surgeons must recognize inherent risks associated with major and severe bleeding, dysphagia, and minor complications, including injury to nerves, mucosal surfaces, teeth, and the eyes. This article briefly discusses prevention and management strategies for common complications.

Oropharyngeal cancers and their treatment can exquisitely affect a patient's quality of life and functional outcome. Transoral robotic surgery offers a minimally invasive surgical approach that mitigates injury from traditional open surgical approaches and offers a treatment more likely to have short-term side effects compared with nonsurgical treatment. Feeding tube dependence, oral intake, and swallowing questionnaires, in addition to swallowing evaluations provide a snapshot of a patient's current swallowing function. Investigation of patient-reported quality-of-life outcomes allows for understanding of their symptomatology and the comparison of different treatment strategies.

Transoral robotic surgery (TORS) is a rapidly growing diagnostic and therapeutic modality in otolaryngology–head and neck surgery, having already made a large impact in the short time since its inception. Cost-effectiveness analysis is complex, and a thorough cost-effectiveness inquiry should analyze not only financial consequences but also impact on the health state of the patient. The cost-effectiveness of TORS is still under scrutiny, but the early data suggest that TORS is a cost-effective method compared with other available options when used in appropriately selected patients.

including the pediatric otolaryngology community. This article highlights the unique ramifications of COVID-19 on pediatric otolaryngology, with a focus on the immediate and potential long-term shifts in practice. Specifically, the article is divided into 3 sections (care for the patient, care for the practitioner, and care for the practice) and details the unique effects of the pandemic on the pediatric otolaryngology specialty.

OTOLARYNGOLOGIC CLINICS
OF NORTH AMERICA

SERIES OF RELATED INTEREST

Facial Plastic Surgery Clinics
Available at: https://www.facialplastic.theclinics.com/

THE CLINICS ARE AVAILABLE ONLINE!
Access your subscription at:
www.theclinics.com

Foreword

Domo Arigato, Mister Roboto

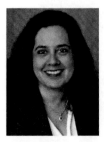

Sujana S. Chandrasekhar, MD, FACS, FAAOHNS
Consulting Editor

The word "robot" was introduced into the English language and into science fiction in 1920 by the Czech playwright Karel Capuk in his work, *Rossum's Universal Robots*, which appeared about 3 years after his brother introduced the concept of an automaton[1,2] (**Figs. 1** and **2**). The word *robot* comes from the Czech word *robota*, which means forced labor or activity. The robots in his play were humanoid in appearance with artificial intelligence and learning capabilities and, like the Terminators of the movie franchise, attempt to overthrow their human controllers and make their own destinies. Robots were popular characters in animated and live-action television shows in the 1950s and onward and are commonly used in many industries. The first robotic surgical procedure was a neurosurgical report of what we would now call stereotactic brain biopsy, by Kwoh and colleagues in 1988.[3] Subsequently, use of robotics in prostatic, gynecourologic, and abdominal and pelvic surgery blossomed and has become commonplace. Otolaryngologists first used robotic techniques in animal models in 2003 and subsequently in humans. Applications have increased exponentially.

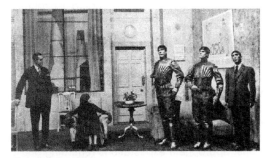

Fig. 1. Capuk's play showing 3 robots.

Otolaryngol Clin N Am 53 (2020) xvii–xix
https://doi.org/10.1016/j.otc.2020.09.007
0030-6665/20/© 2020 Published by Elsevier Inc.

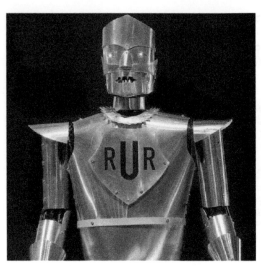

Fig. 2. The original robot from the BBC radio production of Rossum's Universal Robots in 1938.

This issue of *Otolaryngologic Clinics of North America* on Robotics in Otolaryngology, guest edited by Drs Erica Thaler, Arun Sharma, and Umamaheswar Duvvuri, compiles the history, developments, utility, limitations, cost, and potential future of incorporating this technology into Otolaryngology practice. The breadth of information presented by the authors is remarkable.

Most of the otolaryngology applications of robotics involve head and neck surgery. The articles on TORS, or transoral robotic surgery, detail the history, the indications, and the open versus robotic discussions that must be undertaken by the surgeon when counseling patients. What began for adults has grown to encompass children as well. Reaching into a difficult-to-access place, such as the oropharynx, hypopharynx, and larynx, with a robot makes inherent intellectual sense. Salvage surgery in these areas can be made less traumatic with robots, in certain cases. The advantages of using robots for more easily accessible cases, such as thyroidectomy, salivary gland excision, and neck dissection, are harder to see. The authors of each of these articles make the case for both when to and when not to use robotic technology safely and effectively.

Ear surgery is already performed with technology: microscopes and endoscopes, lasers, drills. Adding robotics for atraumatic insertion of a cochlear implant electrode, for example, can be the next step in achieving hearing and structure preservation surgery and setting the stage for future hair cell and natural hearing restoration. Similarly, reaching into the anterior or lateral skull base as atraumatically as possible possible took a giant leap forward with the development of endoscopes; moving on to robotic procedures is a next logical step.

Finally, no discussion of technique or technology is complete without understanding potential complications, appropriate expectations regarding quality of life, and what the patient, physician, and health care system should know regarding costs. All of the aforementioned are covered well in this issue.

Drs Thaler, Sharma, and Duvvuri have compiled a comprehensive list of topics and authors with robust experience to provide the reader with an outstanding self-contained resource to understand robotics and how they may consider implementing their use or expanding their use, in their own practice settings. As always, the more knowledgeable the physician and health care team are about technology, the better they can counsel patients for ideal shared decision making.

It is an exciting time to be an Otolaryngologist. Technological advances are helping us do more in smaller and harder-to-reach spaces than ever before. As Dennis DeYoung wrote and the band Styx recorded on their 1983 album "Kilroy Was Here," *dōmo arigatō misutā robotto*. This translates from the Japanese to "thank you very much, Mr Roboto," and we can say it is for allowing us to be better surgeons and offer our patients effective and minimally invasive surgery.

Sujana S. Chandrasekhar, MD, FACS, FAAOHNS
Consulting Editor, *Otolaryngologic Clinics of North America*

Past President, American Academy of Otolaryngology–Head and Neck Surgery

Secretary-Treasurer, American Otological Society
Vice President, Eastern Section, Triological Society

Partner, ENT & Allergy Associates LLP
18 East 48th Street, 2nd Floor
New York, NY 10017, USA

Clinical Professor, Department of Otolaryngology–Head and Neck Surgery
Zucker School of Medicine at Hofstra-Northwell
Hempstead, NY, USA

Clinical Associate Professor, Department of Otolaryngology–HNS
Icahn School of Medicine at Mount Sinai
New York, NY, USA

E-mail address:
ssc@nyotology.com

REFERENCES

1. Lane T. A short history of robotic surgery. Ann R Coll Surg Engl 2018;100(6 suppl): 5–7.
2. Hockstein NG, Gourin CG, Faust RA, et al. A history of robots: from science fiction to surgical robotics. J Robotic Surg 2007;1:113–8.
3. Kwoh YS, Hou J, Jonckheere EA, et al. A robot with improved absolute positioning accuracy for CT guided stereotactic brain surgery. IEEE. Trans Biomed Eng 1988 Feb;35(2):153–60.

Preface

Robotics in Otolaryngology

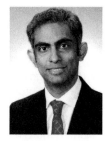 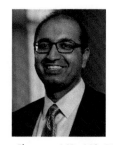 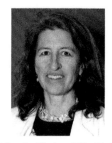

Umamaheswar Duvvuri, Arun Sharma, MD, MS, FACS Erica R. Thaler, MD, FACS
MD, PhD, FACS

Editors

The use of robotics in otolaryngology has dramatically accelerated over the last one and a half decades. In 2020, robotic surgery has left a mark in many subspecialties within the field of otolaryngology–head and neck surgery. In some subspecialties, such as in head and neck surgical oncology, there is over a decade of experience with robotics; as a result, it has broad acceptance and a large body of evidence, although areas of controversy certainly exist. In other subspecialties, robotic surgery is more nascent. Regardless, the current status of robotics in our specialty is un-doubtedly one of exciting potential with plentiful opportunities for continued innovation.

In this issue of *Otolaryngologic Clinics of North America*, we explore the history, cur-rent applications, best evidence, limitations, and future potential of robotic surgery within our specialty. The issue is not intended to be a technical guide to performing ro-botic surgery, but instead is an up-to-date summary of state-of-the-art within otolaryn-gology. The history of robotic surgery in otolaryngology highlights that innovations can come by learning from the experiences of physicians in other specialties. Similarly, one of our intentions with the current issue is to highlight aspects of robotics across the various subspecialties within otolaryngology–head and neck surgery. Doing so allows for continued opportunities to learn from other surgeons, even when they are in other disciplines.

As with any technologic device or surgical instrument, it is important to remember that there are certain clinical situations that merit the use of robotics and others that do not. So, instead of thinking of robotics as its own discipline, it is more appropriate to think of it as another tool in the armamentarium of otolaryngologists–head and neck surgeons. Nevertheless, proficiency in its use in the appropriate clinical setting will allow for the best possible outcomes for our patients.

Otolaryngol Clin N Am 53 (2020) xxi–xxii
https://doi.org/10.1016/j.otc.2020.09.006
0030-6665/20/© 2020 Published by Elsevier Inc.

oto.theclinics.com

The goal of the current issue is to provide a comprehensive and up-to-date overview of robotic surgery in otolaryngology–head and neck surgery. It is our hope that this will be of benefit to practicing physicians, trainees, and our patients.

Umamaheswar Duvvuri, MD, PhD, FACS
University of Pittsburgh
Eye & Ear Institute
203 Lothrop Street, Suite 500
Pittsburgh, PA 15213, USA

Arun Sharma, MD, MS, FACS
Department of Otolaryngology–
Head and Neck Surgery
Southern Illinois University
School of Medicine
720 North Bond Street
Springfield, IL 62702, USA

Erica R. Thaler, MD, FACS
Department of Otorhinolaryngology:
Head and Neck Surgery
5 Silverstein
3400 Spruce Street
Philadelphia, PA 19104, USA

E-mail addresses:
duvvuriu@upmc.edu (U. Duvvuri)
asharma74@siumed.edu (A. Sharma)
Erica.Thaler@uphs.upenn.edu (E.R. Thaler)

Past, Present, and Future of Robotic Surgery

Guillermo Maza, MD, Arun Sharma, MD, MS*

KEYWORDS

- Robotic surgery • Transoral robotic surgery • TORS • History of robotic surgery

KEY POINTS

- Robotic-assisted surgery is the latest form of minimally invasive surgery, building on microsurgical, laparoscopic, and endoscopic techniques.
- Transoral robotic surgery (TORS) takes advantage of the natural oral orifice and allows for en bloc resection of oropharyngeal, hypopharyngeal, and laryngeal tumors.
- Although the cost-effectiveness of robot-assisted surgery is an evolving point of discussion, robotic systems have successfully expanded into the US health care system.
- Introduction of new robotic systems could decrease costs, facilitate wider adoption, and accelerate technological innovation.

INTRODUCTION

The current concept of robotic surgery involves the performance of surgical procedures by using small wristed instruments attached to a robotic arm. The surgeon controls the system obtaining high-definition magnification while taking advantage of the robotic arm's capabilities for precision and miniaturization. Their introduction to medical fields started 30 years ago and now represents one of the fastest areas of growth in the surgical field. Transoral robotic surgery (TORS) has become an effective and safe tool for head and neck surgeons.

PAST

Early Conceptions of Robots

Robots, by definition,[1] are mechanical contraptions able to carry out complex actions automatically. A machine performing a function automatically was firstly described in the myth of Hephaestus, a Greek god that built Talos, a giant made of bronze, to defend the island of Crete.[2] Evidence of human-built machines is found in relics traced as far back as 1500 BC in Egypt, in the form of human figurines striking bells inside water-powered clocks. Nonetheless, the concept of robots as subservient of humanity

Department of Otolaryngology–Head and Neck Surgery, Southern Illinois University School of Medicine, 720 North Bond Street, Springfield, IL 62702, USA
* Corresponding author.
E-mail address: asharma74@siumed.edu
Twitter: @ArunSharmaMDMS (A.S.)

Otolaryngol Clin N Am 53 (2020) 935–941
https://doi.org/10.1016/j.otc.2020.07.005
0030-6665/20/© 2020 Elsevier Inc. All rights reserved.

has always been ingrained to its name. The word "robot" derives from robota, a Czech word for serf or forced labor. It was coined in 1921, in a Czech play by Čapek,[3] centered on a factory that manufactured artificial, human-shaped workers, to do unwanted labor.

In 1495, under the patronage of the Duke of Milan, Leonardo da Vinci built a mechanical knight (Leonardo's Automa Cavaliere) able to perform humanoid movements, such as sitting and lifting his visor. It was believed to be human-powered and controlled through a crank, linked to a system of pulleys and internal gears.[4] Thus, not exactly a robot, but one impressive prototype design for the many automata later created to entertain the higher classes and royalty, during almost half a millennium. Currently, popular culture influences the collective conception of modern robots, from undisputedly mechanical models, such as C-3PO in the Star Wars movies, or lifelike cyborgs from Blade Runner.

Early Robotic Systems

In 1949, Raymond Goerz patented the "master-slave manipulator," an articulated arm intended to safely manipulate radioactive materials from a distance. Goerz's work gave rise to telerobotics, which involves teleoperation (the control of any machine at a distance) and telepresence (capability of remotely exerting effects).[5] Soon afterward, Unimation, the world's first robotic company, created the Unimate, a reprogrammable hydraulic robotic arm that was able to repeatedly perform dangerous transfer tasks.[4] It was the first mass-produced robotic arm for factory automation, and in 1961 it was installed at a General Motors assembly line.[6]

Early Surgical Robotic Systems

The 1980s brought the rise of minimally invasive surgery and its war-horse, the laparoscopic technique, changing the landscape of operating rooms worldwide. But surgery in these ever-decreasing spaces was accompanied by newly discovered limitations to maneuverability and accuracy. These conditions were perfect for the introduction of robots into the nascent field of robotic surgery. In reality, this term is becoming a misnomer, and robot-assisted surgery is a more accurate term, because most systems are not autonomous, but almost completely dependent on an operator.

The early medical robots were specialty-oriented and favored a shared autonomy between surgeon and machine. In 1985, the Unimation Programmable Universal Manipulation Arm (PUMA) 200 used computed tomography (CT) scans to define the trajectory of a brain needle biopsy, in the first documented robot-assisted surgical procedure,[7] with the help of a 6° of freedom manipulator (human wrist has 3° of freedom). Soon after, the PUMA 560 was used to assist with transurethral resection of the prostate.[8] Later in 1989, the Imperial of College in London developed the Pro-Bot, a PUMA robot with a liquidizer blade and aspirator.[9] By preprograming it with transrectal scans, it could automatically perform a transurethral resection of the prostate, within the enclosed prostate's space. Although never commercialized, it was the first truly automatic robot used in medicine.[10] The RoboDoc (a collaboration of University of California, Davis and IBM) was able to automatically perform precise computer-guided femur drilling during hip surgeries, and it was successfully commercialized in Europe and Asia since 1994, gaining Food and Drug Administration (FDA) approval in 2008.[11]

These accomplishments garnered the attention of US government agencies, which were interested in achieving remote surgery capabilities, potentially for astronauts in space and wounded soldiers on the battlefield. A National Aeronautics and Space Administration scientist, Scott Fisher, and Joe Rosen, a plastic surgeon from Stanford

University, collaborated with Phil Green, of the Stanford Research Institute (now SRI International, Menlo Park, CA) and used National Institutes of Health funding to build a new robotic arm.[12]

Computer Motion, Inc (Goleta, CA), created Automated Endoscopic System for Optimal Positioning (AESOP), the first robotic surgery system approved by the FDA, in 1994. It consisted of a voice-controlled robotic arm capable of moving an endoscope during laparoscopy. Meanwhile, the licensing rights from the SRI system were sold to Fredrick Moll, John Freund, and Robert Younge, forming Intuitive Surgical, Inc (Sunnyvale, CA). They updated their acquisition to "Lenny," an early prototype of the da Vinci, followed by other prototypes "Leonardo," "Mona," and finally, the da Vinci surgical system.[13]

Computer Motion went on to build the ZEUS robotic surgical system using AESOP's technology and focused on cardiovascular and gynecologic procedures. In 2001, the Zeus was used for the famous Lindbergh operation, where surgeons in New York performed a cholecystectomy on a patient in Strasbourg, France. Although the system received FDA approval for limited use in 2001,[14] its production was phased out, along with the AESOP, when the company was bought by Intuitive in 2003.

Multiple other robots have been developed, such as the Neuromate (Integrated Surgical Systems, Sacramento, CA), which received FDA approval in 1999 for stereotactic neurosurgical procedures, or the Steady Hand Robot, developed at Johns Hopkins University (1999), to offer counterforce to the movement of the hand to cancel tremor during retinal surgery.

Advent and Use of the da Vinci System

Although the da Vinci is currently the most commonly used surgical robotic system, it completely lacks autonomy, providentially more akin to Leonardo da Vinci's human-powered automata, than other earlier surgical robots. The original da Vinci robotic system had three arms and was commercialized in Europe since 1998 for coronary surgery, before receiving FDA clearance in 2000 for general surgery procedures.[15] In 2001 it was approved for prostate surgery,[16] followed by clearance for gynecologic, thoracoscopic, and cardiovascular procedures.[17,18]

The system consists of a master console with a magnified ($\times$10), high-definition, three-dimensional view of the surgical field; a video platform/laparoscopic insufflator; and a patient-side cart with movable robotic arms. Each arm holds detachable surgical tips through wristed technology, allowing 6° of freedom (3° of translation, 3° of rotation) and 90° articulation, providing human handlike rotation, with an additional degree of freedom given by the attached tool (cutting, grasping). The surgeon can operate the robotic arms, through scaled, finger-controlled cuffs. The most immediate advantages were the annulment of hand tremor and improved dexterity in minimally invasive accesses while maintaining optimal vision.[19]

In 2003 it was upgraded with a fourth arm, for optimal retraction, suction, and irrigation. In 2006 the da Vinci S HD (second generation) added improved resolution, swifter instruments exchange, fewer cable connections, extended-reach instruments (for multiquadrant access), and interactive multi-image displays (TilePro). In 2009 the da Vinci Si HD added shared-control capacity between dual consoles, for training and collaboration, along with improvements to the user interface, digital OR integration, and video resolution.[20]

In 2014, the da Vinci Xi (fourth generation) brought thinner, longer arms; the capability of using fluorescent imaging (Firefly); and a changed setup to an overhead arrangement. It can be connected to a special operating table, for integrated table motion, which allows the repositioning of the patient without having to undock the robotic arms during multiquadrant surgery.[21] A lower-cost version, the X, was released in 2017, with the upgrades of the Xi (also voice and laser guidance, and a lightweight endoscope) but with reduced versatility, because it is installed in a side cart.[22]

PRESENT
Current State of Robot-Assisted Surgery

The presence of robots in the hospital system has grown impressively, despite steep entry costs. Nowadays, the popular perception is favorable to the use of surgical robots and the hospitals that have them.[23,24] Correspondingly, an institution looking to promote minimally invasive surgery capability needs to have a robot. The market is currently dominated by the da Vinci, and approximately 5000 active systems perform more than a million robotic surgeries each year.[25] Robot-assisted surgery is currently used within the fields of breast surgery, obstetrics and gynecology, endocrine surgery, hepatobiliary, thoracic, colorectal and general surgery, urology, and otolaryngology. The latter is mostly through TORS.

TORS takes advantage of the natural oral orifice, permitting en bloc resection of pharyngeal and laryngeal tumors.[26,27] The da Vinci Si was FDA approved in 2009 for malignant and nonmalignant diseases of the tongue base, oropharynx, and supraglottic larynx. The fourth arm is not used because of anatomic constraints. In selected patients (stage II to IVa) with oropharyngeal cancer, TORS could be more cost-effective than nonsurgical treatment.[28]

In 2016 the FDA approved the da Vinci Xi for general laparoscopic surgical, urologic, and gynecologic procedures, but not for head and neck procedures. Thus, most of the literature for TORS is based on the Si Model. Still, the off-label use of the Xi model in TORS has been reported in the United States.[29]

The use of the robotic systems has also been reported in the parapharyngeal space, the nasopharynx, clivus, and upper cervical vertebrae, sometimes aided by open approaches to gain the necessary exposure.[30] Additional evolving applications of robotic technology in otolaryngology include use for neck procedures (eg, neck dissection), endocrine (ie, thyroid/parathyroid) surgery, salivary gland surgery, sleep surgery, sinus and anterior skull base surgery, otology/neurotology, and pediatric surgeries.

Other Robotic Models in Use

In 2013 Stryker (Kalamazoo, MI) became the first major surgical instrument company to get involved in robotics through its acquisition of Mako Surgical, and its Robotic-arm Interactive Orthopedic System, approved for knee and hip replacements (MAKO-plasty). Through preoperative CT scan modeling, an area of safe surgery is delineated, and haptic boundaries limit the robotic arm.[31]

A novel robotic technology that is observed in current operative rooms is robot-assisted flexible endoscopy. The Monarch (Auris Health Inc, Redwood City, CA) was approved by the FDA for diagnostic and therapeutic bronchoscopy procedures in 2018. Through flexible endoscopes, radial endobronchial ultrasound and a videogame-like controller, needle biopsies are taken under direct vision. Recently, Johnson & Johnson (New Brunswick, NJ) acquired Auris Health, led by Fred Moll, and more than 1000 procedures have been performed in multiple US hospitals.[32] In 2019, Intuitive Surgical obtained FDA approval for the Ion endoluminal system. A robotic-assisted lung biopsy platform includes a thin, fully maneuverable robotic catheter of 3.5 mm with a 2-mm working channel. The Ion allows direct vision while able to integrate other imaging technologies, such as fluoroscopy, radial endobronchial ultrasound, and cone-beam CT. The future aim is to expand robot-assisted flexible endoscopy to gastrointestinal[33] and urologic procedures.[34]

Single-port robotic systems include the use of a single robotic arm containing an endoscope and instruments. Currently, single-port systems are available through Intuitive (Single Port) and Medrobotics (Flex Robotic System). The surgical system by Titan Medical is currently in development and features a single-port robotic system, with multiarticulated instruments.

There have also been efforts to unify the operative room system with robotic technology. This includes the Renaissance Surgical System, a bone-mounted guidance system for accurate spinal surgery, and the Mazor X, a robotic arm able to hold surgical wires or be accommodated to Medtronic (Minneapolis, MN) StealthStation software. It is commercialized as a fully integrated experience of preoperative planning, live intraoperative three-dimensional imaging, and powered surgical tools.[35]

FUTURE

The continuous growth of robot-assisted surgery depends on the concept that they will become essential to operative environments in the time to come, in a way not dissimilar to laparoscopic and endoscopic techniques. Because the da Vinci is the most commercially successful model, it also sets the standard for improvement of the current weaknesses of robot-assisted surgery. Its large, rigid arms hinder the ability to obtain an adequate site of exposure. Its cutting tools are limited, and its set-up is time-consuming. A well-trained team is required, to compensate for the time loss of placing the sterile draping, arranging the carts, and attaching and positioning the instruments.

The da Vinci performs well in anatomically enclosed spaces (prostate, uterus), but its lack of haptic feedback results in a well-known risk of tissue-manipulation damage. The open and dynamic anatomic barriers of the head and neck could be more forgiving. Nevertheless, the system and its rigid instruments could benefit from enhanced sensorial input and instruments adapted to the surgery type, to refine surgical capabilities and exposure.

However, the most important barrier to wider adoption is the financial burden, not only of the machine but also its maintenance and consumables. Some of the earliest Intuitive patents started expiring in 2016, and the increasing competition should contribute to decreasing costs.

Potential Improvements to Robotic Technology

Certain developments are needed, such as an improved, validated curriculum, and better delineation of indications, especially in oncologic scenarios. The system could immensely benefit from additional tools (ie, ultrasound guidance) and smaller surgical tips with upgraded abilities, such as bone drilling capacity. The latter would allow bringing robotic surgery to the skull base, cervical spine, and beyond.

Multiple efforts have focused on creating a more streamlined experience in the operative room, by integrating surgical robotics to other new technologies. Image guidance and navigation could become the next frontier for advancements, by overlaying key clinical imaging (augmented or virtual reality) on the surgical field and incorporating machine learning.

Other projections are the expansion of uses of telesurgery, either for telesurgery in rural remote areas or within the confines of a single hospital. This could potentially allow performing multiple procedures in parallel, increasing efficiency.

Nano-robots are another area of potential future applications. These small robots are projected to be able to travel the bloodstream, locally delivering medication and even performing cellular-level surgery.

SUMMARY

Robotic-assisted surgery embodies the latest in technological advancement, applied to the operating management of a patient. Its extension to otolaryngology seems only natural because natural orifices are exploited for access while minimizing disruption to normal structures and optimizing function. Its recent growth and the imminent addition of novel technology could signal the advent of a new era in surgery.

DISCLOSURE

The authors have nothing to disclose.

REFERENCES

1. Definition of ROBOTICS. Merriam-webster.com. Available at: https://www.merriam-webster.com/dictionary/robotics. Accessed February 25, 2020.
2. Mayor A. Gods and robots: myths, machines, and ancient dreams of technology. Princeton (NJ): Princeton University Press; 2018.
3. Moran ME. Rossum's universal robots: not the machines. J Endourol 2007;21(12): 1399–402.
4. Rosheim ME. Leonardo's lost robots. Berlin: Springer; 2006. p. 24.
5. Angelo JA Jr. Robotics: a reference guide to new technology. New York: Greenwood Press; 2006.
6. Moran ME. Evolution of robotic arms. J Robot Surg 2007;1(2):103–11.
7. Kwoh YS, Hou J, Jonckheere EA, et al. A robot with improved absolute positioning accuracy for CT guided stereotactic brain surgery. IEEE Trans Biomed Eng 1988;35(2):153–60.
8. Davies BL, Hibberd RD, Ng WS, et al. The development of a surgeon robot for prostatectomies. Proc Inst Mech Eng H 1991;205(1):35–8.
9. Challacombe BJ, Khan MS, Murphy D, et al. The history of robotics in urology. World J Urol 2006;24(2):120–7.
10. Elhage O, Murphy D, Challacombe B, et al. Robotic urology in the UK: experience and overview of robotic-assisted cystectomy. J Robot Surg 2008;1(4):235–42.
11. Bargar WL. Robots in orthopaedic surgery: past, present, and future. Clin Orthop Relat Res 2007;463:31–6.
12. Hockstein NG, Gourin CG, Faust RA, et al. A history of robots: from science fiction to surgical robotics. J Robot Surg 2007;1(2):113–8.
13. George EI, Brand TC, Laporta A, et al. Origins of robotic surgery: from skepticism to standard of care. JSLS 2018;22(4). e2018.00039.
14. Marescaux J, Rubino F. The ZEUS robotic system: experimental and clinical applications. Surg Clin North Am 2003;83(6):1305–15, vii-viii.
15. FDA approves new robotic surgery device. ScienceDaily 2000. Available at: https://www.sciencedaily.com/releases/2000/07/000717072719.htm. Accessed February 23, 2020.
16. Thiel DD, Winfield HN. Robotics in urology: past, present, and future. J Endourol 2008;22(4):825–30.
17. Kypson AP, Nifong LW, Chitwood WR. Robot-assisted surgery: training and retraining surgeons. Int J Med Robot 2004;1(1):70–6.

18. Canales M. Intuitive Surgical receives FDA clearance for gynecological laparo-scopic procedures. Intuitive surgical. 2005. Available at: https://isrg.intuitive.com/news-releases/news-release-details/intuitive-surgical-receives-fda-clearance-gynecological. Accessed February 29, 2020.
19. Leal ghezzi T, Campos corleta O. 30 years of robotic surgery. World J Surg 2016; 40(10):2550–7.
20. Hagen ME, et al. Introduction to the robotics system. In: Kim KC, editor. Robotics in general surgery. New York: Springer; 2014. p. 10–2.
21. Ngu JC, Tsang CB, Koh DC. The da Vinci Xi: a review of its capabilities, versatility, and potential role in robotic colorectal surgery. Robot Surg 2017;4:77–85.
22. Azizian M, Liu M, Khalaji I, et al. Chapter 1 - The Da Vinci Surgical System. In: Desai JP, Patel RV, editors. Encyclopedia of medical robotics. Singapore: World Scientific; 2008. p. 287–328.
23. Boys JA, Alicuben ET, Demeester MJ, et al. Public perceptions on robotic sur-gery, hospitals with robots, and surgeons that use them. Surg Endosc 2016; 30(4):1310–6.
24. Ahmad A, Ahmad ZF, Carleton JD, et al. Robotic surgery: current perceptions and the clinical evidence. Surg Endosc 2017;31(1):255–63.
25. Annual Report 2018. Intuitive Surgical, Inc. 2018. Available at: http://www.annualreports.com/HostedData/AnnualReports/PDF/NASDAQ_ISRG_2018.pdf. Accessed January 20, 2020.
26. Nakayama M, Holsinger FC, Chevalier D, et al. The dawn of robotic surgery in otolaryngology-head and neck surgery. Jpn J Clin Oncol 2019;49(5):404–11.
27. Mcleod IK, Melder PC. Da Vinci robot-assisted excision of a vallecular cyst: a case report. Ear Nose Throat J 2005;84(3):170–2.
28. Tam K, Orosco RK, Dimitrios colevas A, et al. Cost comparison of treatment for oropharyngeal carcinoma. Laryngoscope 2019;129(7):1604–9.
29. Gabrysz-forget F, Mur T, Dolan R, et al. Perioperative safety, feasibility, and onco-logic utility of transoral robotic surgery with da Vinci Xi platform. J Robot Surg 2020;14(1):85–9.
30. Ozer E, Durmus K, Carrau RL, et al. Applications of transoral, transcervical, trans-nasal, and transpalatal corridors for robotic surgery of the skull base. Laryngo-scope 2013;123(9):2176–9.
31. Roche M. Robotic-assisted unicompartmental knee arthroplasty: the MAKO experience. Orthop Clin North Am 2015;46(1):125–31.
32. Auris Health celebrates 1,000 cases with the Monarch™ Platform - Auris Health. Auris Health. 2019. Available at: https://www.aurishealth.com/about/press-releases/Auris-Health-Celebrates-thousand-Cases-Monarch-Platform. Accessed December 13, 2019.
33. Yeung BP, Chiu PW. Application of robotics in gastrointestinal endoscopy: a re-view. World J Gastroenterol 2016;22(5):1811–25.
34. Navaratnam A, Abdul-Muhsin H, Humphreys M. Updates in urologic robot assis-ted surgery. F1000Res 2018;7:F1000.
35. Malham GM, Wells-quinn T. What should my hospital buy next? Guidelines for the acquisition and application of imaging, navigation, and robotics for spine surgery. J Spine Surg 2019;5(1):155–65.

History and Acceptance of Transoral Robotic Surgery

Erica R. Thaler, MD

KEYWORDS

- Robotic surgery • Head and neck cancer • Surgical innovation

KEY POINTS

- Development of TORS was swift.
- Education and training was key to broad use and acceptance.
- Surgical innovation is a specialty-wide process, and acceptance takes time.

HISTORY OF ROBOTIC SURGERY

Transoral robotic surgery (TORS) in current parlance generally refers to any transoral surgery involving the da Vinci surgical system. Although other robotic systems have been trialed and many are in development currently, these are beyond the scope of this retrospective article. The purpose of this article is to trace the history and evolution of TORS to its current practice. This is worth considering as an exercise in understanding surgical innovation and a medical specialty's adaptation to rapid and marked change in surgical practice.

The term "robot" is credited to the Czech playwright, Karel Capek, in his 1920 play, Rossom's Universal Robots ("rabota" in Czech means forced labor). The development of robotics and computer science took off some decades later, with integration of robots in industry in the 1960s. Medical implementation of robotics was somewhat slower to evolve. Robotic surgery was first performed by Kwoh and colleagues[1] in 1985, to perform precision neurosurgical biopsies. These surgeons used a device called the Puma 560, which was simply an adapted industrial robotic arm. This and other systems were further developed in a collaborative effort that included the National Air and Space Administration, the Stanford Research Institute, and the Department of Defense. Extensive research and development in the 1990s led to the creation of Intuitive Surgical (founded in 1995 in Mountain View, CA), which built on Stanford Research Institute's designs and other companies' developments through mergers, to produce several early prototype surgical robots, first used in humans in the late 1990s. The da Vinci system uses a console where the operating surgeon controls the robot through grips that mimic movement of the robotic arms, a moveable "robot"

Department of Otorhinolaryngology: Head and Neck Surgery, University of Pennsylvania, 3400 Spruce Street, Philadelphia, PA 19003, USA
E-mail address: Erica.thaler@uphs.upenn.edu

Otolaryngol Clin N Am 53 (2020) 943–948
https://doi.org/10.1016/j.otc.2020.07.006
0030-6665/20/© 2020 Elsevier Inc. All rights reserved.

with a light source, camera, and multiple robotic arms, and a video tower with visual display of the surgical procedure. The da Vinci system has gone through multiple generations, including the S, Si, SIHD, X, XI, SP, and ION, with improvements in technology and instrumentation along the way, and some adaptations especially designed for particular surgical specialties.

DEVELOPMENT OF TRANSORAL ROBOTIC SURGERY

The development of TORS occurred in the early 2000s. Early on, this was done largely through the work of Drs O'Malley and Weinstein at the University of Pennsylvania. At Penn, as was the case in many institutions, the da Vinci robot was initially used for some cardiac procedures, then more broadly adopted by urology for prostatectomy and by gynecology for various procedures. The Penn Otolaryngology Department's interest was stimulated by resident physician, Dr Neil Hockstein, and many otorhinolaryngology applications were considered. The concept of transoral use of the robot, particularly for head and neck cancer, seemed most appropriate, particularly because traditional methods for access to site of pathology were limited; technically difficult; or involved extensive, open procedures. A research strategy was put in place involving sequential testing of mannequin and cadaver models, to assess feasibility, accessibility, and safety of the use of the robot in surgery on the pharynx and glottis.[2] The results of this, reported by Hockstein and colleagues,[3] showed that TORS had a safety profile similar to conventional transoral surgery in assessing for risks, such as skin laceration, dental injury, mucosal laceration, mandible fracture, and ocular injury.

Next, a canine model was used to assess live surgery, with attention to secretions and hemostasis. In 2005, Weinstein and coworkers[4] published their findings on this phase of their research. In this paper, they described a successful canine supraglottic partial laryngectomy, with excellent hemostasis and visualization. Furthermore, the robotic system allowed for tremor abolition, motion scaling, and three-dimensional vision. Finally, with institutional review board approval, a human clinical trial was undertaken to assess exposure and safety of the robotic approach. This was undertaken for patients with supraglottic and base of tongue neoplasms. In these efforts, it was determined that key anatomic structures, such as the regional cranial nerves and arteries, could be identified and preserved. In addition, techniques for control of hemostasis, including arterial, were established. In the human subjects, complete resection with negative margins were accomplished.[5] Some other refinements in technique were accomplished in these early efforts. For example, Dingman and Crowe-Davis retractors were not found to be ideal. An FK-WO laryngopharyngoscope retractor was developed by Drs O'Malley and Weinstein, specifically for TORS, to better facilitate visualization and access. In their first three supraglottic partial laryngectomy patients, Weinstein and colleagues[6] were able to complete the procedure in 120 minutes, with no intraoperative or postoperative complications and with complete tumor resection, suggesting the TORS approach may be an alternative to open or conventional approaches.

With these early successes, Weinstein and O'Malley began to expand their efforts, using TORS for radical tonsillectomy in 27 patients with previously untreated squamous cell carcinoma of the tonsillar region. In these patients, final negative margins were achieved in 93% of patients with limited acute morbidity and 96% recovery of normal swallowing function.[7] Further prospective investigation showed similar results, with the addition of concomitant neck dissection and in some cases, intraoral reconstruction. A rapid decrease in the setup time was noted over the time course of the study.[8]

An important part of the development of TORS was the early recognition that training and teaching of fellow head and neck surgeons was important to the adoption of this approach. The first training workshop for TORS was held at Intuitive Surgical in 2006, at which 12 head and neck surgeons attended didactic sessions and laboratory cadaver dissections. Nearly all of these surgeons went on to develop their own TORS programs. This model was brought to Penn in 2007, where surgeons from around the world have come for a week-long experience, including observation in the clinic and operating room and robotic certification in a training laboratory. After Food and Drug Administration approval was obtained in 2009 for transoral use of the da Vinci robot for T1 and T2 oral cavity, pharyngeal, laryngeal cancer, and benign disease, American surgeons started training at Penn in a TORS Masters Training Program in 2010 with a combination of hands-on porcine robotic training, observation of cadaver and live surgery TORS cases, and didactics.

With world-wide dissemination of TORS in progress, other institutions began to report on their experiences with the surgery. Iseli, and colleagues[9] reported on functional outcomes after TORS in their case series of 54 patients. They looked at airway management, swallowing function, and enterogastric feeding, and found that: all patients were either extubated (78%), or decannulated by 14 days; 83% commenced oral intake by 2 weeks; and 17% retained a feeding tube at 12 months postoperative. Complications were limited and managed without major sequelae. Moore and colleagues[10] reported on TORS for oropharyngeal carcinoma of all stages in a prospective case study of 45 patients. In their group, previously untreated patients with oropharyngeal squamous cell carcinoma (T1-T4a) underwent TORS with negative margins and no reported major complications. All patients were extubated or decannulated and of the 22% of patients who required a feeding tube of some sort, all eventually had these removed.

About the same time as these case series were published, articles started to appear on a paradigm shift in the management of patients with head and neck cancer with the advent of TORS.[11,12] These papers suggested that TORS allows for comparable or improved oncologic and functional outcomes over traditional therapies: open and other transoral techniques, and primary chemotherapy and radiation. That this paradigm shift was beginning to occur only 5 years after the first reported canine experimentation is truly remarkable. Also reflective of the beginning of more widespread adoption of TORS as a surgical innovation for the management of pharyngeal and laryngeal cancer, was the rapid increase in number of peer-reviewed publications on the topic per year. Using a PubMed search: in 2009, three English language papers regarding its use were published; in 2010, eight such papers were published; in 2011, 13 papers were published; in 2012, 24 papers were published; and in 2013, 39 papers were published.

In addition, head and neck surgeons were beginning to explore further applications of TORS in surgical tumor management. O'Malley[13] reported on the use of TORS for management of benign and malignant parapharyngeal space tumors with no carotid encasement or bone erosion. In their series, 9 of 10 patients were able to have resection of their tumors with acceptable operative time and blood loss, no significant complications, and with 100% local control of the seven patients in the series with pleomorphic adenomas. Selber[14] wrote about the benefit of using the robot to reconstruct defects left from large oropharyngeal tumor resections, using either free flaps or a facial artery myomucosal flap based on the facial artery to provide tissue coverage. Microvascular anastomoses were performed successfully, transorally with the robot.[14] Weinstein and colleagues[15] reported on TORS for advanced oropharyngeal carcinoma. In their series of 47 patients with stage III and IV cancer of the oropharynx, resection margins were positive in one patient, and disease-specific survival was 90% at 2 years. Using risk stratification, 38% of patients avoided chemotherapy, and 11% of patients did not require adjuvant radiation and concurrent chemotherapy. At 1-year follow-up, only one patient had a gastrostomy tube. Their conclusion was that TORS allowed for disease control, survival, and safety commensurate with traditional therapy, with the added benefit of improved functional outcome.

Although the focus of TORS surgical developments remained predominantly in head and neck cancer management, surgeons began to investigate its' use for other, benign pathologies and disorders. One arena where there was significant early adoption of its use was in the surgical management of obstructive sleep apnea (OSA). Several institutions in America and internationally began investigating the use of TORS for tongue base resection in the surgical management of OSA. Vicini and his group in Italy were the first to publish on this in 2010.[16] In this paper, 10 patients underwent tongue base resection to manage their OSA, with a reduction in apnea-hypopnea index (AHI) from 38.3 ± 23.5 standard deviation to a mean postoperative AHI of 20.6 ± 17.3 standard deviation, with good functional results as measured by pain, swallowing, and quality of life (QOL), and rare or minor complications.[16] Lee and colleagues[17] published a series of 20 patients who reported on robot-assisted lingual tonsillectomy and uvulopalatopharyngoplasty, with reduction of AHI by 56.7% from 55.6 to a mean postoperative value of 24.1 (P<.001), and improvement of minimum arterial oxygen saturation from the mean preoperative value of 75.8% to the mean postoperative value of 81.7% (P = .013). The mean Epworth Sleepiness Scale score improved from 13.4 to 5.9 (P = .003). One patient required postoperative cauterization for a bleeding episode without further sequela. Vicini was instrumental in organizing a consortium of institutions performing this surgery to produce a first major case series on patients with sleep apnea undergoing TORS in 2014. This groups' paper on the clinical outcomes and complications of 243 patients who had undergone TORS for OSA showed that the surgery was safe and effective, with a mean preoperative and postoperative AHI of 43.0 ± 22.6 and 17.9 ± 18.4, respectively (P<.001), and a reduction in Epworth Sleepiness Scale from 12.34 ± 5.19 to 5.7 ± 3.49 (P<.001).[18]

Another clinical domain where application of the surgical technique expanded was the use of TORS for the management of salivary gland neoplasms. Villaneuva and colleagues[19] reported early on the use of TORS for the management of oropharyngeal minor salivary gland tumors. In their series of 10 patients with T1 or T2 malignancies, TORS was used for resection with no surgical complications, negative margins, and excellent functional outcomes. This surgical innovation has expanded to include submandibular gland resection, submandibular stone resection, and resection of salivary gland neoplasms of the parapharyngeal space.

More recently, TORS has been used for resection of skull base neoplasms. A first, cadaveric study investigating the feasibility of a transoral approach to the sella turcica was published by Chauvet and colleagues[20] in 2014. Other clinical studies have followed, but perhaps reflective of the limited utility of TORS in this region, have not abounded. For example, it was not until 3 years later, in 2017, that a clinical study was reported by Chauvet and colleagues[21] on a series of four patients who had undergone a TORS approach for resection of pituitary neoplasm.

ACCEPTANCE OF TRANSORAL ROBOTIC SURGERY

As with all surgical innovation, the ultimate test of the technique is in whether there is sufficient added benefit in outcomes to justify its incorporation in treatment paradigms. This takes years after implementation, because data can only be slowly collected over time to assess outcomes. In the case of head and neck cancer, the outcomes are adjudicated in terms of disease (survivorship) and function. In these regards, TORS for the management of pharyngeal and laryngeal cancer has passed the test of time.

In recent years, numerous studies have been published on survivorship and functional outcomes of patients who underwent TORS as part of their treatment of head and neck cancer. For example, in 2015, de Almeida and colleagues[22] looked at 410 patients who had undergone TORS for laryngeal and pharyngeal cancers, in terms of locoregional control, disease-specific survival, and overall survival. Their 2-year locoregional control rate was 91.8%, disease-specific survival was 94.5%, and overall survival was 91%, which they concluded supported the role of TORS within the multidisciplinary treatment paradigm for head and neck cancer. A more recent systemic review of QOL outcomes after TORS looked at 103 articles assessing QOL and/or swallow outcomes for 659 patients after treatment. Their conclusion was that patients have good QOL and swallowing outcomes after treatment.[23] These outcomes studies have compared favorably with prior treatment paradigms for such patients with head and neck cancer supporting the use of primary chemotherapy and radiation. Although the latter remains the primary treatment of many patients with pharyngeal and laryngeal head and neck cancer, the use of TORS as a component of primary treatment seems to provide comparable or better survivorship and better functional outcomes.[24,25]

Over the course of the past 15 years, TORS has cemented its' place in the treatment of pharyngeal and laryngeal cancer, and has been advocated for as an important surgical innovation in other disease states. The use of robots in otorhinolaryngologic surgery is here to stay.

DISCLOSURE

Research grant funding from Inspire Medical Systems.

REFERENCES

1. Kwoh Y, Hou J, Jonckheere E, et al. A robot with improved absolute positioning accuracy for CT guided stereotactic brain surgery. IEEE Trans Biomed Eng 1988;35(2):153–61.

2. Weinstein G, O'Malley B, Diaz J. TransOral robotic surgery: from the robotics lab to the bedside. In: Weinstein G, O'Malley B, editors. Transoral robotic surgery (TORS). San Diego (CA): Plural Publishing, Inc; 2012. p. 1–6.

3. Hockstein NG, O'Malley BW Jr, Weinstein GS. Assessment of intraoperative safety in transoral robotic surgery. Laryngoscope 2006;116(2):165–8.

4. Weinstein G, O'Malley B, Hockstein N. Transoral robotic surgery: supraglottic laryngectomy in a canine model. Laryngoscope 2005;115(7):1315–9.

5. O'Malley BW Jr, Weinstein GS, Snyder W, et al. Transoral robotic surgery (TORS) for base of tongue neoplasms. Laryngoscope 2006;116(8):1465–72.

6. Weinstein G, O'Malley BW Jr, Snyder W, et al. Transoral robotic surgery: supraglottic partial laryngectomy. Ann Otol Rhinol Laryngol 2007;116(1):19–23.

7. Weinstein G, O'Malley BW Jr, Snyder W, et al. Transoral robotic surgery: radical tonsillectomy. Arch Otolaryngol Head Neck Surg 2007;133(12):1220–6.

8. Genden EM, Desai S, Sung CK. Transoral robotic surgery for the management of head and neck cancer: a preliminary experience. Head Neck 2009;19(1):67–71.

9. Iseli TA, Kulbersh BD, Iseli CE, et al. Functional outcomes after transoral robotic surgery for head and neck cancer. Otolaryngol Head Neck Surg 2009;141(2): 166–71.

10. Moore EJ, Olsen KD, Kasperbauer JL. Transoral robotic surgery for oropharyngeal squamous cell carcinoma: a prospective study of feasibility and functional outcomes. Laryngoscope 2009;119(11):2156–64.

11. Bhayani MK, Holsinger FC, Lai SY. A shifting paradigm for patients with head and neck cancer: transoral robotic surgery (TORS). Oncology (Williston Park) 2010; 24(11):1010–5.

12. Chen AA. Shifting paradigm for patients with head and neck cancer: transoral robotic surgery. Oncology 2010;24(11):1030, 1032.

13. O'Malley B. Transoral robotic surgery for parapharyngeal space tumors. ORL J Otorhinolaryngol Relat Spec 2010;72(6):332–6.

14. Selber JC. Transoral robotic reconstruction of oropharyngeal defects: a case series. Plast Reconstr Surg 2010;126(6):1978–87.

15. Weinstein GS, O'Malley BW Jr, Cohen MA, et al. Transoral robotic surgery for advanced oropharyngeal carcinoma. Arch Otolaryngol Head Neck Surg 2010; 136(11):1079–85.

16. Vicini C, Dallan I, Canzi P, et al. Transoral robotic tongue base resection in obstructive sleep apnoea-hypopnoea syndrome: a preliminary report. ORL J Otorhinolaryngol Relat Spec 2010;72(1):22–7.

17. Lee JM, Weinstein GS, O'Malley BW Jr, et al. Transoral robot-assisted lingual tonsillectomy and uvulopalatopharyngoplasty for obstructive sleep apnea. Ann Otol Rhinol Laryngol 2012;121(10):635–9.

18. Vicini C, Montevecchi F, Campanini A, et al. Clinical outcomes and complications associated with TORS for OSAHS: a benchmark for evaluating an emerging surgical technology in a targeted application for benign disease. ORL J Otorhinolaryngol Relat Spec 2014;76(2):63–9.

19. Villanueva NL, de Almeida JR, Sikora AG, et al. Transoral robotic surgery for the management of oropharyngeal minor salivary gland tumors. Head Neck 2014; 36(1):28–33.

20. Chauvet D, Missistrano A, Hivelin M, et al. Transoral robotic-assisted skull base surgery to approach the sella turcica: cadaveric study. Neurosurg Rev 2014; 37(4):609–17.

21. Chauvet D, Hans S, Missistrano A, et al. Transoral robotic surgery for sellar tumors: first clinical study. J Neurosurg 2017;127(4):941–8.

22. de Almeida JR, Li R, Magnuson JS, et al. Oncologic outcomes after transoral robotic surgery: a multi-institutional study. JAMA Otolaryngol Head Neck Surg 2015;141(12):1043–51.

23. Castellano A, Sharma A. Systematic review of validated quality of life and swallow outcomes after transoral robotic surgery. Otolaryngol Head Neck Surg 2019; 161(4):561–7.

24. Golusinski W. Functional organ preservation surgery in head and neck cancer: transoral robotic surgery and beyond. Front Oncol 2019;9:293.

25. Golusinski W, Golusinski-Kardach E. Current roll of surgery in the management of oropharyngeal cancer. Front Oncol 2019;9:388.

Current Indications for Transoral Robotic Surgery in Oropharyngeal Cancer

Harman S. Parhar, MD, MPH, Christina M. Yver, MD, Robert M. Brody, MD*

KEYWORDS

- Oropharyngeal cancer • Transoral robotic surgery • Throat cancer
- Human papillomavirus

KEY POINTS

- The incidence of oropharyngeal squamous cell carcinoma (OPSCC) is increasing dramatically and is conclusively linked to increasing rates of human papillomavirus (HPV) infection.
- HPV-related oropharyngeal cancers have been shown to occur in a unique demographic group and show favorable oncologic outcomes compared with HPV-negative OPSCC.
- There has been a paradigm shift in the treatment of early-stage OPSCC, with most patients now undergoing primary surgery in the United States.
- Transoral robotic surgery is associated with excellent oncologic and functional outcomes in the treatment of OPSCC and is increasingly being used for a broader range of oropharyngeal indications.

 Video content accompanies this article at http://www.oto.theclinics.com.

INTRODUCTION

This article discusses the changing epidemiology of oropharyngeal squamous cell carcinoma (OPSCC), which has become a key factor in the development of robotics in otolaryngology. It discusses the evolution of the treatment paradigm of OPSCC, from historical open procedures, to advances in radiotherapy and chemoradiation, to the contemporary development of novel transoral procedures, including robotic surgery. In so doing, it describes the shift in patient demographics and outcomes in the human papilloma virus era of OPSCC and how this has affected the landscape of therapy. A detailed review of the current oncologic indications for transoral robotic

Department of Otorhinolaryngology–Head & Neck Surgery, University of Pennsylvania Health System, 3400 Spruce Street, 5th Floor Silverstein Building, Philadelphia, PA 19104, USA
* Corresponding author.
E-mail address: Robert.Brody@uphs.upenn.edu

Otolaryngol Clin N Am 53 (2020) 949–964
https://doi.org/10.1016/j.otc.2020.07.007   oto.theclinics.com
0030-6665/20/© 2020 Elsevier Inc. All rights reserved.

surgery (TORS) is presented as well as a description of the most common surgical procedures: radical tonsillectomy and base of tongue resection.

EPIDEMIOLOGY

Head and neck cancer represents the sixth most common cancer worldwide, with more than 700,000 new cases in 2018.[1] Among them, there has been a notable increase in the incidence of OPSCC, with an estimated annual incidence of 92,887 worldwide.[1] In contrast, the rates of cancer in other subsites of the head and neck have decreased, likely because of lower rates of smoking and alcohol use over the past several decades.[2,3] The increasing incidence of OPSCC has been most pronounced in North America, northern Europe, and Australia.[4-11]

The dramatic increase has been shown, through epidemiologic, molecular, and case-control studies, to be conclusively linked to human papillomavirus (HPV) coinfection.[12-15] In the United States alone, the incidence of HPV-mediated OPSCC increased by 225% between 1998 and 2004.[12] The proportion of OPSCC related to HPV infection varies around the world, with HPV implicated in up to 80% of US cases of OPSCC, but fewer than 20% of OPSCCs in countries with higher rates of tobacco use.[16] The variable global distribution has led some to propose that changes in sexual behaviors (eg, oral sex, multiple sexual partners) among contemporary cohorts have led to increased oral HPV exposure and associated cancer risk.[4,9,12,16-19] The increased incidence of OPSCC is associated not only with certain geographic locations but also with a unique demographic cohort: young (between 40 and 55 years of age) white men, often without a strong history of alcohol or tobacco use.[10,16]

Another distinct feature of HPV-mediated OPSCC is its tendency to originate in the lingual and palatine tonsil subsites, because the virus is thought to preferentially target the reticulated epithelium lining the tonsillar crypts.[20,21] Importantly, HPV-associated OPSCC is associated with a more favorable prognosis compared with HPV-negative OPSCC.[21,22] This prognosis is thought to be related not only to higher response rates to therapy but also to the absence of field cancerization from tobacco and alcohol. HPV-positive patients are also more likely to have excellent performance status and fewer comorbidities.[16,23-25]

HISTORICAL PERSPECTIVE ON OROPHARYNGEAL CANCER TREATMENT

Waldeyer's[26] nineteenth century microscopic studies were the first to show that squamous cancers in the head and neck originated from epithelial surfaces. One early well-documented case occurred in 1884 when America's 18th President, Ulysses S. Grant, developed a right tonsillar carcinoma.[27,28] He underwent a subtotal resection and topical cocaine therapy, which provided some degree of palliation but did not arrest tumor growth, eventually eroding through his palate.[27] He had a sentinel bleed in the spring of 1885 and passed away shortly thereafter.[27,28]

Advances in aseptic technique, general anesthesia, and airway management allowed nineteenth century innovation in head and neck surgery. In 1846 at Harvard, John Warren was the first to remove a cervical tumor under general anesthesia.[29,30] In 1862, Theodore Billroth[31] described the transmandibular approach to the oral cavity and oropharynx.[31,32] Subsequently, in 1880, Theodor Kocher[33] described transcervical techniques to obtain arterial control of head and neck tumors.[29,30,33]

Despite advances, head and neck surgery was associated with prohibitive morbidity, and the treatment of head and neck cancer in the early to mid-twentieth century was therefore dominated by radiotherapy, a new and promising entity.[29,32] However, failure rates of single-modality radiotherapy (up to 95%) and the complications associated with salvage surgery prompted a revival of surgical efforts.[29,32] In the 1940s and 1950s, New York surgeon Hayes Martin popularized the so-called commando operation, which involved a lip split, segmental mandibulectomy, and in-continuity neck dissection for oral cavity and oropharyngeal malignancy.[29] Despite subsequent refinements, such as mandibular lingual release and transpharyngeal approaches, radical approaches continued to dominate the oropharyngeal landscape despite high levels of morbidity and stagnating cure rates.[34–36] Between the 1970s and 1990s, radiotherapy again gained prominence, initially as an adjunct, and later as primary therapy alongside new chemotherapeutics (eg, chemoradiotherapy [CRT]).[37] Eventually, CRT became routinely used as primary therapy for because it was thought to offer similar oncologic results with preservation of form and function.[38,39] However, CRT came with its own set of morbidities, including mucositis and dysphagia, and many patients later required salvage procedures.[40,41]

CURRENT TECHNIQUES IN OROPHARYNGEAL SURGERY

In the late twentieth and early twenty-first century, the dramatic increase in OPSCC incidence driven by HPV oncogenicity became an impetus for innovation in minimally invasive techniques. Although radical tonsillectomy had been described as early as 1951 by Huet[42] and the technique had been practiced by head and neck surgeons throughout the late twentieth century, there were no published studies assessing clinical outcomes in these patients. In the early twenty-first century, Laccourreye and colleagues[43] and Holsinger and colleagues[44] developed a standardized technique for radical tonsillectomy using cold knife and electrocautery. However, these techniques were limited by a lack of adequate visualization of the tongue base and limited access to reliably obtain negative margins. Haughey and colleagues[45] and other investigators described transoral laser microsurgery (TLM) as an alternative surgical technique that provides improved visualization and hemostasis with excellent oncologic outcomes; however, this technique did not become widely adopted.

The limitations of existing techniques for transoral access to the oropharynx prompted the development of a novel application of robotics. Initially used in general surgery, obstetrics and gynecology, and urology, the da Vinci Surgical System (Intuitive Surgical Inc, Sunnyvale, CA) was pioneered for use in transoral surgery at the University of Pennsylvania. In 2005, initial studies on human cadavers and canines confirmed the feasibility of its application.[46,47] Excellent visualization, decreased line of sight issues (using a 30° endoscope), and the addition of an assistant at the head of the bed allowed modification of the Huet procedure to perform a reliable radical tonsillectomy without the limitations associated with the original technique.[48] A standardized radical base of tongue resection technique was subsequently developed.[49] With these 2 standardized TORS procedures, most early-stage oropharyngeal tumors could be reliably treated with primary surgery.

Additional robotic systems, including the Medrobotic Flex system (Medrobotics, Raynham, MA) and accompanying oropharyngeal retractors, have since been pioneered and tested successfully.[50,51] The da Vinci robot now hosts the Si (US Food and Drug Administration [FDA] approved), Xi (off-label), and new SP (off-label, single port) systems.[52]

OROPHARYNGEAL INDICATIONS FOR TRANSORAL ROBOTIC SURGERY
Early-Stage Oropharyngeal Cancers

Outcomes from successful multi-institutional retrospective trials led to the FDA approval of TORS for benign and T1/T2 malignant otolaryngologic tumors in 2009.[53] Although TORS has been used to manage numerous disorders, it is most commonly used for resection of early-stage OPSCC. American population-based data have shown that the percentage of patients undergoing primary surgery for T1/T2 OPSCC increased from 56% in 2004 to 82% in 2013. This shift has been driven by patient preference, excellent oncologic results, encouraging functional results, and advances in surgical robotic technology.[54,55] To better understand which patients with OPSCC are best suited to an upfront surgical approach, it is important to consider contraindications.

Contraindications to TORS can be categorized as vascular, functional, oncologic, and nononcologic.[56] Vascular contraindications include tonsillar cancer with a retropharyngeal carotid artery, tumor in the midline tongue base putting both lingual arteries at risk, tumor adjacent to carotid bulb or internal carotid artery, and tumor or metastatic node encasing carotid artery.[56,57] Functional contraindications include tumor resection requiring more than 50% of the deep tongue base musculature, the posterior pharyngeal wall, the tongue base, or the entire epiglottis.[56] Oncologic contraindications include unresectable tumor (involving lateral pterygoid muscle, pterygoid plates, lateral nasopharynx, skull base, prevertebral fascia), unresectable neck disease, neoplastic-related trismus, and multifocal distant metastases.[56] Additional nononcologic contraindications include systemic disease associated with unacceptable morbidity in the perioperative period, non–cancer-related trismus preventing robotic access, and cervical spine disease interfering with patient positioning and neck extension.[56]

Many investigators advocate that patients with T1/T2 OPSCC who are able to minimize or avoid postoperative adjuvant therapy are best suited to an upfront TORS approach. Upfront TORS has the potential to reduce and/or eliminate the need for adjuvant therapy in certain cases, and numerous encouraging treatment deescalation trials are currently underway. A full discussion of treatment deescalation can be found in a separate Benjamin Wahle and Jose Zevallos' article, "Transoral Robotic Surgery and De-escalation of Cancer Treatment," in this series.

Oncologic results for early-stage OPSCC treated with upfront TORS have been very favorable (**Table 1**). Early studies published by Weinstein and colleagues[48] showed a 100% locoregional control rate for selected T1 to T3 tonsillar cancers (N = 27), as well as a 93% 2-year disease-specific survival rate in a subsequent study including all oropharyngeal subsites (N = 50, T1–T4).[58] Moore and colleagues[59] showed 3-year local and regional disease control rates of 97% and 94%, respectively, as well as 2-year disease-free and recurrence-free survival rates of 95% and 92%, respectively (N = 66; 84.9% T1/T2). A recent large multicenter study of 410 patients undergoing TORS (89% OPSCC) showed 2-year disease-specific and overall survival rates of 95% and 91% respectively.[60] Of these patients, 84% were T1/T2, 70% were HPV positive (of those with known status), and 47% underwent surgery alone without need for adjuvant therapy. This finding was also consistent with a recent systematic review of 772 patients that showed 2-year survival estimates of 82% to 94% for early-stage OPSCC treated with upfront TORS.[61]

Functional outcomes following TORS are also encouraging (**Table 2**). In a study of 38 patients with OPSCC treated with upfront TORS (86.9% T1/T2), Leonhardt and colleagues[62] showed that although decreases in diet-related indices were observed early

Table 1
Oncologic outcomes following transoral robotic surgery for oropharyngeal squamous cell carcinoma

Study	N	T Stage	p16+ (%)	Negative Margins (%)	Adjuvant Therapy (%)			Overall Survival (%)			Disease-Specific Survival (%)			Recurrence-Free Survival (%)		
					S Alone (%)	S + XRT (%)	S + CRT (%)	1-y	2-y	5-y	1-y	2-y	5-y	1-y	2-y	5-y
Weinstein et al,[48] 2007	27	T1–T3	—	92.6	7.4	33.3	55.6	No survival data provided			—	—	—	—	—	—
Cohen et al,[58] 2011	50	T1–T4a	74.0	94.0	18.0	24.0	54.0	95.7	80.6	—	97.8	92.6	—	—	—	—
Moore et al,[59] 2012	66	T1–T4a	66.7	98.0	16.7	21.2	62.0	—	—	—	—	95.1	—	—	92.4	—
De Almeida et al,[60] 2015	410	T1–T4a	69.4	69.1	47.3	31.4	21.3	—	91.0	—	—	94.5	—	—	—	—
Sharma et al,[99] 2016	39	T1–T3	97.0	—	10.3	61.5	28.2	Survival comparable to matched controls (CRT)								
Moore et al,[100] 2018	314	T1–T4a	93.0	98.0	24.0	28.0	48.0	98.0	—	86.0	99.0	—	94.0	98.0	—	98.0
Dhanireddy et al,[101] 2019	65	T1–T2	80.0	—	25.0	37.5	37.5	—	82.3	70.2	—	—	—	—	—	—
Total	971	—	—	—	—	—	—	—	—	—	—	—	—	—	—	—

Abbreviations: S, surgery; XRT, radiotherapy.
Data from Refs.[48,58–60,99–101]

Table 2
Functional outcomes following transoral robotic surgery for oropharyngeal squamous cell carcinoma

Study	N	T Stage	Tumor Site	Tracheostomy Temporary (%)	Tracheostomy Permanent (%)	Gastrostomy Tube Temporary (%)	Gastrostomy Tube Permanent (%)	HRQOL (Overall QOL) Baseline	HRQOL (Overall QOL) 6 mo	HRQOL (Overall QOL) 12 mo
Weinstein et al,[48] 2007	27	T1–T3	Tonsil	—	—	—	3.7	—	—	—
Moore et al,[59] 2012	66	T1–T4a	Tonsil, BOT	25.8	1.5	27.2	4.5	—	—	—
Dziegielewski et al,[102] 2013	81	T1–T4a	Tonsil, BOT, SP	1	0	21	11	76.3 (21.7)	66.0 (25.8)	76.8 (20.5)
Kelly et al,[63] 2014	190	T1–T2	—	—	0	—	5	—	—	—
Sharma et al,[99] 2016	39	T–T3	Tonsil, BOT	—	—	9	3	—	—	—
Achim et al,[103] 2018	74	T1–T2	Tonsil, BOT	1.4	0	9	1	—	—	—
Sethia et al,[104] 2018	111	T1–T4a	Tonsil, BOT	0	0	44.1	10.8	—	—	—
Van Abel et al,[105] 2019	267	T1–T4	—	11	0.7	28.8	2.2	—	—	—

QOL reported as mean (standard deviation).
Permanent is defined as more than 12 months postoperative.
Abbreviations: BOT, base of tongue; HRQOL, health-related quality of life; QOL, quality of life; SP, soft palate.
Data from Refs.[48,59,63,99,102–105]

after TORS, all patients returned to baseline quality of life and functional status at 12 months after surgery. Similar results were shown by Dziegielewski and colleagues, who reviewed a series of 81 patients who had TORS and found that patients had high levels of aesthetic, social and overall quality of life at 1 year after surgery.[102] A recent randomized trial comparing primary TORS and primary radiotherapy (N = 34 per arm) showed comparable oncologic outcomes, differing side effect profile depending on treatment modality, and non–clinically meaningful differences in swallowing-related quality of life.[64]

Complication rates have been found to be acceptably low following TORS for early-stage OPSCC. A recent systematic review found that, among patients undergoing TORS for early OPSCC, the rate of postoperative hemorrhage was 2.4%, the rate of neck hematoma was 0.4%, and the rate of pharyngocutaneous fistula was 2.5%.[61] Other studies have found rates of postoperative hemorrhage ranging from 2.4% to 7.4%, which is similar to hemorrhage following palatine tonsillectomy (3.5%–4.8%).[61,65–69]

Advanced-Stage Oropharyngeal Cancers

Although most of the TORS literature focuses on outcomes of upfront surgery for early-stage OPSCC, there is also a growing body of evidence that TORS may have applications for upfront surgical management of more advanced disease. A 2011 study by Cohen and colleagues[58] reviewed 50 patients with OPSCC undergoing TORS and neck dissection, of whom 89% had stage 3 or stage 4 disease, and found 2-year overall survival and disease-specific survival for the entire cohort to be 81% and 93%, respectively. A recent National Cancer Database study examined 16,891 patients with stage 3 or 4 disease (excluding American Joint Committee on Cancer, Seventh Edition, T4b) and stratified by whether they received primary chemoradiation (N = 8123), surgery followed by radiation (N = 3519), or surgery followed by chemoradiation (N = 5249).[70] Patients receiving triple-modality therapy had the highest 3-year overall survival (90% overall survival for triple modality therapy compared with 85% overall survival for surgery followed by radiation and 82% overall survival for primary chemoradiation; P<.01).[70]

An additional benefit to upfront surgery in advanced OPSCC is the ability to obtain a pathologic specimen for restaging. In many cases, this leads to downstaging and reduces the needed radiation dose, and possibly avoids chemotherapy altogether.[45,70,71] One study of 64 patients showed that upfront TORS resulted in the avoidance of chemotherapy in 34% of patients who presented with T3/T4 tumors, and another study of 76 patients showed that chemotherapy was able to be avoided in 46% of T3/T4 tumors.[71,72]

Unknown Primary

Approximately 2% to 5% of all head and neck malignancies present as metastatic cervical squamous cell carcinoma with an unknown primary site.[73,74] However, a traditional work-up involving history and physical examination, preoperative imaging studies, and selective operative endoscopy has been shown to identify primary malignancy in only 47% to 59% of patients.[73,75] Primary identification is important because it helps to target therapy and also potentially reduce radiotherapy dosage, thus reducing radiation-related morbidity, and improve survival.[76–78] Several institutions have described protocols generally involving TORS-assisted resection of ipsilateral palatine and possible lingual tonsillectomy with immediate frozen-section pathologic examination.[79–82] If the primary is located, an oncologic procedure will proceed. If not, a contralateral diagnostic surgery will occur.[79] These TORS-assisted strategies successfully identify the primary in 72% to 80% of cases.[79–82] A full discussion of TORS for work-up of primary unknown malignancy, including a detailed surgical algorithm, can be found in a separate John R. de Almeida's article, "Role of TORS in the Work-Up of The Unknown Primary," of this series.

Salvage Oropharyngeal Surgery

Although surgery has been regarded as a salvage option following a partial response or local recurrence following primary radiotherapy or chemoradiotherapy for OPSCC, oncologic results have been disappointing. Five-year disease-free survival rates range from 19% to 22% in multiple large cohorts after traditional salvage surgery.[83–85] In addition, major complication rates approach 50%, and include orocutaneous fistulae, neck abscess, systemic complications, and carotid rupture.[84,85] In addition, traditional approaches to salvage oropharyngeal surgery are more invasive and often necessitate segmental mandibulectomy (44%–76%), total laryngectomy (6%–17%), and microvascular reconstruction (68%–82%).[83–85] Permanent tracheostomy and gastrostomy tube rates following open salvage surgery have been found to vary between 7% and 15% and 4% and 65%, respectively.[83–85]

The TORS approach to oropharyngeal salvage has shown encouraging early results compared with traditional techniques for salvage surgery. White and colleagues[86] described a 128-patient cohort of patients matched by TNM (tumor, node, metastasis) and evenly split between TORS and open salvage from a multi-institution study. TORS was found to significantly reduce rates of permanent gastrostomy (3% vs 31%) as well as reduce hospital length of stay (4 vs 8 days), blood loss (49 vs 331 mL), operative time (111 vs 350 minutes), and rates of positive margin (9% vs 29%).[86] Two-year disease-free survival was 74% and 43% in the TORS and open groups, respectively.[86] In a survival analysis of 30 patients who underwent TORS surgical salvage for OPSCC, Meulemans and colleagues[87] described a 2-year overall survival rate of 74% and disease-free survival of 76%. There are currently additional multi-institution cohort studies underway to further corroborate the benefits of TORS in the salvage setting.

Minor Salivary Gland Malignancies in the Oropharynx

Although minor salivary gland tumors vary greatly in their clinical behavior and appearance, most are malignant.[88] Standard therapy includes upfront surgery followed by pathology-driven adjuvant therapy because they tend to be radioresistant and therefore do poorly with radiation alone.[89–91] Adjuvant radiation is recommended if the tumor is incompletely resected, is of an advanced stage, or if there are other adverse pathologic features.[90–92]

Margin status is of the utmost importance, because negative margins have been shown to be an independent predictor for survival in numerous series.[88,93–95] This finding poses a unique challenge to surgeons, because minor salivary tumors in the oropharynx have a propensity for submucosal growth and are located in a region that is traditionally difficult to access.[88] It is therefore unsurprising that efforts to resect tumors using traditional open approaches are associated with high rates of positive margins. For example, in a large series of 61 patients who underwent upfront open surgery for oropharyngeal minor salivary tumors (20 transoral, 4 transcervical, and 37 transmandibular), 28 (46%) patients had a positive margin on pathologic review.[88] In contrast, the TORS approach is well suited to the resection of oropharyngeal salivary malignancy because of improved access and visualization. Villaneueva and colleagues[96] reviewed a series of 10 patients who underwent TORS for oropharyngeal minor salivary gland tumors and reported that no patients in the cohort had a positive margin on final pathology. Similarly, Schoppy and colleagues[97] performed either

TORS or TLM on a group of 20 patients with oropharyngeal minor salivary tumors (18 TORS and 2 TLM) and reported a negative margin rate of 95%.

SURGICAL TECHNIQUES
Preoperative Evaluation

Evaluation begins with detailed history and physical examination, with an emphasis on the presence and degree of trismus and assessment of cervical spine mobility.[98] Cross-sectional imaging is performed for staging, to assess resectability and to rule out internal carotid artery involvement.[98] An examination under anesthesia is performed to assess the extent of the tumor and whether there exists any contraindication for surgery (listed earlier).[98] In addition, patients are presented at a multidisciplinary tumor board to discuss options for treatment.

Radical Tonsillectomy

Setup: the nurse sits to the left of the patient, the robotic cart is positioned to the right of the patient, and the bedside surgical assistant sits at the patient's head. The patient is paralyzed. A tongue retraction suture is placed. A Crow-Davis mouth gag provides pharyngeal exposure and the patient is suspended via a Storz arm (Karl Storz, Tuttlingen, Germany). The 0° endoscope is placed in the central robotic arm and the lateral arms are loaded with a 5-mm monopolar cautery and Maryland retractor. The bedside assistant also has access to 2 suctions, a bayonet-style bipolar cautery, and an endoscopic clip applier with medium clip houses.[48,98]
 Step 1: an incision is made at the level of the pterygomandibular raphe through the buccal mucosa between the upper and lower molars using cautery. Step 2: dissection proceeds lateral to the constrictor muscles, bluntly dissecting the parapharyngeal fat pad laterally, identifying the pterygoid musculature laterally, and is carried down to the styloglossus and stylopharyngeus. Step 3: the soft palate and superior aspect of pharyngeal constrictors are transected through to the prevertebral fascia. Step 4: the constrictor muscles are bluntly elevated off the prevertebral fascia. Step 5: an index cut is made through the mucosa of the posterior pharyngeal wall. Step 6: a tongue base margin is taken by making an incision across the posterior floor of the mouth to the lateral tongue base down to the level of the vallecula. Step 7: care is taken to avoid transecting the lingual artery, but, if encountered, it is ligated with surgical clips. Step 8: the posterior pharyngeal wall is then resected from the vallecula up to the level of the soft palate along the previously made index cut. Care is taken on the lateral cuts as well as the pharyngeal cuts to protect the carotid arterial system.[48,98] Step 9: pathologic analysis, final hemostasis, and reconstruction as required.[48,98] Step 10: neck dissection occurs either concurrently or in a staged manner. A case example of TORS radical tonsillectomy is shown in Video 1.

Base of Tongue Resection

Setup: the setup for tongue base resection is similar to a radical tonsillectomy except an FK-WO retractor (with short Weinstein-O'Malley blade) is used and suspension is achieved with a Mayo stand. A Storz arm attaches to the bedside frame and supports the FK-WO retractor.[49,98] The procedure is generally started with a 0° scope but is occasionally changed to a 30° scope later in the procedure.[49,98]
 Step 1: a pharyngeal cut is made in the tonsillar fossa. If the tumor is located in the glossotonsillar sulcus, a radical tonsillectomy will accompany the tongue base resection. If not, a small amount of tonsillar fossa is resected.[49,98] Step 2: a partial horizontal tongue base mucosal cut is carried adjacent to retractor blade. Step 3: a midline

tongue base incision is made to an appropriate depth to account for tumor and margin. Step 4: the deep musculature transection is completed to an appropriate depth horizontally. Step 5: a lateral tongue base incision is made to bridge the pharyngeal cut and the lateral muscular cut. Step 7: the ipsilateral lingual artery and/or branches are identified and ligated with surgical clips. Step 8: the final dissection involves cutting through the remaining deep muscle and the underlying vallecular mucosa. Step 9: pathologic analysis, final hemostasis, and reconstruction as required. Step 10: neck dissection occurs either concurrently or in a staged manner.[49,98] A case example of TORS tongue base resection is shown in Video 2.

SUMMARY

The dramatic increase in the incidence of OPSCC has been conclusively linked to HPV oncogenicity. These cancers, defined by a unique demographic profile and favorable outcomes, served as an impetus for the development of minimally invasive surgical techniques, including TORS. TORS has shown excellent oncologic and functional outcomes in the treatment of OPSCC and is also being increasingly used for other oropharyngeal indications.

DISCLOSURE

The authors have nothing to disclose.

SUPPLEMENTARY DATA

Supplementary data related to this article can be found online at https://doi.org/10.1016/j.otc.2020.07.007.

REFERENCES

1. Bray F, Ferlay J, Soerjomataram I, et al. Global cancer statistics 2018: GLOBOCAN estimates of incidence and mortality worldwide for 36 cancers in 185 countries. CA Cancer J Clin 2018;68(6):394–424.
2. Blot WJ, Devesa SS, McLaughlin JK, et al. Oral and pharyngeal cancers. Cancer Surv 1994;19-20:23–42.
3. Franceschi S, Bidoli E, Herrero R, et al. Comparison of cancers of the oral cavity and pharynx worldwide: etiological clues. Oral Oncol 2000;36(1):106–15.
4. Hong AM, Grulich AE, Jones D, et al. Squamous cell carcinoma of the oropharynx in Australian males induced by human papillomavirus vaccine targets. Vaccine 2010;28(19):3269–72.
5. Auluck A, Hislop G, Bajdik C, et al. Trends in oropharyngeal and oral cavity cancer incidence of human papillomavirus (HPV)-related and HPV-unrelated sites in a multicultural population: the British Columbia experience. Cancer 2010; 116(11):2635–44.
6. Blomberg M, Nielsen A, Munk C, et al. Trends in head and neck cancer incidence in Denmark, 1978-2007: focus on human papillomavirus associated sites. Int J Cancer 2011;129(3):733–41.
7. Braakhuis BJM, Visser O, Leemans CR. Oral and oropharyngeal cancer in The Netherlands between 1989 and 2006: Increasing incidence, but not in young adults. Oral Oncol 2009;45(9):e85–9.
8. Mork J, Møller B, Dahl T, et al. Time trends in pharyngeal cancer incidence in Norway 1981-2005: a subsite analysis based on a reabstraction and recoding of registered cases. Cancer Causes Control 2010;21(9):1397–405.

9. Hammarstedt L, Lindquist D, Dahlstrand H, et al. Human papillomavirus as a risk factor for the increase in incidence of tonsillar cancer. Int J Cancer 2006; 119(11):2620–3.
10. Chaturvedi AK, Engels EA, Anderson WF, et al. Incidence trends for human papillomavirus-related and -unrelated oral squamous cell carcinomas in the United States. J Clin Oncol 2008;26(4):612–9.
11. Reddy VM, Cundall-Curry D, Bridger MWM. Trends in the incidence rates of tonsil and base of tongue cancer in England, 1985-2006. Ann R Coll Surg Engl 2010;92(8):655–9.
12. Chaturvedi AK, Engels EA, Pfeiffer RM, et al. Human papillomavirus and rising oropharyngeal cancer incidence in the United States. J Clin Oncol 2011;29(32): 4294–301.
13. D'Souza G, Kreimer AR, Viscidi R, et al. Case-control study of human papillomavirus and oropharyngeal cancer. N Engl J Med 2007;356(19):1944–56.
14. Ryerson AB, Peters ES, Coughlin SS, et al. Burden of potentially human papillomavirus-associated cancers of the oropharynx and oral cavity in the US, 1998-2003. Cancer 2008;113(10 Suppl):2901–9.
15. Gillison ML. Human papillomavirus-associated head and neck cancer is a distinct epidemiologic, clinical, and molecular entity. Semin Oncol 2004;31(6): 744–54.
16. Marur S, D'Souza G, Westra WH, et al. HPV-associated head and neck cancer: a virus-related cancer epidemic. Lancet Oncol 2010;11(8):781–9.
17. Majchrzak E, Szybiak B, Wegner A, et al. Oral cavity and oropharyngeal squamous cell carcinoma in young adults: a review of the literature. Radiol Oncol 2014;48(1):1–10.
18. Schnelle C, Whiteman DC, Porceddu SV, et al. Past sexual behaviors and risks of oropharyngeal squamous cell carcinoma: a case-case comparison. Int J Cancer 2017;140(5):1027–34.
19. D'Souza G, Agrawal Y, Halpern J, et al. Oral sexual behaviors associated with prevalent oral human papillomavirus infection. J Infect Dis 2009;199(9):1263–9.
20. Pai SI, Westra WH. Molecular pathology of head and neck cancer: implications for diagnosis, prognosis, and treatment. Annu Rev Pathol 2009;4:49–70.
21. Fakhry C, Westra WH, Li S, et al. Improved survival of patients with human papillomavirus-positive head and neck squamous cell carcinoma in a prospective clinical trial. J Natl Cancer Inst 2008;100(4):261–9.
22. Ang KK, Harris J, Wheeler R, et al. Human papillomavirus and survival of patients with oropharyngeal cancer. N Engl J Med 2010;363(1):24–35.
23. Bristow RG, Benchimol S, Hill RP. The p53 gene as a modifier of intrinsic radiosensitivity: implications for radiotherapy. Radiother Oncol 1996;40(3):197–223.
24. Butz K, Geisen C, Ullmann A, et al. Cellular responses of HPV-positive cancer cells to genotoxic anti-cancer agents: repression of E6/E7-oncogene expression and induction of apoptosis. Int J Cancer 1996;68(4):506–13.
25. Lindel K, Beer KT, Laissue J, et al. Human papillomavirus positive squamous cell carcinoma of the oropharynx: a radiosensitive subgroup of head and neck carcinoma. Cancer 2001;92(4):805–13.
26. Waldeyer W. Die Entwicklung der Carcinome. Arch Pathol Anat 1867;41: 470–522.
27. Steckler RM, Shedd DP. General Grant: his physicians and his cancer. Am J Surg 1976;132(4):508–14.
28. Renehan A, Lowry JC. The oral tumours of two American presidents: what if they were alive today? J R Soc Med 1995;88(7):377–83.

29. Folz BJ, Silver CE, Rinaldo A, et al. An outline of the history of head and neck oncology. Oral Oncol 2008;44(1):2–9.
30. Folz BJ, Ferlito A, Silver CE, et al. Neck dissection in the nineteenth century. Eur Arch Otorhinolaryngol 2007;264(5):455–60.
31. Billroth T. Osteoplastiche Resectionen des Unterkiefers nach Eigener Methode. Arch Klin Chri 1862;2:651–7.
32. McGurk M, Goodger NM. Head and neck cancer and its treatment: historical review. Br J Oral Maxillofac Surg 2000;38(3):209–20.
33. Kocher T. Ueber Radicalheilung des Krebses. Dtsch Z Chir 1880;13:134–66.
34. Holsinger FC, Weber RS. Swing of the surgical pendulum: a return to surgery for treatment of head and neck cancer in the 21st century? Int J Radiat Oncol Biol Phys 2007;69(2 Suppl):S129–31.
35. Christopoulos E, Carrau R, Segas J, et al. Transmandibular approaches to the oral cavity and oropharynx. A functional assessment. Arch Otolaryngol Head Neck Surg 1992;118(11):1164–7.
36. Stanley RB. Mandibular lingual releasing approach to oral and oropharyngeal carcinomas. Laryngoscope 1984;94(5 Pt 1):596–600.
37. Vikram B, Strong EW, Shah J, et al. Elective postoperative radiation therapy in stages III and IV epidermoid carcinoma of the head and neck. Am J Surg 1980;140(4):580–4.
38. Calais G, Alfonsi M, Bardet E, et al. Randomized trial of radiation therapy versus concomitant chemotherapy and radiation therapy for advanced-stage oropharynx carcinoma. J Natl Cancer Inst 1999;91(24):2081–6.
39. Pignon J-P, le Maître A, Maillard E, et al, MACH-NC Collaborative Group. Meta-analysis of chemotherapy in head and neck cancer (MACH-NC): an update on 93 randomised trials and 17,346 patients. Radiother Oncol 2009;92(1):4–14.
40. Caudell JJ, Schaner PE, Meredith RF, et al. Factors associated with long-term dysphagia after definitive radiotherapy for locally advanced head-and-neck cancer. Int J Radiat Oncol Biol Phys 2009;73(2):410–5.
41. Machtay M, Moughan J, Trotti A, et al. Factors associated with severe late toxicity after concurrent chemoradiation for locally advanced head and neck cancer: an RTOG analysis. J Clin Oncol 2008;26(21):3582–9.
42. Huet PC. [Electrocoagulation in epitheliomas of the tonsils]. Ann Otolaryngol 1951;68(7):433–42.
43. Laccourreye O, Hans S, Ménard M, et al. Transoral lateral oropharyngectomy for squamous cell carcinoma of the tonsillar region: II. An analysis of the incidence, related variables, and consequences of local recurrence. Arch Otolaryngol Head Neck Surg 2005;131(7):592–9.
44. Holsinger FC, McWhorter AJ, Ménard M, et al. Transoral lateral oropharyngectomy for squamous cell carcinoma of the tonsillar region: I. Technique, complications, and functional results. Arch Otolaryngol Head Neck Surg 2005;131(7):583–91.
45. Haughey BH, Hinni ML, Salassa JR, et al. Transoral laser microsurgery as primary treatment for advanced-stage oropharyngeal cancer: a United States multicenter study. Head Neck 2011;33(12):1683–94.
46. Hockstein NG, O'Malley BW, Weinstein GS. Assessment of intraoperative safety in transoral robotic surgery. Laryngoscope 2006;116(2):165–8.
47. Weinstein GS, O'malley BW, Hockstein NG. Transoral robotic surgery: supraglottic laryngectomy in a canine model. Laryngoscope 2005;115(7):1315–9.
48. Weinstein GS, O'Malley BW, Snyder W, et al. Transoral robotic surgery: radical tonsillectomy. Arch Otolaryngol Head Neck Surg 2007;133(12):1220–6.

49. O'Malley BW, Weinstein GS, Snyder W, et al. Transoral robotic surgery (TORS) for base of tongue neoplasms. Laryngoscope 2006;116(8):1465–72.

50. Mandapathil M, Duvvuri U, Güldner C, et al. Transoral surgery for oropharyngeal tumors using the Medrobotics(®) Flex(®) System - a case report. Int J Surg Case Rep 2015;10:173–5.

51. Persky MJ, Issa M, Bonfili JR, et al. Transoral surgery using the Flex Robotic System: Initial experience in the United States. Head Neck 2018;40(11):2482–6.

52. Holsinger FC, Magnuson JS, Weinstein GS, et al. A next-generation single-port robotic surgical system for transoral robotic surgery: results from prospective nonrandomized clinical trials. JAMA Otolaryngol Head Neck Surg 2019. https://doi.org/10.1001/jamaoto.2019.2654.

53. Weinstein GS, O'Malley BW, Magnuson JS, et al. Transoral robotic surgery: a multicenter study to assess feasibility, safety, and surgical margins. Laryngoscope 2012;122(8):1701–7.

54. Cracchiolo JR, Roman BR, Kutler DI, et al. Adoption of transoral robotic surgery compared with other surgical modalities for treatment of oropharyngeal squamous cell carcinoma. J Surg Oncol 2016;114(4):405–11.

55. Lam JS, Scott GM, Palma DA, et al. Development of an online, patient-centred decision aid for patients with oropharyngeal cancer in the transoral robotic surgery era. Curr Oncol 2017;24(5):318–23.

56. Weinstein GS, O'Malley BW, Rinaldo A, et al. Understanding contraindications for transoral robotic surgery (TORS) for oropharyngeal cancer. Eur Arch Otorhinolaryngol 2015;272(7):1551–2.

57. Loevner LA, Learned KO, Mohan S, et al. Transoral robotic surgery in head and neck cancer: what radiologists need to know about the cutting edge. Radiographics 2013;33(6):1759–79.

58. Cohen MA, Weinstein GS, O'Malley BW, et al. Transoral robotic surgery and human papillomavirus status: Oncologic results. Head Neck 2011;33(4):573–80.

59. Moore EJ, Olsen SM, Laborde RR, et al. Long-term functional and oncologic results of transoral robotic surgery for oropharyngeal squamous cell carcinoma. Mayo Clin Proc 2012;87(3):219–25.

60. de Almeida JR, Li R, Magnuson JS, et al. Oncologic Outcomes After Transoral Robotic Surgery: A Multi-institutional Study. JAMA Otolaryngol Head Neck Surg 2015;141(12):1043–51.

61. de Almeida JR, Byrd JK, Wu R, et al. A systematic review of transoral robotic surgery and radiotherapy for early oropharynx cancer: a systematic review. Laryngoscope 2014;124(9):2096–102.

62. Leonhardt FD, Quon H, Abrahão M, et al. Transoral robotic surgery for oropharyngeal carcinoma and its impact on patient-reported quality of life and function. Head Neck 2012;34(2):146–54.

63. Kelly K, Johnson-Obaseki S, Lumingu J, et al. Oncologic, functional and surgical outcomes of primary Transoral Robotic Surgery for early squamous cell cancer of the oropharynx: a systematic review. Oral Oncol 2014;50(8):696–703.

64. Nichols AC, Theurer J, Prisman E, et al. Radiotherapy versus transoral robotic surgery and neck dissection for oropharyngeal squamous cell carcinoma (ORATOR): an open-label, phase 2, randomised trial. Lancet Oncol 2019. https://doi.org/10.1016/S1470-2045(19)30410-3.

65. Asher SA, White HN, Kejner AE, et al. Hemorrhage after transoral robotic-assisted surgery. Otolaryngol Head Neck Surg 2013;149(1):112–7.

66. Parhar HS, Gausden E, Patel J, et al. Analysis of readmissions after transoral robotic surgery for oropharyngeal squamous cell carcinoma. Head Neck 2018; 40(11):2416–23.

67. Stokes W, Ramadan J, Lawson G, et al. Bleeding complications after transoral robotic surgery: a meta-analysis and systematic review. Laryngoscope 2020. https://doi.org/10.1002/lary.28580.

68. Lowe D, van der Meulen J, Cromwell D, et al. Key messages from the National Prospective Tonsillectomy Audit. Laryngoscope 2007;117(4):717–24.

69. Bhattacharyya N, Kepnes LJ. Revisits and postoperative hemorrhage after adult tonsillectomy. Laryngoscope 2014;124(7):1554–6.

70. Roden DF, Schreiber D, Givi B. Triple-modality treatment in patients with advanced stage tonsil cancer. Cancer 2017;123(17):3269–76.

71. Hurtuk A, Agrawal A, Old M, et al. Outcomes of transoral robotic surgery: a preliminary clinical experience. Otolaryngol Head Neck Surg 2011;145(2):248–53.

72. Gildener-Leapman N, Kim J, Abberbock S, et al. Utility of up-front transoral robotic surgery in tailoring adjuvant therapy. Head Neck 2016;38(8):1201–7.

73. Waltonen JD, Ozer E, Hall NC, et al. Metastatic carcinoma of the neck of unknown primary origin: evolution and efficacy of the modern workup. Arch Otolaryngol Head Neck Surg 2009;135(10):1024–9.

74. Schmalbach CE, Miller FR. Occult primary head and neck carcinoma. Curr Oncol Rep 2007;9(2):139–46.

75. Keller F, Psychogios G, Linke R, et al. Carcinoma of unknown primary in the head and neck: comparison between positron emission tomography (PET) and PET/CT. Head Neck 2011;33(11):1569–75.

76. Grewal AS, Rajasekaran K, Cannady SB, et al. Pharyngeal-sparing radiation for head and neck carcinoma of unknown primary following TORS assisted workup. Laryngoscope 2020;130(3):691–7.

77. Haas I, Hoffmann TK, Engers R, et al. Diagnostic strategies in cervical carcinoma of an unknown primary (CUP). Eur Arch Otorhinolaryngol 2002;259(6):325–33.

78. Davis KS, Byrd JK, Mehta V, et al. Occult Primary Head and Neck Squamous Cell Carcinoma: Utility of Discovering Primary Lesions. Otolaryngol Head Neck Surg 2014;151(2):272–8.

79. Hatten KM, O'Malley BW, Bur AM, et al. Transoral Robotic Surgery-Assisted Endoscopy With Primary Site Detection and Treatment in Occult Mucosal Primaries. JAMA Otolaryngol Head Neck Surg 2017;143(3):267–73.

80. Patel SA, Magnuson JS, Holsinger FC, et al. Robotic surgery for primary head and neck squamous cell carcinoma of unknown site. JAMA Otolaryngol Head Neck Surg 2013;139(11):1203–11.

81. Fu TS, Foreman A, Goldstein DP, et al. The role of transoral robotic surgery, transoral laser microsurgery, and lingual tonsillectomy in the identification of head and neck squamous cell carcinoma of unknown primary origin: a systematic review. J Otolaryngol Head Neck Surg 2016;45(1):28.

82. Geltzeiler M, Doerfler S, Turner M, et al. Transoral robotic surgery for management of cervical unknown primary squamous cell carcinoma: Updates on efficacy, surgical technique and margin status. Oral Oncol 2017;66:9–13.

83. Zafereo ME, Hanasono MM, Rosenthal DI, et al. The role of salvage surgery in patients with recurrent squamous cell carcinoma of the oropharynx. Cancer 2009;115(24):5723–33.

84. Righini C-A, Nadour K, Faure C, et al. Salvage surgery after radiotherapy for oropharyngeal cancer. Treatment complications and oncological results. Eur Ann Otorhinolaryngol Head Neck Dis 2012;129(1):11–6.

85. Patel SN, Cohen MA, Givi B, et al. Salvage surgery for locally recurrent oropharyngeal cancer. Head Neck 2016;38(Suppl 1):E658–64.

86. White H, Ford S, Bush B, et al. Salvage surgery for recurrent cancers of the oropharynx: comparing TORS with standard open surgical approaches. JAMA Otolaryngol Head Neck Surg 2013;139(8):773–8.

87. Meulemans J, Vanclooster C, Vauterin T, et al. Up-front and Salvage Transoral Robotic Surgery for Head and Neck Cancer: A Belgian Multicenter Retrospective Case Series. Front Oncol 2017;7:15.

88. Iyer NG, Kim L, Nixon IJ, et al. Factors predicting outcome in malignant minor salivary gland tumors of the oropharynx. Arch Otolaryngol Head Neck Surg 2010;136(12):1240–7.

89. Guzzo M, Locati LD, Prott FJ, et al. Major and minor salivary gland tumors. Crit Rev Oncol Hematol 2010;74(2):134–48.

90. Mendenhall WM, Morris CG, Amdur RJ, et al. Radiotherapy alone or combined with surgery for salivary gland carcinoma. Cancer 2005;103(12):2544–50.

91. Parsons JT, Mendenhall WM, Stringer SP, et al. Management of minor salivary gland carcinomas. Int J Radiat Oncol Biol Phys 1996;35(3):443–54.

92. Spiro RH. Salivary neoplasms: overview of a 35-year experience with 2,807 patients. Head Neck Surg 1986;8(3):177–84.

93. Copelli C, Bianchi B, Ferrari S, et al. Malignant tumors of intraoral minor salivary glands. Oral Oncol 2008;44(7):658–63.

94. Carrillo JF, Maldonado F, Carrillo LC, et al. Prognostic factors in patients with minor salivary gland carcinoma of the oral cavity and oropharynx. Head Neck 2011;33(10):1406–12.

95. Hay AJ, Migliacci J, Karassawa Zanoni D, et al. Minor salivary gland tumors of the head and neck-Memorial Sloan Kettering experience: Incidence and outcomes by site and histological type. Cancer 2019;125(19):3354–66.

96. Villanueva NL, de Almeida JR, Sikora AG, et al. Transoral robotic surgery for the management of oropharyngeal minor salivary gland tumors. Head Neck 2014; 36(1):28–33.

97. Schoppy DW, Kupferman ME, Hessel AC, et al. Transoral endoscopic head and neck surgery (eHNS) for minor salivary gland tumors of the oropharynx. Cancers Head Neck 2017;2:5.

98. Weinstein GS, O'Malley BW. TransOral robotic surgery (TORS). San Diego (CA): Plural Pub; 2012.

99. Sharma A, Patel S, Baik FM, et al. Survival and gastrostomy prevalence in patients with oropharyngeal cancer treated with transoral robotic surgery vs chemoradiotherapy. JAMA Otolaryngol Head Neck Surg 2016;142(7):691–7.

100. Moore EJ, Van Abel KM, Price DL, et al. Transoral robotic surgery for oropharyngeal carcinoma: Surgical margins and oncologic outcomes. Head Neck 2018; 40(4):747–55.

101. Dhanireddy B, Burnett NP, Sanampudi S, et al. Outcomes in surgically resectable oropharynx cancer treated with transoral robotic surgery versus definitive chemoradiation. Am J Otolaryngol 2019;40(5):673–7.

102. Dziegielewski PT, Teknos TN, Durmus K, et al. Transoral robotic surgery for oropharyngeal cancer: long-term quality of life and functional outcomes. JAMA Otolaryngol Head Neck Surg 2013;139(11):1099–108.

103. Achim V, Bolognone RK, Palmer AD, et al. Long-term functional and quality-of-life outcomes after transoral robotic surgery in patients with oropharyngeal cancer. JAMA Otolaryngol Head Neck Surg 2018;144(1):18–27.

104. Sethia R, Yumusakhuylu AC, Ozbay I, et al. Quality of life outcomes of transoral robotic surgery with or without adjuvant therapy for oropharyngeal cancer. Laryngoscope 2018;128(2):403–11.

105. Van Abel KM, Quick MH, Graner DE, et al. Outcomes following TORS for HPV-positive oropharyngeal carcinoma: PEGs, tracheostomies, and beyond. Am J Otolaryngol 2019;40(5):729–34.

Role of Transoral Robotic Surgery in the Work-up of the Unknown Primary

John R. de Almeida, MD, MSc, FRCSC[a,b,*]

KEYWORDS

- Unknown primary • Tongue base mucosectomy • Lingual tonsillectomy
- Transoral robotic surgery

KEY POINTS

- Transoral robotic surgery may be used to increase the diagnostic yield of identifying a primary tumor in the tongue base.
- Identifying a primary tumor may help tailor radiotherapy volumes or eliminate pharyngeal radiotherapy in patients whose primary tumors are completely excised.
- A small percentage of primary tumors may be identified in the contralateral pharynx or with multiple primary sites, which may require intensive adjuvant therapy.

INTRODUCTION/HISTORY/DEFINITIONS/BACKGROUND

Head and neck squamous cell carcinoma of unknown primary site (CUP) comprises a relatively small proportion of all head and neck cancers. The historical diagnostic work-up for these tumors included clinical examination, imaging of the head and neck, and operative examination under anesthesia, which includes a panendoscopy and directed biopsies of suspicious sites with palatine tonsillectomy. Imaging with fludeoxyglucose [1] fluorodeoxyglucose (FDG)-PET as well as new surgical diagnostic techniques, such as transoral lingual tonsillectomy with robotic or laser-assisted technology may improve the likelihood of identifying a primary tumor. This article reviews the role of transoral robotic surgery (TORS) in the diagnostic evaluation and therapeutic paradigm in the management of CUP and hidden, small-volume oropharyngeal cancers.

[a] Department of Otolaryngology–Head and Neck Surgery, Princess Margaret Cancer Centre/University Health Network, University of Toronto, Toronto General Hospital, 200 Elizabeth Street, 8NU-883, Toronto, Ontario, Canada; [b] Department of Surgical Oncology, Princess Margaret Cancer Centre/University Health Network, University of Toronto, Toronto General Hospital, 200 Elizabeth Street, 8NU-883, Toronto, Ontario, Canada
* Department of Surgical Oncology, Princess Margaret Cancer Centre/University Health Network, University of Toronto, Toronto General Hospital, 200 Elizabeth Street, 8NU-883, Toronto, Ontario, Canada.
E-mail address: john.dealmeida@uhn.ca

Otolaryngol Clin N Am 53 (2020) 965–980
https://doi.org/10.1016/j.otc.2020.07.008
0030-6665/20/Crown Copyright © 2020 Published by Elsevier Inc. All rights reserved.

oto.theclinics.com

DISCUSSION
Epidemiology

CUP is a rare disease entity accounting for only 1.5% to 9% of all head and neck cancers.[2–4] Historically, patients with CUP were believed to harbor either a small occult malignancy in a putative mucosal site, such as the tonsil, tongue base, piriform sinuses, or nasopharynx, or to have a primary tumor that has involuted over time due to an antitumor response by the immune system.[5] Recent studies, however, have shown that a vast majority of patients who present with an unknown primary and metastatic nodal disease and who ultimately have a primary tumor identified at the time of operative examination under anesthesia have a primary tumor in the oropharynx.[6] In a study by Cianchetti and colleagues,[6] 89% of all tumors eventually identified were in the oropharynx, of which 45% were in the tonsil and 44% were in the tongue base.

Like oropharyngeal squamous cell carcinomas (OPCs), CUP commonly is associated with the human papillomavirus (HPV).[7–9] Although it has not been demonstrated clearly in population-level studies, it is likely that the rising incidence of OPC is paralleled closely in CUP.[10] One multi-institutional study demonstrated that the prevalence of HPV-mediated CUP has risen over time.[11] This finding is consistent with the observation that HPV-mediated oropharyngeal cancers typically present with larger nodal burden than HPV-negative oropharyngeal cancers,[12] further supporting the notion that CUP is increasing in incidence.

Diagnostic Work-up

Nodal biomarkers

With the recent changes in the 8th edition of TNM staging by the American Joint Committee on Cancer and the Union for International Cancer Control, patients with CUP potentially are assigned a specific anatomic site based on their nodal biomarker status.[13] Patients whose lymph nodes indicate HPV-mediated disease by overexpression of the tumor suppressor protein p16 (cyclin-dependent kinase 2A) on immunohistochemistry may harbor a possible HPV-mediated primary tumor in the oropharynx. Studies have shown, however, that other primary sites, such as cutaneous primaries, may overexpress p16.[14] Because non-HPV–mediated cancers also may overexpress p16, confirmatory testing with in situ hybridization should be performed. In this setting, a T0 category of the oropharynx is assigned after careful evaluation of the patient with examination, imaging, and biopsies to rule out a primary. Similarly, patients with nodal disease that stains positive for Epstein-Barr virus–encoded RNA (EBER) may harbor a nasopharyngeal primary and, if examination, imaging, and biopsies are negative, they are assigned a nasopharyngeal primary site. Patients whose lymph nodes are negative for both biomarkers cannot be assigned a primary tumor site. Nodal biomarkers may have both diagnostic and therapeutic implications. These biomarkers may help surgeons direct diagnostic biopsies and/or excisions as well as radiation oncologists tailor their treatment volumes. Future research in novel biomarkers, such as nodal microRNA, may further help predict and localize primary tumors by tumor subsite.[15]

Axial Imaging (Computed Tomography and Magnetic Resonance Imaging)

All patients with a head and neck malignancy should routinely undergo axial imaging with computed tomography (CT) and/or magnetic resonance imaging (MRI). These imaging modalities may reveal subtle anatomic abnormalities that may help guided surgical biopsy at the time of operative endoscopy. These modalities are limited, however, in that many occult neoplasms may be hidden in small crypts of Waldeyer ring. One study reported a sensitivity, specificity, positive predictive value, and negative predictive value of 70%, 62%, 84%, 42%, respectively, for conventional imaging.[16] Specific sequences on MRI, such as diffusion-weighted imaging, may help improve diagnostic properties, although further research is needed to confirm these findings.[17]

Ultrasound

A recent guideline issued by the French Society of Otorhinolaryngology recommended the use of ultrasound in the setting of unknown primary in order to characterize and evaluate lymph nodes architecture as well as the thyroid gland to rule out a primary tumor in the thyroid and to evaluate cystic or necrotic components of a node that may further point to a oropharyngeal primary lesion.[18] Small series also have demonstrated that transcervical ultrasound may be used to identify small tongue base primary tumors.[2,19] In a single-institutional case series, in patients with no primary lesion identified on PET, ultrasound identified a hypoechoic target in 9 out of 10 patients, most of whom were in the tongue base, and of whom 7 eventually were identified by biopsy.[19] Further larger-scale evaluation of this approach may be needed.

PET/Computed Tomography

The advent of functional imaging with FDG PET/CE has improved the ability to identify candidate primary tumor sites in patients presenting with unknown primary carcinomas. In 1 systematic review and meta-analysis of 28 studies and 910 patients, the detection rate, sensitivity, and specificity of PET/CT were 29%, 78% and 79%, respectively.[20] In a subsequent systematic review and meta-analysis of 7 studies and 246 patients with unknown primary and cervical nodal metastases, the detection rate, sensitivity, and specificity were 44%, 97%, and 68%, respectively (**Table 1**).[21] In these studies, care must be taken in interpreting a high test sensitivity because this property may be artificially inflated in cases of no primary tumor found at the time of operative examination under anesthesia. A false-negative test is a test in which a PET/CT does not reveal a primary tumor and one is found at the time of operative examination under anesthesia. As such, when techniques, such as panendoscopy alone, are employed, fewer tumors are found at the time of operative examination under anesthesia. A more representative measure of the test properties is the diagnostic identification rate of a primary tumor.

Another caveat to interpretation of PET/CT imaging is that they may be associated with false-positive test results and lack specificity. The lingual tonsil commonly is an anatomic site with PET avidity and this may lead to misinterpretation of a primary site. In the former of the 2 meta-analyses, primary tumors identified in the tongue base on PET were associated with false-positive rate of 28.6%.[20] Furthermore, the same investigators suggest that PET exhibits a lower sensitivity for identifying primary tumors of the tongue base (68%) and tonsil (76%), respectively. Taken together, these data suggest that although PET/CT may provide additional information compared with

Table 1
Diagnostic test properties for evaluation of the unknown primary

	Sensitivity	Specificity	Identification Rate
Panendoscopy and tonsillectomy[22]	N/A	N/A	31% in PET-negative patients
Tonsillectomy[24]	N/A	N/A	34%
PET[20,21]	78%–97%	68%–79%	29%–44%
NBI[26,27]	74%–83%	76%–88%	32%–35%
TORS/TLM-guided approach[36,38]	N/A	N/A	70%–78%

physical examination and conventional imaging in order to inform potential biopsy targets at the time of operative examination under anesthesia, this imaging modality still may not replace biopsy confirmation of a primary site in order to determine therapeutic targets.

Pandendoscopy and Biopsy

Traditional work-up of the unknown primary involves operative examination under anesthesia with a combination of different endoscopic techniques, such as nasopharyngoscopy, laryngoscopy, esophagoscopy, and bronchoscopy. Regardless of the endoscopic instruments used, the ultimate goal is to carefully evaluate the putative mucosal sites of the upper aerodigestive tract, including the nasopharynx, oropharynx, larynx, and hypopharynx, to rule out a primary in one of the putative mucosal sites. This examination involves direct visualization and palpation, where possible. Surface irregularities, such as erythema, prominent vasculature, and ulceration, may help identify targets for biopsy. A systematic approach is required with careful evaluation of the palatine tonsil and pillars, glossotonsillar sulci, tongue base, vallecula, piriform sinuses, and postcricoid space. The evaluation may be informed by findings on nodal biomarkers (eg, p16 and EBER status of the node) or by areas of PET avidity. Primary tumors may be hidden in the tonsillar crypts or lymphoid tissue or have significant submucosal extension and palpation may help identify these tumors that may escape visual identification. Targeted biopsies of irregular areas based on a combination of the inspection, palpation, and PET findings may help identify a primary tumor. In a recent study, a primary tumor was found at the time of panendoscopy even in 32 of 103 (31%) patients with a negative PET scan.[22,23] Of the primary tumors identified, a majority were in the palatine tonsil (56%), with a smaller proportion identified in the tongue base (25%), likely due to the fact that the investigators performed bilateral palatine tonsillectomy at the time of panendoscopy if no primary tumor was identified with panendoscopy.

Palatine Tonsillectomy

Palatine tonsillectomy has been incorporated as part of the standard work-up of the unknown primary carcinoma with cervical nodal metastases. Clinical practice guidelines from the National Comprehensive Cancer Network recommend routine palatine tonsillectomy in patients who present with metastatic squamous cell carcinoma to lymph nodes in the upper neck (levels I, II, II, and upper V).[22] A recent systematic review and meta-analysis summarized results from 14 studies and 673 patients of whom 416 underwent palatine tonsillectomies. The overall primary tumor detection rate in this study was 34%, of which 89% were ipsilateral, 10% synchronous bilateral and 1% unilateral.[24] These data suggest that providers should consider bilateral palatine tonsillectomy or comprehensive sampling of the contralateral palatine tonsil in the work-up of the unknown primary carcinoma. Deep biopsies of the tonsil alone may not be adequate if they are negative, and surgeons evaluating these cancers should consider complete palatine tonsillectomy on the ipsilateral side at least and possibly bilateral palatine tonsillectomy. Waltonen and colleagues[25] demonstrated that the likelihood of finding an occult primary in the tonsil with deep biopsy alone was 3% compared with 29% with complete excision of the palatine tonsil. These findings were confirmed in a subsequent meta-analysis where the odds ratio of finding a primary was more than 10-fold higher in patients undergoing tonsillectomy compared with those undergoing deep biopsies.[24] If a lesion is suspected, however, based on visualization or palpation, a deep biopsy may be performed to identify the primary tumor. This approach with deep biopsy first of suspicious lesions prior to palatine tonsillectomy may be preferable, particularly in the setting when one may consider definitive surgical resection through a transoral approach.

Narrow Band Imaging

Narrow band imaging (NBI) is an adjunctive technique to standard white light illumination of surface anatomy. With this technique, white light illumination through an endoscope can be filtered, such that all but 2 wavelengths, 1 band centered at 415 nm and a second band centered at 540 nm.[26] The former of these 2 bands may penetrate the superficial mucosa to visualize submucosal capillaries and is visualized as a brown color whereas the latter penetrates through the submucosal layer to visualize prominent vessels as a cyan color.[26] Data from previous systematic review and meta-analysis suggest that the use of this imaging modality is associated with a pooled sensitivity of 74% and pooled specificity of 86% across 4 studies.[26] Based on this systematic review, however, the identification rate of primary tumors across 5 studies was 36 of 144 (32%), suggesting that many small primary tumors may be missed with this technique. These data were corroborated in an updated systematic-review and meta-analysis published a by another group demonstrating a pooled detection rate, sensitivity, and specificity of 35%, 83%, and 88%, respectively, across 5 studies and 169 patients.[27] Perhaps one of the biggest benefits of NBI is the ability to offer this technique as an adjunctive office-based procedure that may guide biopsies and rapid detection and thus may avoid operative intervention.[28]

Lingual Tonsillectomy

Several cases series have demonstrated incremental benefit of the addition of a transoral lingual tonsillectomy to the traditional operative diagnostic work-up of the unknown primary.[29–35] In these case-series, the addition of lingual tonsillectomy either with a transoral laser microsurgery (TLM) or a TORS approach resulted in improved identification of an occult primary tumor. Preliminary reports described that that many of these unknown primary tumors may be harbored in the tongue base. Karni and colleagues[29] demonstrated that with a TLM approach, an occult primary can be found in 94% of cases, of which 63% were identified in the tongue base. This finding was corroborated by a subsequent series demonstrating that with a TORS lingual tonsillectomy in patients that have previously not had a primary tumor identified with conventional work-up, the detection rate of an occult primary tumor was 90%.[30] Subsequent systematic reviews by our group and others have demonstrated that a transoral lingual tonsillectomy and mucosal resection may identify a primary tumor in 70% to 78% of cases.[36–38] Even in the absence of suspicious findings on clinical examination, axial imaging and PET, a primary tumor may still be found in 64% to 67% of cases.[36,37]

Extent of Lingual Tonsillectomy A lingual tonsillectomy typically is defined by mucosal and lymphoid resection of the superficial surface of the tongue base starting at the circumvallate papilla anteriorly and extending posteriorly to the vallecula with the lateral extent of the excision extending bilaterally to the glossotonsillar sulci. Typically, the deep plane of resection is the plane between the lingual tonsillar tissue and the tongue base musculature. Some consideration may be given, however, to minimal muscular resection in order to avoid positive deep margins if a definitive removal is planned. Different surgeons advocate different approaches ranging from an ipsilateral or hemilingual tonsillectomy to subtotal to total lingual tonsillectomy. The decision to proceed with a less than total lingual tonsillectomy assumes that a vast majority of primary tumors are located on the side of the nodal burden, assuming that the patient presents with unilateral lymphadenopathy. Secondly, the decision to avoid extensive mucosal and lymphoid resection is to minimize postoperative pain and the possibility of downstream pharyngeal stenosis.

Emerging data, however, suggest although a hemilingual tonsillectomy may identify a majority of primary tumors, that contralateral and midline tumors may be missed or incompletely excised. Geltzeiller and colleagues[39] demonstrated that the identification rate with bilateral lingual tonsillectomy is 80% compared with 68% in patients undergoing a unilateral hemi lingual tonsillectomy. In patients undergoing bilateral lingual tonsillectomy, a primary tumor was found on the contralateral side in 12% of patients.[39] As such, incremental detection rate must be weighed against the added morbidity of the procedure when deciding on a subtotal versus a total lingual tonsillectomy.

Rationale for Lingual Tonsillectomy Because of the relatively small size of the majority of tumors identified in the tongue base by a lingual tonsillectomy, it is conceivable to achieve a negative margin resection with this diagnostic procedure. In 1 systematic review, the positive margin rate after diagnostic lingual tonsillectomy was 19%.[38] In a large single-institutional series, however, the rate of positive margins was 49%, with a majority of positive margins occurring at the deep margin.[39] For this reason the authors' institutional practice is to take a small margin of muscle during the resection to minimize this risk of a positive margin.

The authors' group has further shown that if a small-volume (T1) tongue base primary tumor is identified, and a patient requires adjuvant therapy for close or positive margins to the primary tumor, the size of the radiation volumes is significantly less than in patients where the tumor is treated as a true unknown primary (T0) and the patient receives elective radiotherapy to the pharyngeal axis.[40] Furthermore, recent retrospective studies have shown that in patients who had an extensive diagnostic work-up to investigate an known primary with a TORs approach, and in whom no primary tumor was identified (ie, T0 tumors), avoidance of elective radiotherapy to the pharyngeal axis is associated with similar local control as those who received elective radiotherapy to the pharyngeal axis.[41,42]

Lingual Tonsillectomy in Human Papilloma Virus–Negative Unknown Primary Although it is unclear at the present moment whether transoral lingual tonsillectomy is equally effective in identifying a small-volume primary tumor in the tongue base in patients with HPV-negative disease, 1 recent study suggests that the likelihood of identifying a primary tumor is low (13%) in patients with HPV-negative disease.[43]

Therapeutic Considerations for Transoral Robotic Surgery for Unknown Primary

TORS also may be used as a therapeutic procedure for patients presenting with an unknown primary. In patients with a primary tumor identified at the time of diagnostic endoscopy, a definitive resection may be performed. For example, if a primary palatine tonsil is identified by intraoperative biopsy, a definitive TORS pharyngectomy can be completed in addition to a neck dissection. In patients where no obvious primary tumor is identified at the time of examination under anesthesia, excision of the palatine tonsil on the side of the disease may be considered and evaluating the contents of the tonsil evaluated with intraoperative serial frozen sectioning of the tonsil (ie, bread-loafing). Then, a therapeutic procedure may be considered if a primary tumor is identified on frozen section analysis. In the authors' institutional clinical trial, procedures are offered for patients with limited nodal disease and in the absence of radiographic signs of extranodal extension so as to minimize the need for adjuvant concurrent chemoradiotherapy.

Radiotherapy Considerations for Management of the Unknown Primary

The management of the unknown primary with radiotherapy, much like the diagnostic surgical work-up, is heterogenous. Many experts advocate elective radiotherapy to putative mucosal sites and the neck.[43] The exact mucosal targets vary across institutional practices, although many would advocate elective mucosal radiotherapy to high-risk targets, depending on nodal biomarkers (eg, nodal p16 and EBER status), risk factors, such as smoking status, ethnicity, and other features. For patients with EBER-positive nodes, radiotherapy target volumes include the nasopharynx and bilateral neck nodes. For patients with p16-positive nodes and a suspected oropharyngeal primary, radiotherapy target volumes include at least the mucosal surfaces of the oropharynx and the lymph nodes of the neck.[44] When no primary site is suspected based on nodal biomarkers and other clinical and demographic features, a primary tumor typically is suspected in the oropharynx, larynx, or hypopharynx. Some studies suggest that, in these cases, unilateral neck radiotherapy may be feasible in patients with limited nodal disease (eg, patients with a single node <6 cm).[44] It is still unclear, however, if patients treated in this manner may be at increased risk of contralateral nodal failures,[45] although in selected series unilateral techniques may offer similar disease control in carefully selected patients.[46-48] Delivery of radiotherapy to the mucosal sites also is variable between institutions, with some providers avoiding elective radiotherapy to candidate mucosal sites,[46] whereas others perform elective radiation to mucosal surfaces.[45] Even if mucosal targets are not deliberately covered, however, nodal targets may result in coverage of the lateral tonsil and tongue base between 50 Gy and 60 Gy.[46]

Treatment Toxicities

Transoral robotic lingual tonsillectomy is associated with a risk of hemorrhage approximately 5%.[36,37] In 1 systematic review, only 1 procedure-related mortality was reported in 556 patients who underwent either a TORS-based or TLM-based diagnostic evaluation.[37] Other complications include tongue sensitivity and numbness, hospital readmission due to pain, and dehydration.[37] Tracheostomy tubes typically are not required and no tracheostomies were required in 220 patients reviewed, whereas 2 of 300 patients reviewed (0.7%) required a gastrostomy tube.[37]

Although there is a scarcity of long-term outcomes with this approach, 1 study demonstrated a deterioration of eating and social disruption domains of the Head and Neck Cancer Inventory at 1 year after completion of treatment, whereas speech and appearance remain similar to baseline.[49]

Avoidance of radiotherapy to the pharyngeal axis in patients with T0 tumors or in patients with primary sites excised and with clear margins may reduce the overall treatment-related toxicity. Preliminary evidence from single institutional studies demonstrates that radiotherapy can be avoided to the pharyngeal axis in patients with true unknown primaries or with primaries excised with margins greater than or equal to 2 mm.[41,50] These approaches may be associated with less requirement for narcotic medication, fewer feeding tubes, less mucositis and fewer unplanned treatment-related hospitalizations.[41]

Treatment Paradigm

Incorporation of transoral techniques, such as TORS or TLM, to increase the diagnostic yield depends on the availability of this technology and a multidisciplinary discussion on how this technology may benefit each individual patient. This discussion must weigh the burden of nodal disease, the potential benefit of identifying a hidden primary tumor, and the side effects of incremental surgery. **Fig. 1** describes a potential treatment algorithm that accounts for these various factors. In patients with advanced nodal disease such as nodes greater than 6 cm or bilateral lymphadenopathy, the incorporation of a lingual tonsillectomy as a diagnostic procedure may help to tailor pharyngeal radiation or avoid it altogether if the tumor is completely excised. This, however, must be weighed against the potential harm of surgery with short-term discomfort as well as the potential delay of proceeding with definitive chemoradiotherapy. If a lingual tonsillectomy were incorporated with neck dissection(s), the added morbidity of neck dissection(s) in patients who are likely to received chemoradiotherapy in the adjuvant setting must be weighted. Results of current and future clinical trials will help define algorithms for management of patients based on extent of disease and with the goals of reducing treatment toxicity and maintaining disease control.

Disease Prognosis

Patients presenting with CUP generally have a good prognosis. As with oropharyngeal cancer, patients with HPV-mediated CUP have a better prognosis than those with HPV-negative disease. In patients with HPV-positive disease and in whom no primary is identified, the prognosis is similar to those patients with small-volume tongue base tumors, with a 3-year survival of 91% in 1 study.[40] Studies have suggested that there is no difference in survival when comparing patients in whom a primary is found and those in whom a primary is not found.[40,51,52]

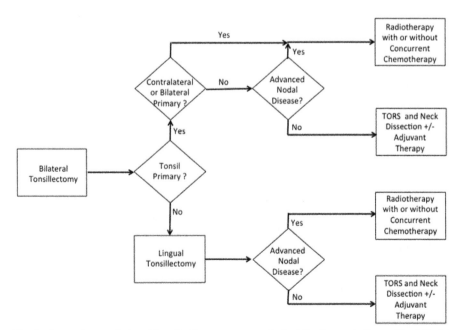

Fig. 1. A management algorithm for the management of patients presenting with metastatic disease to the neck with no obvious primary tumor.

CASE PRESENTATIONS
Case 1

Clinical presentation

A 66-year-old gentleman with a 50 pack-year smoking history presented with a left-sided neck mass and a CT scan showing a 3.6-cm × 1.9-cm left neck mass with no obvious primary tumor (**Fig. 2**). A fine-needle aspiration revealed metastatic squamous cell carcinoma and p16 status could not be determined. He underwent a left tonsillectomy and panendoscopy by another head and neck surgeon and no primary tumor was identified. Further imaging with an MRI reported an asymmetric right palatine tonsil and subtle asymmetry in the left lateral tongue base. A PET scan reported PET avidity in the left tongue base with a standardized uptake value (SUV) of 7.5.

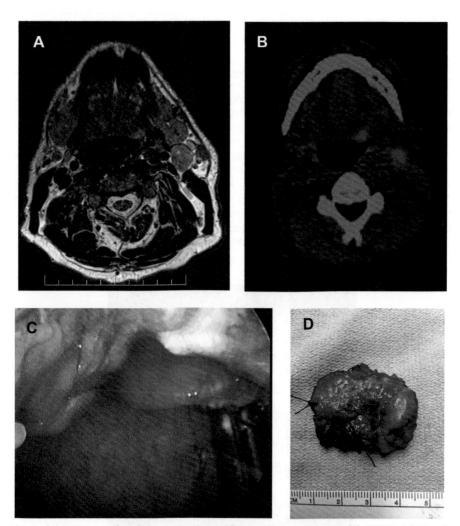

Fig. 2. (*A*) MRI scan of patient presenting with an unknown primary. (*B*) PET/CT. (*C*) Visualization of a suspicious primary site at the time of panendoscopy/examination under anesthesia. (*D*) Resection specimen after transoral robotic tongue base resection.

The patient underwent an examination under anesthesia where a small lesion identified in the left lateral tongue base was biopsied and confirmed to be the primary tumor. The patient underwent a TORS left tongue base resection and left neck dissection. The final pathology demonstrated a 1.2-cm primary tumor with lymphovascular invasion, no perineural invasion, and circumferential clear margins (>5 mm). He had a single metastatic node out of 46 nodes excised measuring 2.7 cm with no extranodal extension. He did not receive adjuvant therapy and has been free of disease for 3 years.

Discussion

The definition of CUP is highly variable and depends on the expertise of the clinicians evaluating the patient, the absence of a clear primary tumor on clinical examination and on imaging. In this case, the patient was previously evaluated with a panendoscopy and imaging at an outside institution but subsequently was noted to have highly suspicious MRI and PET findings, which were confirmed at the time of a second examination under anesthesia. Because of limited primary site disease and nodal disease, this patient was treated with surgery alone.

Case 2

Clinical presentation

A 49-year-old gentleman with a 40 pack-year smoking history presented with a rapidly enlarging right neck mass (**Fig. 3**). On clinical examination, he had a soft tissue mass measuring 7 cm with skin invasion and muscle invasion. A fine-needle aspiration biopsy confirmed p16-positive metastatic squamous cell carcinoma. An MRI demonstrated a 5.7 × 5.1 coalescent neck mass invading the sternocleidomastoid muscle and external skin but no visible primary tumor. PET imaging demonstrated FDG avidity, measuring with an SUV measuring 13.2 in the right with a coalescent mass measuring 6.6 cm × 4.5 cm. No obvious primary tumor was seen. Given the extent of his nodal disease and concern about regional control with definitive chemoradiotherapy, he underwent an upfront surgical approach with radical neck dissection with skin excision and soft tissue reconstruction and a lingual tonsillectomy. His final

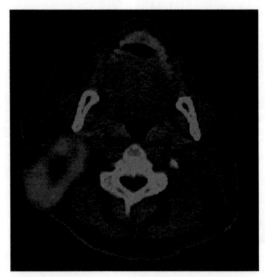

Fig. 3. PET/CT of patient with advanced nodal disease and no obvious primary tumor.

pathology demonstrated a 9-mm right tongue base tumor with the closest margin 3 mm on the lateral deep margin. His nodal dissection revealed 5/38 positive nodes with clear soft tissue margins but major extranodal extension. He underwent planned adjuvant chemoradiotherapy. He has been disease-free for 15 months.

Discussion

In this case, management of the nodal burden and regional control are likely the most important goals of care. With N3 disease at presentation, the authors' multidisciplinary opinion was to treat the patient with triple-modality treatment and with surgery upfront. The addition of a lingual tonsillectomy helped confirm the primary site and, in this case, definitively resect it.

Case 3

Clinical presentation

A 53-year-old otherwise healthy lady with a 25 pack-year smoking history presented with a p16-positive metastatic squamous cell carcinoma to the left neck (**Fig. 4**). The MRI scan demonstrated metastatic node with radiographic extranodal extension. A PET/CT demonstrated FDG uptake in the left neck nodes and asymmetric uptake in the left palatine tonsil with a maximum SUV of 9.1 in the left palatine tonsil and 8.0 in the right. She underwent bilateral palatine tonsillectomy, which were negative for malignancy, and subsequently underwent a lingual tonsillectomy and left neck dissection. No primary tumor was found. Her neck dissection pathology revealed 1 out of 53 nodes, the largest measuring 4.3 cm with no extranodal extension. She underwent adjuvant therapy to the left neck alone sparing the pharyngeal axis and is disease-free at 12 months post-treatment.

Discussion

In this case, the challenges of interpreting a PET/CT are illustrated. This patient demonstrated PET avidity in both palatine tonsils arguably suggestive of either an

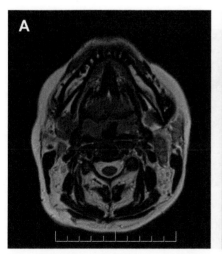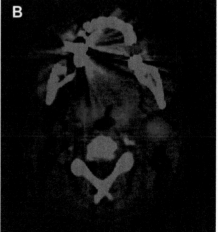

Fig. 4. (*A*) MRI scan of patient presenting with large volume palatine and lingual tonsil tissue with suspicious primary site on the side of nodal disease. (*B*) PET/CT of the same patients showing PET avidity in the both palatine tonsils with mild asymmetric uptake on the side of the nodal disease.

ipsilateral primary tumor in the palatine tonsil or bilateral tonsil primaries. Similar PET avidity was noted in the lingual tonsil. This case demonstrates the challenges of interpretation of PET/CT in the absence of a tissue evaluation. In this case, no primary tumor was found and the pharyngeal axis was spared radiotherapy. This approach is not universally accepted as a standard of care and may require further study.

Case 4

Clinical presentation

A 65-year-old man suffering from atrial fibrillation and history of transient ischemic attacks and a 10 pack-year smoking history presented with a biopsy-confirmed p16-positive left neck mass (**Fig. 5**). An MRI demonstrated multiple left neck nodes, the largest of which measured 3.2 cm × 2.2 cm, with other 0.7-cm and 0.8-cm nodes in levels 2a/b and 3, with no evidence of extranodal extension with no obvious primary tumor. PET/CT demonstrated metabolically active level 2/3 nodes and asymmetric uptake in the left tongue base suspicious for a left tongue base primary. The patient underwent a palatine tonsillectomy with intraoperative frozen section analysis, which failed to identify a primary tumor. The patient then underwent a lingual tonsillectomy and left neck dissection. The final pathology identified a palatine tonsil tumor measuring 8 mm and involving the deep margin and a separate 0.4-cm contralateral right tongue base primary tumor with the closest margin measuring 3 mm posteriorly. There were 4 positive metastatic nodes in the left neck out of 50 removed, the largest of which was 3.5 cm with major extranodal extension greater than 2 mm. The patient received bilateral neck and pharyngeal irradiation with concurrent chemotherapy in the adjuvant setting. He has been disease-free for 3 months.

Discussion

This case demonstrates the potential intensification of treatment with a surgical approach incorporating transoral techniques. If this patient had undergone a tonsillectomy and panendoscopy alone, an ipsilateral primary tumor would have been identified and the patient then treated with radiotherapy. Instead, with a lingual

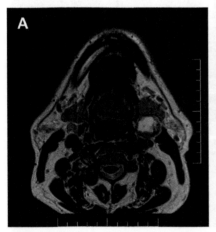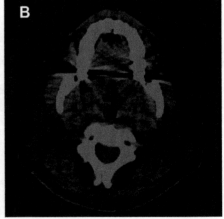

Fig. 5. (A) MRI scan of patient with left-sided nodal disease and no obvious primary site. (B) PET/CT of the same patient with a report suggestive of a tongue base primary tumor. The final pathology demonstrated a palatine tonsil and contralateral tongue base synchronous primary tumors.

tonsillectomy, a synchronous tongue base tumor was identified and extranodal extension identified at the time of neck dissection and as such required adjuvant chemoradiotherapy.

SUMMARY

Transoral techniques, including lingual tonsillectomy, may improve the identification of primary tumors in patients presenting with unknown primary squamous cell carcinomas of the neck. The increase in the identification rate of these tumors may be associated with short-term morbidity of pain and risk of bleeding. Toxicity must be weighed against the long-term benefits and the potential to spare mucosal radiation. Further trials may help better define the risks and benefits of these techniques.

CLINICS CARE POINTS

- Transoral techniques, such as TORS and TLM, may increase the identification rate of hidden primary tumors in the oropharynx to more than 70%.
- The addition of a lingual tonsillectomy may be associated with short-term pain, acute swallowing impairment, risk of bleeding, and potentially longer hospital stay.
- Identifying these tumors may help to tailor adjuvant therapies and reduce radiotherapy volumes to the pharyngeal axis and, in some instances, avoid radiotherapy altogether.
- Preliminary case series suggest that incorporating transoral techniques is associated with disease control rates similar to those with standard panendoscopy and tonsillectomy as part of the diagnostic work-up.

DISCLOSURE

The author has nothing to disclose.

REFERENCES

1. Mydlarz WK, Liu J, Blanco R, et al. Transcervical ultrasound identifies primary tumor site of unknown primary head and neck squamous cell carcinoma. Otolaryngol Head Surg 2014;151(6):1090–2.
2. Strojan P, Ferlito A, Medina JE, et al. Contemporary management of lymph node metastases from an unknown primary to the neck: 1: A review of diagnostic approaches. Head Neck 2013;35(1):123–32.
3. Rodel RM, Matthias C, Blomeyer BD, et al. Impact of distant metastasis in patients with cervical lymph node metastases from cancer of an unknown primary site. Ann Otol Rhinol Laryngol 2009;118:662–9.
4. Waltonen JD, Ozer E, Hall NC, et al. Metastatic carcinoma of the neck of unknown primary origin: evaluation and efficacy of the modern workup. Arch Otolaryngol Head Neck Surg 2009;135:1024–9.
5. Jones AS, Cook J, Phillips DE, et al. Squamous carcinoma presenting as an enlarged cervical lymph node. Cancer 1993;72:1756–61.
6. Cianchetti M, Mancuso AA, Amdur RJ, et al. Diagnostic evaluation of squamous cell carcinoma metastatic to cervical lymph nodes from an unknown head and neck primary site. Laryngoscope 2009;119:2348–54.
7. Ren J, Xu W, Su J, et al. HPV status improves classification of head and neck gray zone cancers. J Dent Res 2019;98(8):879–87.

8. Ren J, Yang W, Su J, et al. Human papillomavirus and p16 immunostraining, prevalence and prognosis of squamous carcinoma of unkown primary in the head and neck region. Int J Cancer 2019;145(6):1465–74.

9. Dixon PR, Au M, Hosni A, et al. Impact of p16 expression, nodal status, and smoking on oncologic outcomes of patients with head and neck unknown primary squamous cell carcinoma. Head Neck 2016;38(98):1347–53.

10. Chaturvedi AK, Engels EA, Pfeiffer RM, et al. Human papillomavirus and rising oropharyngeal cancer incidence in the United States. J Clin Oncol 2011; 29(32):4294–301.

11. Schroeder L, Boscolo-Rizzo P, Dal Cin E, et al. Human papillomavirus as prognostic marker with rising prevalence in neck squamous cell carcinoma of unknown primary: A retrospective multicenter study. Eur J Cancer 2017;74:73–81.

12. Stenmark MH, Shumway D, Guo C, et al. Influence of human papillomavirus on the clinical presentation of oropharyngeal carcinoma in the United States. Laryngoscope 2017;127(10):2270–8.

13. Lydiatt WM, Patel SG, O'Sullivan B, et al. Head and neck cancers-major changes in the American Joint Committee on cancer eighth edition cancer staging manual. CA Cancer J Clin 2017;67(2):122–37.

14. Beadle BM, William WN Jr, McLemore MS, et al. p16 expression in cutaneous squamous carcinomas with neck metastases: a potential pitfall in identifying unknown primaries of the head and neck. Head Neck 2013;35(11):1527–33.

15. Barker EV, Cervigne NK, Reis PP, et al. microRNA evaluation of unknown primary lesionsin the head and neck. Mol Cancer 2009;23(8):127.

16. Avci NC, Hatipoglu F, Alacacioglu A, et al. FDG PET/CT and Conventional imaging methods in cancer of unknown primary: an approach to overscanning. Nucl Med Mol Imaging 2018;52(6):438–44.

17. Noij DP, Martens RM, Zwezerijnen B, et al. Diagnostic value of diffusion-weighted imaging and 18F-FDG-PET/CT for the detection of unknown primary head and neck cancer in patients presenting with cervical metastasis. Eur J Radiol 2018; 107:20–5.

18. Santini L, Favier V, Benoudiba F, et al. Cystic form of cervical lymphadenopathy in adults. Guidelines of the French Society of Otorhinolaryngology (short verion). Part 2 – etiological diagnosis procedure: Clinical and imaging assessment. Eur Ann Otorhinolaryngol Head Neck Dis 2020;137(2):117–21.

19. Fakhry C, Agrawal N, Califano J, et al. The use of ultrasound in the search for the primary site of unknown primary head and neck squamous cell cancers. Oral Oncol 2014;50(7):640–5.

20. Dong MJ, Zhao K, Lin XT, et al. Role of fluorodeoxygluose-PET versus fluorodeoxyglucose-PET/computed tomography in detection of unknown primary tumor: a meta-analysis of the literature. Nucl Med Commun 2008;29(9):791–802.

21. Zhu L, Wang N. 18F-fluorodeoxyglucose positron emission tomography-computed tomography as a diagnostic tool in patients with cervical nodal metastases of unknown primary site: a meta-analysis. Surg Oncol 2013;22(3):190–4.

22. Sokoya M, Chowdjur F, Kadakia S, et al. Combination of panendoscopy and positron emission tomography/computed tomography increases detection of unknown primary head and neck carcinoma. Laryngoscope 2018;128(11):2573–5.

23. National Comprehensive Cancer Network. Bone cancer (version 2.2019 2019. Available at: https://www.nccn.org/professionals/physician_gls/default.aspx#head-and-neck. Accessed March 20, 2020.

24. Di Maio P, Iocca O, De Virgilio A, et al. Role of palatine tonsillectomy in the diagnostic workup of head and neck squamous cell carcinoma of unknown primary origin: a systematic review and meta-analysis. Head Neck 2019;41(4):1112–21.
25. Waltonen JD, Schuller DE, Agrawal A, et al. Tonsillectomy vs. deep tonsil biopsies in detecting occult tonsil tumors. Laryngoscope 2009;119:102–6.
26. Cosway B, Drinnan M, Paleri V. Narrow band imaging for the diagnosis of head and neck squamous cell carcinoma: a systematic review. Head Neck 2016;38(Suppl 1):E2358–67.
27. Di Maio P, Iocca O, De Virgillio A, et al. Narrow band imaging in head and neck unknown primary carcinoma: systematic review and meta-analysis. Laryngoscope 2019;130(7):1692–700.
28. Filauro M, Paderno A, Perotti P, et al. Role of narrow-band imaging in detection of head and neck unknown primary squamous cell carcinoma. Laryngoscope 2018;128(9):2060–6.
29. Karni RJ, Rich JT, Sinha P, et al. Transoral laser microsurgery: a new approach for unknown primaries of the head and neck. Laryngoscope 2011;121(6):1194–201.
30. Mehta V, Johson P, Tassler A, et al. A new paradigm for the diagnosis and management of unknown primary tumors of the head and neck: a role of transoral robotic surgery. Laryngoscope 2013;123(1):146–51.
31. Nagel TH, Hinni ML, Hayden RE, et al. Transoral laser microsurgery for the unknown primary: role of lingual tonsillectomy. Head Neck 2014;36(7):942–6.
32. Durmus K, Rangarajan SV, Old MO, et al. Transoral robotic approach to carcinoma of unknown primary. Head Neck 2014;36(6):848–52.
33. Patel SA, Magnuson JS, Holsinger FC, et al. Robotic surgery for primary head and neck squamous cell carcinoma of unknown site. JAMA Otolaryngol Head Neck Surg 2013;139(11):1203–11.
34. Channir HI, Rubek N, Nielsen HU, et al. Transoral robotic surgery for the management of head and neck squamous cell carcinoma of unknown primary. Acta Otolaryngol 2015;135(10):1051–7.
35. Hatten KM, O'Malley BW, Bur AM, et al. Transoral robotic surgery-assisted endoscopy with primary site detection and treatment in occult mucosal primaries. JAMA Otolaryngol Head Neck Surg 2017;143(3):267–73.
36. Fu TS, Foreman A, Goldstein DP, et al. The role of transoral robotic surgery, transoral laser microsurgery, and lingual tonsillectomy in the identification of head and neck squamous cell carcinoma of unknown primary origin: a systematic review. J Otolaryngol Head Neck Surg 2016;45(1):28.
37. Farooq S, Khandavalli S, Dretzke J, et al. Transoral tongue base mucosectomy for the identification of the primary site in the work-up of cancers of unknown origin: Systematic review and meta-analysis. Oral Oncol 2019;91:97–106.
38. Meccariello G, Cammaroto G, Ofo E, et al. The emerging role of transoral robotic surgery for the detection of the primary tumour site in patients with head-neck unknown primary cancers: a meta-analysis. Auris Nasus Larynx 2019;46(5):663–71.
39. Geltzeiller M, Doerfler S, Turner M, et al. Transoral robotic surgery for management of cervical unknown primary squamous cell carcinoma: updates on efficacy, surgical technique, and margin status. Oral Oncol 2017;66:9–13.
40. Hosni A, Dixon PR, Rishi A, et al. Radiotherapy characteristics and outcomes for head and neck carcinoma of unknown primary vs. T1 base-of-tongue carcinoma. JAMA Otolaryngol Head Neck Surg 2016;142(12):1208–15.
41. Grewal AS, Rajasekaran K, Cannady SB, et al. Pharyngeal-sparing radiation for head and neck carcinoma of unknown primary following TORS assisted workup. Laryngoscope 2020;130(3):691–7.

42. De Almeida JR, Noel CW, Veigas M, et al. Finding/identifying primaries with neck disease (FIND) clinical trial protocol: a study integrating transoral robotic surgery, histopathologic localization and tailored de-intensification of radiotherapy for unknown primary and small oropharyngeal head and neck squamous cell carcinoma. BMJ Open 2019;9(12):e035431.

43. Kubik MW, Channir HI, Rubek N, et al. TORS base-of-tongue mucosectomy in human papillomavirus-negative carcinoma of unknown primary. Laryngoscope 2020. https://doi.org/10.1002/lary.28617.

44. Biau J, Lapeyre M, Troussier I, et al. Selection of lymph node target volumes for definitive head and neck radiation therapy: a 2019 update. Radiother Oncol 2019;134:1–9.

45. Pflumio C, Troussier I, Sun XS. Unilateral or bilateral irradiation in cervical lymph node metastases of unknown primary? A retrospective cohort study. Eur J Cancer 2019;111:69–81.

46. Tiong A, Rischin D, Young RJ, et al. Unilateral radiotherapy treatment for p16/human papillomavirus-positive squamous cell carcinoma of unknown primary in the head and neck. Laryngoscope 2018;128(9):2076–83.

47. Straetmans JMJAA, Stuut M, Wagemakers S, et al. Tumor control of cervical lymph node metastases of unknown primary origin: the impact of the radiotherapy target volume. Eur Arch Otorhinolaryngol 2020;277(6):1753–61.

48. Ligey A, Gentil J, Crehange G, et al. Impact of target volumes and radiation technique on loco-regional control and survival for patietns with unilateral cervical lymph node metastases from an unknown primary. Radiother Oncol 2009;93(3):483–7.

49. Ozbay I, Yumusakhuylu AC, Sethia R, et al. One-year quality of life and functional outcomes of transoral robotic surgery for carcinoma of unknown primary. Head Neck 2017;39(8):1596–602.

50. Swisher-McClure S, Lukens JN, Aggarwal C, et al. A Phase 2 Trial of Alternative volumes of oropharyngeal irradiation for de-intensification (AVOID): omission of the resected primary tumor bed after transoral robotic surgery for human papilloma virus-related squamous cell carcinoma of the oropharynx. Int J Radiat Oncol Phys 2020;106(4):725–32.

51. Ryan JF, Motz KM, Rooper LM, et al. The impact of a stepwise approach to primary tumor detection in squamous cell carcinoma of the neck with unknown primary. Laryngoscope 2019;129(7):1610–6.

52. Graboyes EM, Sinha P, Thorstad WL, et al. Management of human papillomavirus-related unknown primaries of the head and neck with a transoral surgical approach. Head Neck 2015;37(11):1603–11.

Transoral Robotic Surgery and De-escalation of Cancer Treatment

Benjamin Wahle, MD, Jose Zevallos, MD, MPH*

KEYWORDS

- Transoral robotic surgery • Transoral laser microsurgery
- Squamous cell carcinoma of the oropharynx
- Human papillomavirus–associated oropharynx cancer • Treatment de-escalation
- Treatment deintensification

KEY POINTS

- By improving access and exposure of tumors, transoral robotic surgery (TORS) and transoral laser microsurgery (TLM) have expanded the number of patients that can be successfully treated with primary surgery transorally, thus avoiding the high morbidity associated with historical open surgical approaches to tumors of the oropharynx.
- Compared with human papillomavirus (HPV)-negative oropharynx squamous cell carcinoma (OPSCC), HPV(+) disease is molecularly and clinically distinct, responding more favorably to treatment and affecting a younger and healthier population of patients. Because HPV(+) OPSCC patients may survive for decades after diagnosis, an important goal is to establish appropriate treatment regimens that reduce treatment morbidity without affecting oncologic success.
- Recent trials indicate that transoral surgery may have an important role in future HPV(+) treatment deintensification by providing pathologic staging data, which may justify the use of de-escalated adjuvant therapeutic regimens.
- Ongoing prospective trials addressing HPV(+) OPSCC treatment de-escalation and choice of primary treatment modality are more numerous than those that have been completed to date. Over the coming decade, these trials will greatly expand the understanding of the roles of TORS, radiation, and chemotherapy in the primary treatment of HPV(+) OPSCC.

Research reported in this publication was supported by the National Institute of Deafness and Other Communication Disorders within the National Institutes of Health, through the "Development of Clinician/Researchers in Academic ENT" training grant number T32DC000022. The content is solely the responsibility of the authors and does not necessarily represent the official views of the National Institutes of Health.

Division of Head and Neck Surgery, Department of Otolaryngology–Head and Neck Surgery, Washington University School of Medicine, 660 South Euclid Avenue, Campus Box 8115, St Louis, MO 63110, USA
* Corresponding author.
E-mail address: jpzevallos@wustl.edu

Otolaryngol Clin N Am 53 (2020) 981–994
https://doi.org/10.1016/j.otc.2020.07.009
0030-6665/20/© 2020 Elsevier Inc. All rights reserved.

BACKGROUND

In this article, we explore transoral robotic surgery (TORS) as it relates to the de-escalation of therapy for oropharyngeal squamous cell carcinoma (OPSCC). We define treatment de-escalation as the alteration of primary and/or adjuvant therapies with the goal of reducing treatment morbidity and mortality without sacrificing oncologic outcomes. TORS and transoral laser microsurgery (TLM) are minimally invasive surgical approaches to the tonsils and tongue base that represent an important platform for treatment de-escalation on two fronts. First, these surgical techniques have expanded candidacy for primary transoral surgical therapy, reducing the use of highly morbid open surgical approaches to tumors of the oropharynx. Second, the increasing prevalence of human papillomavirus–related (HPV[+]) tumors has changed the landscape of OPSCC and has presented a new arena in which primary surgery therapy now competes with primary chemoradiation as a viable primary treatment modality.

Historical Context

Treatment modalities for OPSCC, surgical and nonsurgical, have transformed significantly over the past three decades. Given that many are completing residency training in an era where transoral surgical approaches to the oropharynx are common, the historical context that produced these techniques is important to understand. Advancements in TORS, TLM, and intensity-modulated radiation therapy (IMRT) have all occurred in parallel with one other. Furthermore, these advancements have coincided with an epidemiologic shift toward most OPSCC tumors being HPV(+).

Historically, treatment of OPSCC has consisted of surgery, radiation therapy (RT), and/or chemotherapy, often in combination as dictated by the stage of disease. In many instances, the choice of primary treatment modality that patients received was dictated by institutional patterns of practice. By the 1990s, the question of whether to use of surgery or radiotherapy as the primary treatment modality for OPSCC was not settled. Given the increasing use of morbidity-reducing RTs, such as IMRT in the late 1990s and early 2000s,[1] it was not clear that surgery to the primary site was noninferior to primary RT especially when treatment morbidity and mortality was concerned.

In 2002, a review of studies between 1970 and 2000 was performed exploring outcomes in primary surgery plus RT versus primary RT plus neck dissection. Although oncologic outcomes were similar between groups, authors reported strikingly higher severe (25% vs 6%) and fatal complications (3.2% vs 0.8%) in patients treated with primary surgery.[2] It must be noted that the surgical approaches to the oropharynx during this study period often involved transcervical and/or transmandibular exposure and free flap reconstruction. Based on these findings, primary chemoradiation therapy (CRT) became an increasingly preferred primary treatment modality in many centers around this period of time.[3]

As it became clear that the open surgical approaches described previously would carry unacceptably high complication rates when compared with primary CRT, minimally invasive techniques to address tumors of the oropharynx were developed and gained popularity. TLM was initially performed in the early 1970s by Strong and Jako,[4] who were the first to combine the CO_2 laser with microlaryngoscopy. Over the subsequent decades, the role of TLM in treating upper aerodigestive tract malignancies expanded beyond its initial use in small laryngeal tumors.[5] By the 2000s it was clear that TLM could be used successfully to treat tumors of the tongue base and pharynx.[6]

Around the same time that TLM was becoming established as a minimally invasive modality for treatment of OPSCC, the use of the da Vinci Surgical System was expanding in other surgical fields, notably urology and general surgery.[7] It was quickly recognized by multiple groups as a technology whose utility could be translated for use in head and neck surgery.[8–10] Work by Hockstein, Weinstein, and O'Malley brought this technology from initial simulations on mannequins and cadavers to demonstrating the safety and efficacy of TORS in human clinical trials.[11–14] TORS received US Food and Drug Administration approval in 2009 for use in pharyngeal and laryngeal tumors.[15] TORS and TLM are now frequently used at several centers for smaller primary tumors of the oropharynx.

DISCUSSION
Transoral Robotic Surgery as a De-escalated Surgical Therapy

Before TORS and TLM, tumors that could not be approached transorally required much more invasive surgery. Historically, only select tumors of the tonsil, posterior pharyngeal wall, and soft palate were routinely removed transorally. The limited ability to properly expose base of tongue tumors and tonsil and posterior pharyngeal wall tumors with inferior extension prevented many modestly sized tumors from being resected transorally. In these instances, open surgical exposure was required. Although open techniques did result in good exposure of tumors, dissection and division of anatomic structures not affected by tumor is required in these approaches. Lateral and transhyoid pharyngotomies were often used to access tumors with inferior extent. Muscular attachments to the hyoid are divided in the latter approach, which may contribute to postoperative dysphagia. The pharyngotomy required in both approaches results in fistula formation in a subset of patients, and the hypoglossal and recurrent laryngeal nerves are placed at risk in this approach. Midline mandibulotomy, also known as mandibular swing, was another common means of exposing tumors of the oropharynx. This involves splitting the mandible and dividing the floor of mouth musculature. Complications associated with this technique included increased blood loss, mandibular malunion, hardware infections, fistula, inferior alveolar nerve injuries, and dysphagia.[16]

TORS and TLM may be considered treatment de-escalation because they have limited the morbidity and mortality associated with primary surgical treatment of OPSCC without sacrificing oncologic outcomes.[17–19] By improving access and exposure of tumors, these techniques have expanded the share of patients that are successfully treated with a primary surgical approach while avoiding the risks of open approaches. Transoral approaches significantly reduce the occurrence of postoperative fistulas even when a neck dissection is performed simultaneously.[20] Because the neck and/or mandible are not disassembled during surgery and disrupted tissues are limited to an area immediately surrounding the tumor, TORS and TLM better preserve blood and nervous supply to unresected tissues of the oropharynx. This may explain the generally favorable swallowing outcomes observed with minimally invasive approaches.[17] For the same reason, defects in TORS and TLM are more amenable to healing by secondary intention, allowing many more OPSCC patients to be treated with primary surgery while avoiding the morbidity associated with locoregional flaps or free tissue transfer.[21]

Despite the advantages of transoral approaches compared with open approaches, the ability to successfully perform transoral surgery in a way that limits patient morbidity depends on individual patient factors, many of which are available preoperatively through physical examination and routine imaging. Aside from comorbidities that would limit ability to safely tolerate general anesthesia, one must consider factors related to the patient's normal anatomy and the patient's tumor. Patients must not have significant trismus; the tongue must be able to be retracted to an extent that the field can be exposed; and other structures in the oral cavity, such as the teeth and mandibular arch, must accommodate retractors. Tumors that are exophytic and mobile are generally preferred to tumors that are endophytic and fixed. Removing more than 50% of the base of tongue or 75% of the soft palate may result in significant velopharyngeal insufficiency and dysphagia, respectively.[22,23] Even in the absence of absolute contraindications to transoral surgery, there remain instances where primary CRT is preferable to surgery, especially given both approaches are sound from an oncologic standpoint.

Treatment De-escalation in Human Papillomavirus–Positive Disease

Although the development of less invasive surgical approaches, such as TORS and TLM, has represented a de-escalation in primary surgical therapy for tumors of the oropharynx, these techniques also exist as part of a broader effort to de-escalate therapy specifically for patients with HPV(+) OPSCC. Although traditionally regarded as a disease caused by tobacco and alcohol use, a shift toward HPV infection representing the causative event in OPSCC has occurred since the 1980s.[24] It is estimated that 60% to 70% of new OPSCC diagnoses are attributable to HPV,[25] and OPSCC has surpassed cervical cancer as the most common HPV-related malignancy in the United States.[26]

Compared with HPV(−) OPSCC, HPV(+) disease has a markedly more favorable prognosis.[25–27] The observed differences in clinical outcomes are most likely explained by the fact that, despite sharing a similar macroscopic phenotype, HPV(+) and HPV(−) tumors are molecularly distinct entities.[28,29] HPV(+) tumors seem to respond well to RT and primary surgical therapy. Sinha and colleagues[27] performed a systematic review comparing surgical versus nonsurgical treatment of HPV(+) OPSCC, which found that although there is heterogeneity between studies and a lack of randomized trials, there was no clear evidence of a difference between treatment modalities.

The recently published ORATOR trial was a phase 2 randomized controlled trial (RCT) that compared TORS plus neck dissection and indicated adjuvant therapy versus definitive CRT.[30] Patients were AJCC7 T1-2, N0-2, M0, and 88% were p16(+). There were no differences in overall survival or progression-free survival between groups. The study's primary outcome of interest was quality of life related to swallowing as measured by the MD Anderson Dysphagia Inventory. Although patients in the CRT group had significantly higher MD Anderson Dysphagia Inventory scores compared with the TORS group, this did not amount to a clinically significant difference.[30]

Patients with HPV(+) are demographically distinct compared with patients with HPV(−) disease. Compared with HPV(−) patients, HPV(+) patients tend to be male, White, younger, healthier, and are less likely to have a significant smoking history.[25] The typical demographic characteristics of the HPV(+) OPSCC population are an important consideration regarding treatment de-intensification. In HPV(−) OPSCC, the morbidity of treatment may seem justified by the comparatively low rates of survival within an aged population with high rates of medical comorbidities. In contrast, most HPV(+) patients respond well to treatment and because they are younger and healthier at the time of diagnosis, they may survive for decades after successful treatment. Thus, longer term treatment morbidity that is not as frequently observed in HPV(−) patients has become a greater concern within this expanding population.

Each treatment modality brings its own unique set of risks to the OPSCC patient. Inherent risks of transoral surgery include those related to general anesthesia and risks associated with a short postoperative hospitalization. The most potentially severe surgical complication is postoperative bleeding from the primary surgical site. At minimum, these patients must return to the operating room for cauterization. Rarely these bleeds may lead to asphyxiation; the rate of fatal hemorrhage is estimated to be 0.17% of all TORS cases.[31] Prophylactic transcervical arterial ligation reduces the severity of postoperative bleeding events.[32] Other short-term sequalae can include postoperative swelling, which in some cases exacerbates obstructive sleep apnea and rarely produces a need for a temporary tracheostomy. Velopharyngeal insufficiency is a rare long-term complication of transoral surgery but may be minimized when patients are selected carefully. Dysphagia may be a short- or long-term complication, and is significantly more likely in patients treated with adjuvant RT or CRT.[17]

Inherent to primary or adjuvant RT are acute and long-term treatment effects. The most common acute effects are mucositis and candidiasis, both of which may result in pain that limits oral intake. Dysphagia is one of the most significant complications of RT and can occur as an early and late treatment effect. Dysphagia has been shown to be more prevalent in CRT compared with RT alone.[33] Multiple studies have established the relationship between post-treatment dysphagia and the radiation dose to the pharyngeal constrictors, glottis, and supraglottis.[34,35] A substantial proportion of patients treated with RT experience dysphagia years after treatment.[36–38] Other long-term treatment effects include xerostomia and neck fibrosis, both of which may significantly affect patient quality of life and sometimes evolve for years after treatment.[38] In addition to exacerbating dysphagia, platinum-based chemotherapeutics also carry their own known treatment effects including sensorineural hearing loss and peripheral neuropathies.

The ability for primary surgical therapy to yield pathologic specimens distinguishes it from primary CRT. In theory, the tumor's pathologic characteristics reveal potentially important information about the tumor's biologic behavior that are not available from radiologic imaging, physical examination, or biopsy specimens. This in turn should allow for the identification of low-risk patients whose therapies can be safely de-escalated. However, in current practice primary surgical therapy only allows a minority of patients with HPV(+) disease to avoid adjuvant therapy, whereas a sizable portion go on to be treated with all three modalities (surgery + adjuvant CRT).[39] This is the case because in HPV(+) disease, the cervical neck metastasis is most often the first symptom that the patient experiences, thus the regional metastatic extent of the disease is such that adjuvant therapy is usually indicated. Although the currently used adjuvant RT and chemotherapy doses are lower relative to definitive CRT, de-escalation efforts described next aim to further reduce dose-dependent toxicity after surgical therapy.

Our current paradigm for assigning patients adjuvant therapy is largely based on evidence from HPV(−) disease.[40,41] A current source of controversy within the literature relates to whether the histopathologic predictors of adverse oncologic outcomes in HPV(−) disease are also useful in HPV(+) disease for the assignment of adjuvant therapy. For example, multiple groups have provided evidence in the form of retrospective/cohort studies suggesting that extracapsular extension (ECE) is not a predictor of oncologic outcomes in HPV(+) OPSCC.[42–45] However, other authors have found conflicting evidence regarding ECE and advocate its inclusion in future HPV(+) OPSCC staging systems.[46–48] Ongoing prospective trials described next may provide high-quality evidence that clarifies questions regarding traditional histopathologic features and how primary surgical treatment and the use of specimens may be able to guide de-escalations in adjuvant therapy.

Multiple prospective studies are in progress or have been recently completed that investigate treatment de-escalation in HPV(+) disease treated with primary surgery. Two published studies have investigated alteration of RT, either through the exclusion of structures from the radiation field or through limitation of the total radiation dose. The AVOID trial was a single-arm phase 2 trial that investigated the avoidance of primary tumor sites from inclusion in the radiation field if tumors were adequately resected and free of adverse histopathologic features, such as perineural or lymphovascular invasion.[49] In this trial, the 2-year rate of local control was 98.3% and a favorable toxicity profile was observed.[49] MC1273 was a phase II trial that investigated a reduced overall adjuvant RT dose of 30 to 36 Gy as guided by ECE status in p16(+) OPSCC patients.[50] It should be noted that this was investigated in combination with simultaneous docetaxel in all patients.[50] These authors similarly demonstrated a 96.2% locoregional control rate at 2 years and favorable toxicity profile.[50] These single-arm trials provide early prospective evidence that adjuvant therapy may be safely reduced in select HPV(+) OPSCC tumors that are adequately managed with surgery.

ECOG-E3311 is a phase II RCT that has been focused primarily on assessing a reduced RT dose in patients with HPV(+) disease. Although the complete results are not yet in publication, an abstract describing this trial's findings is available.[51] The total number of patients enrolled was 519, and all patients underwent transoral surgery and neck dissection for clinically T1-2 tumors that were AJCC7 stage III or IV without matting of nodes. Intermediate-risk patients were those who had clear or close surgical margins, two to four positive nodes, or had Extranodal Extension (ENE) less than or equal to 1 mm. Intermediate-risk patients were randomized to either 50 or 60 Gy of RT. Low-risk patients avoided RT and high-risk patients were assigned standard of care adjuvant CRT. Authors found that 2-year progression-free survival was similar regardless of RT dose in the intermediate-risk groups. Low-risk patients who did not have adjuvant therapy had similar favorable outcomes. These authors conclude that transoral surgery may be an effective part of surgical de-escalation, with low-risk patients able to avoid adjuvant therapy and selected intermediate-risk patients able to benefit from lower RT doses.

Although the focus of this review is treatment de-escalation as it relates to TORS, it should be noted that substitution of cisplatin with less toxic chemotherapeutic agents has represented a major goal in HPV(+) treatment de-escalation. Recently a large RCT comparing definitive RT + cisplatin versus RT + cetuximab was completed.[52] This trial demonstrated a clear benefit of cisplatin over cetuximab for overall and progression-free survival, suggesting that substitution of cetuximab does not represent a viable option for chemotherapeutic de-escalation in definitive CRT for HPV(+) OPSCC.[52]

Trials in Progress

Multiple RCTs are now in progress that will add to the understanding of the effect of adjuvant treatment de-escalation after primary surgery on oncologic outcomes and treatment toxicity (Table 1). DART-HPV is a phase III RCT that is building on the results of MC1273 described previously. The experimental group will receive 30 to 36 Gy + docetaxel, whereas the experimental arm will receive standard doses of RT + cisplatin (ClinicalTrials.gov: NCT02908477). PATHOS is a phase III RCT that similarly compares 50 versus 60 Gy in intermediate-risk patients. It also compares the removal of cisplatin with standard of care CRT in high-risk patients (ClinicalTrials.gov: NCT02215265).[53] The MINT trial is a phase II RCT that will evaluate reduction of RT and chemotherapy doses. Low-risk patients will receive 42 Gy of IMRT alone,

Table 1
Adjuvant therapy de-escalation trials in progress

Name	Title	Phase	Interventions	Enrollment	Estimated Completion	Primary Outcome Measures	NCT #	Study Sponsor
DART-HPV	DART-HPV: A Phase III Evaluation of De-escalated Adjuvant Radiation Therapy for HPV-Associated Oropharynx Cancer	3	Reduced RT (30–36 Gy, depending on risk group) + docetaxel is compared with 60 Gy ± cisplatin	214	2024	Adverse events rate	NCT02908477	Mayo Clinic
PATHOS	A Phase III Trial of Risk-stratified, Reduced Intensity Adjuvant Treatment in Patients Undergoing Transoral Surgery for Human Papillomavirus (HPV)-Positive Oropharyngeal Cancer	3	Intermediate risk-group: reduced RT (50 Gy) is compared with 60 Gy High-risk group: adjuvant CRT is compared with adjuvant RT alone	1100	2026	MDADI/overall survival coprimary end point	NCT02215265	Lisette Nixon
MINT	Phase II Trial of Surgery Followed by Risk-Directed Post-Operative Adjuvant Therapy for HPV-Related Oropharynx Squamous Cell Carcinoma: "The Minimalist Trial (MINT)"	2	Low-risk group: reduced RT (42 Gy) alone Intermediate-risk group: reduced RT (42 Gy) + one cisplatin dose High-risk group: standard of care (60 Gy + 3 doses cisplatin)	43	2022	Percent weight loss in patients during modified adjuvant CRT	NCT03621696	Washington University School of Medicine

Abbreviation: MDADI, MD Anderson Dysphagia Inventory.
Data from NIH. National Library of Medicine. ClinicalTrials.Gov.

Table 2
Trials in progress comparing primary treatment modalities

Title	Phase	Interventions	Enrollment	Estimated Completion	Primary Outcome Measures	NCT #	Study Sponsor
A Randomized Trial of Treatment De-Escalation for HPV-Associated Oropharyngeal Squamous Cell Carcinoma: Radiotherapy vs Trans-Oral Surgery (ORATOR IIᵃ	2	De-escalated primary CRT (60 Gy ± cisplatin) is compared with transoral surgery, neck dissection, and adjuvant RT (50–60 Gy, depending on risk)	140	2028	Overall survival	NCT03210103	Lawson Health Research Institute
Quality of Life After Primary Transoral Robotic Surgery vs Intensity-modulated Radiotherapy for Patients With Early-stage Oropharyngeal Squamous Cell Carcinoma: A Randomized National Trial (QOLATI)	2	TORS, neck dissection ± CRT is compared with primary CRT	138	2029	Swallowing-related quality of life (MDADI)	NCT04124198	Christian von Buchwald
Phase III Study Assessing The "Best of" Radiotherapy Compared to the "Best of" Surgery (Trans-oral Surgery (TOS)) in Patients With T1-T2, N0 Oropharyngeal Carcinoma	3	Transoral surgery and neck dissection is compared with RT and neck dissection	170	2026	Change in MDADI scores	NCT02984410	European Organization for Research and Treatment of Cancer

Comparative Effectiveness Trial of Transoral Head and Neck Surgery Followed by Adjuvant Radio(Chemo) Therapy vs Primary Radio(chemo)therapy for Oropharyngeal Cancer	4	Transoral surgery, neck dissection ± CRT is compared with primary CRT	280	2023	Time to local or locoregional failure or death from any cause	NCT03691441	Universitätsklinikum Hamburg-Eppendorf

Abbreviation: MDADI, MD Anderson Dysphagia Inventory.
Data from NIH. National Library of Medicine. ClinicalTrials.Gov.

intermediate-risk patients (those with ECE or positive margins) will receive 42 Gy + one dose of cisplatin, and high-risk patients (c/pT4 or cN3) will receive standard of care adjuvant CRT (ClinicalTrials.gov: NCT03621696).

Additionally, there are multiple ongoing RCTs that compare various forms of primary surgical therapy with primary nonsurgical therapy (**Table 2**). Some of these trials also include de-escalated treatment protocols. ORATOR II is an RCT that will compare two modes of de-escalated primary treatment. One group will be randomized to a de-escalated definitive RT regimen (60 Gy ± chemotherapy) and the other to transoral surgery and neck dissection ± adjuvant RT (50–60 Gy) (ClinicalTrials.gov: NCT03210103). The QoLATI study will compare TORS plus neck dissection against IMRT ± chemotherapy (ClinicalTrials.gov: NCT04124198). A trial by the European Organization for Research and Treatment of Cancer of patients with early stage OPSCC is being conducted that will compare IMRT + selective neck dissection against transoral surgery, selective neck dissection, and adjuvant therapy as indicated by risk factors (ClinicalTrails.gov: NCT02984410). A trial by Universitätsklinikum Hamburg-Eppendorf will compare transoral surgery and neck dissection and adjuvant therapy as indicated by risk factors against standard primary CRT (ClinicalTrials.gov: NCT03691441).

SUMMARY

TORS and TLM allow for improved access and exposure to oropharyngeal tumors and have expanded the share of patients that can have adequate surgical resection while avoiding invasive open surgical approaches. Compared with HPV(−) disease, HPV(+) OPSCC is molecularly and clinically distinct. HPV(+) OPSCC patients respond well to therapy and are younger and healthier at the time of diagnosis. Because they can survive for decades after treatment, long-term treatment sequelae are an increasingly important consideration within the growing population of HPV(+) OPSCC survivors. Initial evidence indicates that transoral surgery may have an important role in future HPV(+) treatment de-intensification by providing pathologic staging data, which may justify the avoidance or de-escalation of adjuvant therapeutic regimens. Numerous trials are in progress that investigate strategies for de-escalating adjuvant therapies after surgery or compare outcomes of primary surgery against primary CRT. We expect the evidence that will emerge in the coming decade will better define the roles of TORS, radiation, and chemotherapy in the treatment of HPV(+) OPSCC.

DISCLOSURE

Dr J. Zevallos is the Chief Medical Officer and an Equity Holder in SummitDX, which is developing salivary liquid biopsy tests for the early detection of head and neck cancer. Saliva-based diagnostics are not discussed in this article. Dr B. Wahle has no financial relationships to disclose.

REFERENCES

1. Chao KS, Majhail N, Huang CJ, et al. Intensity-modulated radiation therapy reduces late salivary toxicity without compromising tumor control in patients with oropharyngeal carcinoma: a comparison with conventional techniques. Radiother Oncol 2001;61(3):275–80.

2. Parsons JT, Mendenhall WM, Stringer SP, et al. Squamous cell carcinoma of the oropharynx: surgery, radiation therapy, or both. Cancer 2002;94(11):2967–80.

3. Chen AY, Schrag N, Hao Y, et al. Changes in treatment of advanced oropharyngeal cancer, 1985-2001. Laryngoscope 2007;117(1):16–21.
4. Strong MS, Jako GJ. Laser surgery in the larynx. Early clinical experience with continuous CO 2 laser. Ann Otol Rhinol Laryngol 1972;81(6):791–8.
5. Steiner W. Results of curative laser microsurgery of laryngeal carcinomas. Am J Otolaryngol 1993;14(2):116–21.
6. Steiner W, Fierek O, Ambrosch P, et al. Transoral laser microsurgery for squamous cell carcinoma of the base of the tongue. Arch Otolaryngol Head Neck Surg 2003;129(1):36–43.
7. Shah J, Vyas A, Vyas D. The history of robotics in surgical specialties. Am J Robot Surg 2014;1(1):12–20.
8. Hockstein NG, Nolan JP, O'malley BW, et al. Robotic microlaryngeal surgery: a technical feasibility study using the daVinci surgical robot and an airway mannequin. Laryngoscope 2005;115(5):780–5.
9. Haus BM, Kambham N, Le D, et al. Surgical robotic applications in otolaryngology. Laryngoscope 2003;113(7):1139–44.
10. McLeod IK, Melder PC. Da Vinci robot-assisted excision of a vallecular cyst: a case report. Ear Nose Throat J 2005;84(3):170–2.
11. O'Malley BW, Weinstein GS, Hockstein NG. Transoral robotic surgery (TORS): glottic microsurgery in a canine model. J Voice 2006;20(2):263–8.
12. O'Malley BW, Weinstein GS, Snyder W, et al. Transoral robotic surgery (TORS) for base of tongue neoplasms. Laryngoscope 2006;116(8):1465–72.
13. Weinstein GS, O'Malley BW, Snyder W, et al. Transoral robotic surgery: radical tonsillectomy. Arch Otolaryngol Head Neck Surg 2007;133(12):1220–6.
14. Weinstein GS, O'Malley BWJ, Desai SC, et al. Transoral robotic surgery: does the ends justify the means? Curr Opin Otolaryngol Head Neck Surg 2009;17(2):126–31.
15. Bekeny JR, Ozer E. Transoral robotic surgery frontiers. World J Otorhinolaryngol Head Neck Surg 2016;2(2):130–5.
16. Sinha P, Harreus U. Malignant neoplasms of the oropharynx. In: Flint PW, editor. Cummings otolaryngology. 6th edition. Philadelphia: Saunders; 2015. p. 1432-53.
17. Haughey BH, Hinni ML, Salassa JR, et al. Transoral laser microsurgery as primary treatment for advanced-stage oropharyngeal cancer: a united states multicenter study. Head Neck 2011;33(12):1683–94.
18. Dhanireddy B, Burnett NP, Sanampudi S, et al. Outcomes in surgically resectable oropharynx cancer treated with transoral robotic surgery versus definitive chemoradiation. Am J Otolaryngol 2019;40(5):673–7.
19. Ling DC, Chapman BV, Kim J, et al. Oncologic outcomes and patient-reported quality of life in patients with oropharyngeal squamous cell carcinoma treated with definitive transoral robotic surgery versus definitive chemoradiation. Oral Oncol 2016;61:41–6.
20. Moore EJ, Olsen KD, Martin EJ. Concurrent neck dissection and transoral robotic surgery. Laryngoscope 2011;121(3):541–4.
21. Park DA, Lee MJ, Kim S-H, et al. Comparative safety and effectiveness of transoral robotic surgery versus open surgery for oropharyngeal cancer: a systematic review and meta-analysis. Eur J Surg Oncol 2020;46(4 Pt A):644–9.
22. Abel KMV, Moore EJ. Transoral approaches to malignant neoplasms of the oropharynx. In: Flint PW, editor. Cummings otolaryngology. 6th edition. Philadelphia: Saunders; 2015. p. 1454–78.

23. Gross JH, Townsend M, Hong HY, et al. Predictors of swallow function after transoral surgery for locally advanced oropharyngeal cancer. Laryngoscope 2020;130(1):94–100.
24. Chaturvedi AK, Engels EA, Pfeiffer RM, et al. Human papillomavirus and rising oropharyngeal cancer incidence in the United States. J Clin Oncol 2011; 29(32):4294–301.
25. Ang KK, Harris J, Wheeler R, et al. Human papillomavirus and survival of patients with oropharyngeal cancer. N Engl J Med 2010;363(1):24–35.
26. Chaturvedi AK, Anderson WF, Lortet-Tieulent J, et al. Worldwide trends in incidence rates for oral cavity and oropharyngeal cancers. J Clin Oncol 2013; 31(36):4550–9.
27. Sinha P, Karadaghy OA, Doering MM, et al. Survival for HPV-positive oropharyngeal squamous cell carcinoma with surgical versus non-surgical treatment approach: a systematic review and meta-analysis. Oral Oncol 2018;86: 121–31.
28. Lawrence MS, Sougnez C, Lichtenstein L, et al. Comprehensive genomic characterization of head and neck squamous cell carcinomas. Nature 2015;517(7536): 576–82.
29. Gillison ML, Akagi K, Xiao W, et al. Human papillomavirus and the landscape of secondary genetic alterations in oral cancers. Genome Res 2018. https://doi.org/10.1101/gr.241141.118.
30. Nichols AC, Theurer J, Prisman E, et al. Radiotherapy versus transoral robotic surgery and neck dissection for oropharyngeal squamous cell carcinoma (ORATOR): an open-label, phase 2, randomised trial. Lancet Oncol 2019; 20(10):1349–59.
31. Stokes W, Ramadan J, Lawson G, et al. Bleeding complications after transoral robotic surgery: a meta-analysis and systematic review. Laryngoscope 2020. https://doi.org/10.1002/lary.28580.
32. Kubik M, Mandal R, Albergotti W, et al. Effect of transcervical arterial ligation on the severity of postoperative hemorrhage after transoral robotic surgery. Head Neck 2017;39(8):1510–5.
33. Nuyts S, Dirix P, Clement PMJ, et al. Impact of adding concomitant chemotherapy to hyperfractionated accelerated radiotherapy for advanced head-and-neck squamous cell carcinoma. Int J Radiat Oncol Biol Phys 2009;73(4): 1088–95.
34. Eisbruch A, Schwartz M, Rasch C, et al. Dysphagia and aspiration after chemoradiotherapy for head-and-neck cancer: which anatomic structures are affected and can they be spared by IMRT? Int J Radiat Oncol Biol Phys 2004;60(5): 1425–39.
35. Dirix P, Abbeel S, Vanstraelen B, et al. Dysphagia after chemoradiotherapy for head-and-neck squamous cell carcinoma: dose–effect relationships for the swallowing structures. Int J Radiat Oncol Biol Phys 2009;75(2):385–92.
36. Machtay M, Moughan J, Trotti A, et al. Factors associated with severe late toxicity after concurrent chemoradiation for locally advanced head and neck cancer: an RTOG analysis. J Clin Oncol 2008;26(21):3582–9.
37. Hutcheson KA, Nurgalieva Z, Zhao H, et al. Two-year prevalence of dysphagia and related outcomes in head and neck cancer survivors: an updated SEER-Medicare analysis. Head Neck 2019;41(2):479–87.
38. Baudelet M, Van den Steen L, Tomassen P, et al. Very late xerostomia, dysphagia, and neck fibrosis after head and neck radiotherapy. Head Neck 2019;41(10): 3594–603.

39. Huang SH, Hansen A, Rathod S, et al. Primary surgery versus (chemo)radio-therapy in oropharyngeal cancer: the radiation oncologist's and medical oncol-ogist's perspectives. Curr Opin Otolaryngol Head Neck Surg 2015;23(2): 139–47.

40. Bernier J, Cooper JS, Pajak TF, et al. Defining risk levels in locally advanced head and neck cancers: a comparative analysis of concurrent postoperative radiation plus chemotherapy trials of the EORTC (#22931) and RTOG (# 9501). Head Neck 2005;27(10):843–50.

41. Blanchard P, Baujat B, Holostenco V, et al. Meta-analysis of chemotherapy in head and neck cancer (MACH-NC): a comprehensive analysis by tumour site. Radiother Oncol 2011;100(1):33–40.

42. Lewis JS, Carpenter DH, Thorstad WL, et al. Extracapsular extension is a poor predictor of disease recurrence in surgically treated oropharyngeal squamous cell carcinoma. Mod Pathol 2011;24(11):1413–20.

43. Maxwell JH, Ferris RL, Gooding W, et al. Extracapsular spread in head and neck carcinoma: impact of site and human papillomavirus status. Cancer 2013; 119(18):3302–8.

44. Sinha P, Kallogjeri D, Gay H, et al. High metastatic node number, not extracapsu-lar spread or N-classification is a node-related prognosticator in transorally-resected, neck-dissected p16-positive oropharynx cancer. Oral Oncol 2015; 51(5):514–20.

45. Sinha P, Lewis JS, Kallogjeri D, et al. Soft tissue metastasis in p16-positive oropharynx carcinoma: prevalence and association with distant metastasis. Oral Oncol 2015;51(8):778–86.

46. Shevach J, Bossert A, Bakst RL, et al. Extracapsular extension is associated with worse distant control and progression-free survival in patients with lymph node-positive human papillomavirus-related oropharyngeal carcinoma. Oral Oncol 2017;74:56–61.

47. Kompelli AR, Morgan P, Li H, et al. Prognostic impact of high-risk pathologic fea-tures in HPV-related oropharyngeal squamous cell carcinoma and tobacco use. Otolaryngol Head Neck Surg 2019;160(5):855–61.

48. Bauer E, Mazul A, Chernock R, et al. Extranodal extension is a strong prognosti-cator in HPV-positive oropharyngeal squamous cell carcinoma. Laryngoscope 2020;130(4):939–45.

49. Swisher-McClure S, Lukens JN, Aggarwal C, et al. A phase 2 trial of alternative volumes of oropharyngeal irradiation for de-intensification (AVOID): omission of the resected primary tumor bed after transoral robotic surgery for human papil-loma virus-related squamous cell carcinoma of the oropharynx. Int J Radiat Oncol Biol Phys 2020;106(4):725–32.

50. Ma DJ, Price KA, Moore EJ, et al. Phase II evaluation of aggressive dose de-escalation for adjuvant chemoradiotherapy in human papillomavirus–associated oropharynx squamous cell carcinoma. J Clin Oncol 2019;37(22): 1909–18.

51. Ferris R, Flamand Y, Weinstein G, et al. Transoral robotic surgical resection fol-lowed by randomization to low- or standard-dose IMRT in resectable p16+ locally advanced oropharynx cancer: a trial of the ECOG-ACRIN Cancer Research Group (E3311). Am Soc Clin Oncol 2020. https://doi.org/10.1200/JCO.2020.38. 15_suppl.6500.

52. Gillison ML, Trotti AM, Harris J, et al. Radiotherapy plus cetuximab or cisplatin in human papillomavirus-positive oropharyngeal cancer (NRG Oncology RTOG

1016): a randomised, multicentre, non-inferiority trial. Lancet 2019;393(10166): 40–50.

53. Owadally W, Hurt C, Timmins H, et al. PATHOS: a phase II/III trial of risk-stratified, reduced intensity adjuvant treatment in patients undergoing transoral surgery for human papillomavirus (HPV) positive oropharyngeal cancer. BMC Cancer 2015; 15. https://doi.org/10.1186/s12885-015-1598-x.

Open Versus Robotic Surgery for Oropharyngeal Cancer

Gina D. Jefferson, MD, MPH*, Hudson Frey, MD

KEYWORDS

- Oropharyngeal cancer • Squamous cell carcinoma of the oropharynx
- Oropharyngeal surgery • Transoral robotic surgery • TORS
- Open approach to the oropharynx

KEY POINTS

- Consider transoral robotic surgery (TORS) for human papilloma virus (HPV)-positive and HPV-negative oropharyngeal squamous cell carcinoma in a select group of patients.
- TORS offers minimally invasive technique for achieving adequate oncologic outcomes while also providing good and sometime superior functional outcomes to other treatment.
- TORS is sometimes applicable for patients with persistent or recurrent OPSCC with appropriate patient selection.

INTRODUCTION

Traditionally, patients diagnosed with oropharyngeal squamous cell carcinoma (OPSCC) are treated with open surgical approaches to resect the cancer and to perform the reconstruction. Surgery is then followed by radiation with or without chemotherapy depending on reported pathologic features.[1] Open surgery of the oropharynx is accomplished via a transcervical-transpharyngeal, transmandibular-transpharyngeal, transfacial-transpharyngeal, or even intraoral access to the tumor. These approaches often involve reconstruction by a microvascular free flap, which increases length of recovery time. These open invasive procedures also often ultimately contribute to impediments of speech and breathing, as well as longstanding dysphagia.[2]

The Veterans Administration Laryngeal trial published in 1991[3] demonstrated a role for induction chemotherapy plus definitive concurrent chemotherapy with radiation as an equal means for achieving survival in locoregionally advanced laryngeal cancer in

Department of Otolaryngology-Head & Neck Surgery, University of Mississippi Medical Center, 2500 North State Street, 5 East, Jackson, MS 39216, USA
* Corresponding author.
E-mail address: gjefferson@umc.edu
Twitter: @drginajo (G.D.J.)

Otolaryngol Clin N Am 53 (2020) 995–1003
https://doi.org/10.1016/j.otc.2020.07.010
0030-6665/20/Published by Elsevier Inc.

comparison with surgery followed by radiation. The use of surgery to address oropharyngeal tumors declined due to extrapolation of organ-preserving protocols to the oropharynx. However, the use of concurrent chemoradiation "organ preservation" nonsurgical protocols resulted in an increase of treatment-related toxicities such as dysphagia, xerostomia, stricture, tissue fibrosis, and neuropathy.[4,5]

The work of Weinstein and O'Malley[6–8] to demonstrate feasibility and efficacy of the DaVinci Surgical System (Intuitive Surgical, Inc., Sunnyvale, CA) for transoral "robotic" access to the upper aerodigestive tract led to approval by the US Food and Drug Administration (FDA) in 2009. The Flex Robotic System (MedRobotics, Raynham, MA) offers a platform with flexible working arms and 3-dimensional camera, which subsequently received FDA approval for transoral procedures from the lips to the larynx in 2015. Transoral robot surgery (TORS) is facilitated by exposure to the pharynx and larynx by means of a retractor specifically designed for this purpose that includes a variety of tongue blades to best expose the anatomic subsite of interest. The 3-dimensional view afforded by these robotic platforms provides direct visualization of the surgical field, aids in an often en bloc resection of the tumor, reduces the morbidity associated with transcutaneous access to the anatomic location, and improves patient recovery time.[2]

Transoral Robotic Surgery

Data pooled from a multi-institutional feasibility study suggests the most commonly addressed subsites of the upper aerodigestive tract are the oropharynx and the supraglottic larynx. This study included 177 patients who underwent TORS in which 139 (78%) were for an oropharyngeal lesion and 26 procedures (15%) were performed targeting the larynx. The remainder of procedures were performed for tumors involving the hypopharynx and oral cavity.[9]

Indications

Data from the Surveillance, Epidemiology, End Results (SEER) database demonstrate that during the time period of 1992 to 2014 the incidence of OPSCC tripled.[10] Now during the 2000s approximately 70% of OPSCCs diagnosed in the United States are associated with the human papillomavirus (HPV).[11,12] Patients diagnosed with an HPV-associated OPSCC experience a unique disease presentation, tumor biology, and survival advantage.[13] The unique presentation of HPV-associated OPSCC includes lower T stage in comparison with patients diagnosed with HPV-negative OPSCC, most commonly of the tonsil followed by the base of tongue.[14] HPV-associated OPSCC clinical presentation permits addressing the primary site surgically with ability to achieve negative resection margins.[9] Furthermore, surgical management of the primary site and neck dissection when appropriate may result in avoidance of adjuvant radiation based on the final surgical pathology, or de-intensification of adjuvant radiation. De-intensification protocols and efficacy are still undergoing evaluation in clinical trials such as the Postoperative Adjuvant Treatment for Human Papillomavirus (HPV)-positive Tumors (PATHOS).[15] The anticipated benefit of deescalation is the reduction of treatment regimens without compromise of survival outcomes while maintaining superior functional outcomes. De-intensification incorporates TORS.

Patients with HPV-negative OPSCC are candidates for TORS management in certain instances as well.[16] A recent publication used the National Cancer Data Base to assess survival benefit of primary TORS versus nonsurgical definitive management. The investigators performed subgroup analysis based on HPV status stratified by early stage (T1-2N0-1) and advanced stage (T3-4N0-3 andT1-4N2-3) and found a survival advantage for patients with HPV-negative OPSCC when treated with TORS versus nonsurgical management. In their analysis when accounting for age, stage, and tumor grade, the 206 HPV-negative OPSCC patients did experience significantly better 3-year survival outcomes with TORS treatment "intensification" in comparison with patients addressed by radiation 84% (95% confidence interval [CI] 76%–91%) versus 66% (95% CI 57%–77%), P = .01. The investigators note the established relative radioresistance of HPV-negative OPSCC and surmise that surgical debulking of the radioresistant clones may result in the superior results for TORS basis of treatment in their study, also noting that 71% of all of the patients (both HPV-positive and HPV-negative) required adjuvant radiation therapy and 54% adjuvant chemotherapy.[17]

There is a higher local failure rate for patients with HPV-negative OPSCC than those with HPV-positive disease.[18] No matter the HPV disease status, surgical salvage is considered the best oncologic option for persistent or recurrent disease after primary radiation or chemoradiation therapy. TORS may prove efficacious for the appropriate patient in this setting. Small recurrent or persistent, or second primary OPSCC tumors are those amenable to TORS. However, larger tumors in the face of prior irradiation will benefit from concomitant microvascular reconstruction to minimize bleeding risk, particularly when re-irradiation is considered depending on pathologic findings for locoregional control of disease. It is important to note that plan for microvascular reconstruction of a defect is not mutually exclusive from TORS. TORS-assisted resection with the avoidance of mandibulotomy may prove beneficial coupled with microvascular reconstruction.[2]

Imaging assessment is key in determining patients eligible to undergo TORS anatomically. Imaging studies obtained during the evaluation and staging period for the patient's oropharyngeal cancer by contrast-enhanced computed tomography scan or MRI may demonstrate features that suggest a patient treated surgically may have positive margins or extracapsular spread of cancer involving regional lymph nodes. Both instances are indications for adjuvant chemotherapy with radiation. In selecting patients who are good candidates for TORS, the goal is to achieve R0 resection in a minimally invasive manner while also attempting to deescalate adjuvant therapies to not compromise disease control but to reduce treatment-related morbidity.[19]

When considering TORS to surgically manage tonsillar cancer, physical examination and imaging consistent with disease limitation to the tonsillar fossa are good candidates for achieving negative margins safely. Whether surgical management is open or transoral, presence of tumor surrounding the carotid artery by 270° or more is considered unresectable. Disease involvement of the prevertebral musculature or the bony vertebrae themselves are also considered unresectable. Specific to TORS, a surgical margin that requires extension beyond the periosteum of the mandible is not attainable given inability to perform marginal mandibulectomy with current robotic instrumentation. Similarly, involvement of the masticator space, pterygoids and temporalis muscles are not amenable to TORS, but often are amenable to open surgical resection with reconstruction. Involvement of the parapharyngeal space that lies posterolateral to the tonsillar fossa makes it difficult to achieve negative margins via the transoral robotic approach. Given that the posterior compartment of this space, the post-styloid space, contains the carotid sheath and cranial nerves 9 through 11, an open approach to surgical resection may preserve these vital structures while also enabling complete resection. Imaging that demonstrates medial carotid artery position abutting the tonsillar fossa also makes TORS a challenge for achieving safe surgical resection. Physical examination and imaging showing soft palatal involvement would suggest alternative treatment to achieve superior functional outcome. Surgical resection of the soft palate without reconstruction would result in the quality-of-life changing velopharyngeal insufficiency. When physical examination and imaging demonstrate oropharyngeal tumor extension into the nasopharynx, TORS resection is likely not attainable.[19,20] The flex robotic system is, however, promising in its ability to retroflex, enabling surgeons to potentially address a nasopharyngeal component of disease.

Involvement of the extrinsic tongue musculature, extension of base of tongue disease significantly into the pre-epiglottic space, involvement of bilateral lingual arteries, and tumor extending across midline where both neurovascular bundles would require sacrifice for resection are all better suited for open surgical resection with reconstruction of the defect. These instances would result in tongue devascularization and loss of tongue bulk and structure contributing to poor long-term functional outcomes and may contribute to inadequate resection by a transoral approach.[19]

When anatomic imaging suggests TORS is feasible both with respect to adequate, safe resection and anticipated functional outcome, exposure of the primary site is considered. Adequate exposure is assessed by patient ability to achieve maxillary-mandibular interincisor excursion, flexibility of the neck, the width of the mandibular arch, presence of bony tori of the mandible, and degree of macroglossia if present.[2]

Description of procedures
Briefly, for resection of tonsillar OPSCC via TORS, the Feyh-Kastenbauer (FK) retractor (Gyrus ACMI, Southborough, MA) is used for exposure and suspension. The procedure begins with incision of the pterygomandibular raphe. This incision exposes the superior constrictor, which serves as the lateral resection margin, while elevating the buccopharyngeal fascia. The resection was completed by incising the soft palate medially carried down to the constrictor freeing the muscle from the prevertebral fascia. Inferiorly, the styloglossus and stylopharyngeus muscles are transected and dissection proceeds from superior to the inferior incision (**Fig. 1**).[21]

Access to the base of tongue requires retraction for adequate exposure. Early use of the DaVinci system by O'Malley and colleagues[22] found use of the FK retractor provided advantages over the Crow Davis and Dingman retractors. Namely, the lateral retraction blades as well as the variety of tongue blades provided exposure for complete tumor resection. Utilization of both the 0° and 30° camera enabled adequate visualization of the surgical field to complete resection. These investigators describe exposing the vallecula using the open laryngeal blade to first make these vallecular incisions. The appropriate tongue blade with cut-out is exchanged for the laryngeal blade to enable the superior and lateral cuts next. These incisions are carried deep to the inferior depth desired for margin control enabling en bloc resection. The lingual artery is surgically clipped when it is encountered.[22]

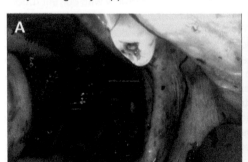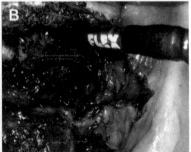

Fig. 1. Transoral robotic radical tonsillectomy and partial pharyngectomy.

Advantages of TORS versus open surgical technique or radiation-based therapies are related to the decreased damage to the pharyngeal musculature or to the major neurovascular structures and surrounding normal tissues. There are multiple reports of decreased hospital stay, decreased dysphagia, and decreased need for tracheostomy and feeding tube dependence. The impact of radiation-based therapies on HPV-positive patients is significant given this demographic is typically younger with greater life expectancy to experience the ongoing consequences of radiation fibrosis, dysphagia, xerostomia, and loss of taste sensation.[23,24]

Disadvantages associated with TORS include the initial cost and maintenance. The cost may preclude institutions from purchase. This in turn leads to subsequent inability of a given patient population to have access to this minimally invasive technique. In addition, disparity among hospital institutions contributes to potentially serious complications for those specialized surgeons using this technology, discharging patients without tracheostomy after a shorter time period where a postoperative hemorrhage at home may lead to death. Yet another potential disadvantage is limitations of robotic instrumentation, whereby access to the more distal upper aerodigestive tract may pose a significant challenge.[25] Flexible robotic systems may improve on this problem.

Open Surgery of the Oropharynx

As described in other sections of this article, the trend for surgical approach to the oropharynx has moved from an open approach to less invasive procedures, including transoral laser microsurgery and TORS.[26,27]

Indications

Indications for an open surgical approach include advanced tumors not amenable to the less invasive procedures given tumor characteristics, body habitus, or need for trimodality therapy. In addition, open surgery is commonly indicated for salvage surgery in previously treated malignancy for which surgery is the only remaining option. In these circumstances, wide surgical margins are advocated, which are readily accomplished through an open approach. This often results in pharyngeal communication with the neck requiring complex tissue inset into the defect.[26]

Description of procedures

The transmandibular-transpharyngeal approach to the oropharynx involves the use of a mandibulotomy or segmental mandibulectomy to gain access accomplished by a traditional lip split incision. An alternative approach is the visor flap whereby a large incision is made in the anterior neck and the skin is elevated superiorly over the mandible (**Fig. 2**).[27] The mandible is then divided with care taken to avoid injury to the mental nerve when oncologically feasible. The tongue musculature is transected permitting direct access to the oropharynx while protecting the neurovascular bundle if desired. If the tumor demands, a segment of involved mandibular bone is accessible for resection or a marginal mandibulectomy performed as needed for margins. Primary closure, adjacent tissue transfer, or microvascular free tissue transfer provide adequate reconstruction methods.[27,28]

Alternative approaches to accesses the oropharynx avoiding the morbidity associated with mandibulotomy include lateral pharyngotomy, transhyoid pharyngotomy, and suprahyoid pharyngotomy. The lateral pharyngotomy approach is facilitated by performing a selective neck dissection, thereby exposing the posterior belly of the digastric, hyoid bone and musculature, and branches of the external branch of the carotid. For tumors of the lateral and posterior pharyngeal wall, the hypoglossal nerve is protected superiorly by releasing the musculature from the superior aspect

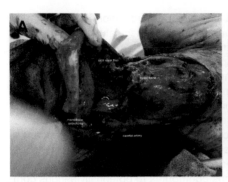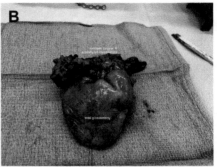

Fig. 2. Open total glossectomy, right partial glossectomy, and bilateral neck dissections via transcervical-transmandibular approach. A visor skin was used rather than lip splitting incision.

of the hyoid bone and reflecting cranially. The inferior muscular attachments to the hyoid are released for access to the ipsilateral vallecula. The lingual artery is ligated at this point and potentially saved for microvascular reconstruction. Resection of the lateral hyoid bone may aid direct visualization. Exposure is facilitated further by transection of the lateral portion of the thyroid cartilage in a vertical plane to access the posterior pharyngeal wall, or anteriorly with transection of the styloglossus and sacrifice of the facial nerve, or by excision of the tip of the angle of mandible. If an isolated posterior pharyngeal wall lesion is encountered, preservation of the hyoid bone is possible while the middle pharyngeal constrictor is incised along the length of the thyroid lamina.[29]

Suprahyoid pharyngotomy is an approach to base of tongue tumors from anterior. This is accomplished through a transcervical incision anteriorly carried down to the hyoid complex. Once isolated, the suprahyoid musculature is released in the midline with care taken to stay directly on the bone, thus avoiding the hypoglossal nerve and lingual vascular pedicle. The hyoepiglottic ligament is followed posteriorly leading to the mucosa of the vallecula, which is then incised. This approach allows for excision with primary closure assuming the tumor does not extend to the anterior tongue or deep tongue musculature. The muscles are then resuspended to the hyoid before closure.[29,30] A variation of this approach is useful to access lateral tongue lesions by transection of the hyoid and excision of the lateral tongue base, lingual vessel, and hypoglossal nerve as dictated by the tumor.[31]

The main advantages of open surgery include wide surgical field and exposure, especially in approaches in which mandibulotomy is performed. An additional advantage of the open surgical approaches is de-intensification of therapy where the tumor is completely excised and no additional treatment is required. This is realized when compared with quality-of-life measures seen in patients treated with primary radiation or chemoradiation where long -erm toxicities are often experienced.[2,26]

Disadvantages of open surgery are well documented and can have a significant impact on quality of life. Alteration of the tongue musculature impacts speech as well as swallowing, which is further impacted by pharyngeal surgery.[26,27] If mandibulotomy is performed, complications include malocclusion, hardware extrusion, osteomyelitis, and osteoradionecrosis in previously radiated bone.[28] Additional disadvantages are prolonged hospitalization, gastrostomy dependence, tracheostomy dependence, need for vascular free flap reconstruction, and cosmetic deformity of the lip if a lip split approach is used.[26,28]

Transoral Robotic Surgery Versus Open Surgery

An early report comparing TORS with open surgical approaches prospectively enrolled TORS patients and retrospectively matched this group to patients with OPSCC treated by open surgery. Patient demographics, tumor staging, and pathologic data including HPV status were similar between the groups. The investigators found patients treated with open surgery fared worse than those treated by TORS, which was not explained by pathologic outcomes of margin status or extracapsular spread. Survival analysis revealed 1-year, 2-year, and 3-year survival rates for TORS patients was 94%, 91%, and 89%, whereas for patients treated with open surgery, the rates were 85%, 75%, and 73% (P = .035). As stated previously, in tumor "debulking" by TORS enough radioresistant cancer cell clones may render adjuvant (chemo)radiation more efficacious in locoregional control of disease.[16] In addition, the period between TORS to adjuvant therapy in comparison with open surgery time to adjuvant therapy may have benefit of shorter period contributing to suboptimal disease control in patients undergoing open surgery.[17]

One major rationale for performing TORS is improved function in comparison with other treatment modalities. A prospective trial comparing oncologic and functional outcomes after TORS versus conventional surgery for T1-3 tonsillar cancer found significant differences in patient return to oral diet, hospital stay, and time to decannulation in favor of TORS. Return to oral diet occurred in 6.5 ± 4.2 days for TORS group versus 16.7 ± 5.3 for mandibulotomy approach (P <.001). Similarly, hospital stay for the TORS group was 14.6 ± 4 days in comparison to mandibulotomy approach of 24.6 ± 5.9 days (P = .001). In addition, time to decannulation in TORS patients occurred at 5 ± 1 days compared with the mandibulotomy approach at 13.2 ± 6. days (P<.001). The investigators also noted that as the study progressed, patients in the TORS group no longer underwent prophylactic tracheostomy at all.[32]

Complications associated with TORS notably occurred more often initially following FDA approval of the DaVinci system in 2009; Memorial Sloan Kettering reported 33% complication rate in 2010, progressively declining to 10% rate in 2015. The investigators reported that resection involving more than 2 subsites as increased odds for complication. Surgical resection involving more than 2 subsites infers a large tumor volume with likely resultant dysphagia contributing to aspiration pneumonia and greater raw surface area that may contribute to postoperative bleeding.[33]

Cost to purchase a robot may provide a significant challenge for many institutions. In 2009, Weinstein and colleagues[34] reported purchase cost for a DaVinci system of $1.5 million, yearly maintenance of $100,000 and $200 cost for each case performed to provide the disposable instrumentation.

In summary, TORS is advantageous when selected for appropriate patients. These patients include HPV-positive patients with OPSCC who may avoid adjuvant therapies in certain instances or who may enjoy adjuvant treatment de-intensification pending clinical trial evidence. Furthermore, some HPV-negative patients may prove good candidates based on tumor anatomy with some reports of improved survival in this patient population compared to open surgery or nonsurgical management.[16,17] Finally, TORS may also serve certain patients undergoing surgical salvage.

DISCLOSURE

The authors have nothing to disclose.

REFERENCES

1. Parsons JT, Mendenhall WM, Stringer SP, et al. Squamous cell carcinoma of the oropharynx: surgery, radiation therapy, or both. Cancer 2002;94(11):2967–80.
2. Sload R, Silver N, Jawad BA, et al. The role of transoral robotic surgery in the management of HPV negative oropharyngeal squamous cell carcinoma. Curr Oncol Rep 2016;18(9):53.
3. Wolf GT, Fisher SG, Hong WK, et al. Induction chemotherapy plus radiation compared with surgery plus radiation in patients with advanced laryngeal cancer. N Engl J Med 1991;324(24):1685–90.
4. Goepfert RP, Yom SS, Ryan WR, et al. Development of a chemoradiation therapy toxicity staging system for oropharyngeal carcinoma. Laryngoscope 2015; 125(4):869–76.
5. Clark JM, Holmes EM, O'Connell DA, et al. Long-term survival and swallowing outcomes in advanced stage oropharyngeal squamous cell carcinomas. Papillomavirus Res 2019;7:1–10.
6. Weinstein GS, O'malley BW, Hockstein NG. Transoral robotic surgery: supraglottic laryngectomy in a canine model. Laryngoscope 2005;115(7):1315–9.
7. O'Malley B, Weinstein GS, Hockstein N. Transoral robotic surgery (TORS): glottic microsurgery in a canine model. J Voice 2006;20:263–8.
8. Weinstein GS, O'Malley BW, Snyder W, et al. Transoral robotic surgery: radical tonsillectomy. Arch Otolaryngol Head Neck Surg 2007;133(12):1220–6.
9. Weinstein GS, O'Malley BW, Magnuson JS, et al. Transoral robotic surgery: a multicenter study to assess feasibility, safety, and surgical margins. Laryngoscope 2012;122(8):1701–7.
10. Fakhry C, Krapcho M, Eisele DW, et al. Head and neck squamous cell cancers in the United States are rare and risk is now higher among whites than blacks for the first time. Cancer 2018;124(10):2125–33.
11. Chaturvedi AK, Engels EA, Pfeiffer RM, et al. Human papillomavirus and rising oropharyngeal cancer incidence in the United States. J Clin Oncol 2011; 29(32):4294–301.
12. Viens LJ, Henley SJ, Watson M, et al. Human papillomavirus-associated cancers - United States, 2008-2012. MMWR Morb Mortal Wkly Rep 2016;65(26):661–6.
13. Posner MR, Lorch JH, Goloubeva O, et al. Survival and human papillomavirus in oropharynx cancer in TAX 324: a subset analysis from an international phase III trial. Ann Oncol 2011;22(5):1071–7.
14. Liederbach E, Kyrillos A, Wang CH, et al. The national landscape of human papillomavirus-associated oropharynx squamous cell carcinoma. Int J Cancer 2017;140(3):504–12.
15. Hargreaves S, Beasley M, Hurt C, et al. Deintensification of adjuvant treatment after transoral surgery in patients with human papillomavirus-positive oropharyngeal cancer: the conception of the PATHOS study and its development. Front Oncol 2019;9:936–45.
16. Ford SE, Brandwein-Gensler M, Carroll WR, et al. Transoral robotic versus open surgical approaches to oropharyngeal squamous cell carcinoma by human papillomavirus status. Otolaryngol Head Neck Surg 2014;151(4):606–11.
17. Mahmoud O, Sung K, Civantos FJ, et al. Transoral robotic surgery for oropharyngeal squamous cell carcinoma in the era of human papillomavirus. Head Neck 2018;40(4):710–21.

18. Fakhry C, Westra WH, Li S, et al. Improved survival of patients with human papillomavirus-positive head and neck squamous cell carcinoma in a prospective clinical trial. J Natl Cancer Inst 2008;100(4):261–9.
19. Kwan BYM, Khan NM, Almeida JR, et al. Transoral robotic surgery for head and neck malignancies: imaging features in presurgical workup. Head Neck 2019; 41(11):4018–25.
20. Gun R, Durmus K, Kucur C, et al. Transoral Surgical Anatomy and Clinical Considerations of Lateral Oropharyngeal Wall, Parapharyngeal Space, and Tongue Base. Otolaryngol Head Neck Surg 2016;154(3):480–5.
21. Moore EJ, Olsen KD, Kasperbauer JL. Transoral robotic surgery for oropharyngeal squamous cell carcinoma: a prospective study of feasibility and functional outcomes. Laryngoscope 2009;119(11):2156–64.
22. O'Malley BW, Weinstein GS, Snyder W, et al. Transoral robotic surgery (TORS) for base of tongue neoplasms. Laryngoscope 2006;116(8):1465–72.
23. Van Abel KM, Quick MH, Graner DE, et al. Outcomes following TORS for HPV-positive oropharyngeal carcinoma: PEGs, tracheostomies, and beyond. Am J Otolaryngol 2019;40(5):729–34.
24. Al-Khudari S, Bendix S, Lindholm J, et al. Gastrostomy tube use after transoral robotic surgery for oropharyngeal cancer. ISRN Otolaryngol 2013;2013:190364.
25. Nakayama M, Holsinger FC, Chevalier D, et al. The dawn of robotic surgery in otolaryngology-head and neck surgery. Jpn J Clin Oncol 2019;49(5):404–11.
26. Golusiński W, Golusińska-Kardach E. Current role of surgery in the management of oropharyngeal cancer. Front Oncol 2019;9:388.
27. Clayburgh DR, Gross N. Surgical innovations. Otolaryngol Clin North Am 2013; 46(4):615–28.
28. Dziegielewski PT, Mlynarek AM, Dimitry J, et al. The mandibulotomy: friend or foe? Safety outcomes and literature review. Laryngoscope 2009;119(12): 2369–75.
29. Laccourreye O, Villeneuve A, Rubin F, et al. Lateral pharyngotomy. Eur Ann Otorhinolaryngol Head Neck Dis 2019;136(2):135–40.
30. Zeitels SM, Vaughan CW, Ruh S. Suprahyoid pharyngotomy for oropharynx cancer including the tongue base. Arch Otolaryngol Head Neck Surg 1991;117(7): 757–60.
31. Civantos F, Wenig BL. Transhyoid resection of tongue base and tonsil tumors. Otolaryngol Head Neck Surg 1994;111(1):59–62.
32. Lee SY, Park YM, Byeon HK, et al. Comparison of oncologic and functional outcomes after transoral robotic lateral oropharyngectomy versus conventional surgery for T1 to T3 tonsillar cancer. Head Neck 2014;36(8):1138–45.
33. Hay A, Migliacci J, Karassawa Zanoni D, et al. Complications following transoral robotic surgery (TORS): a detailed institutional review of complications. Oral Oncol 2017;67:160–6.
34. Weinstein GS, O'Malley BW, Desai SC, et al. Transoral robotic surgery: does the ends justify the means? Curr Opin Otolaryngol Head Neck Surg 2009;17(2): 126–31.

Robotics in Pediatric Otolaryngology-Head and Neck Surgery and Advanced Surgical Planning

Neeraja Konuthula, MD[a], Sanjay R. Parikh, MD[b],
Randall A. Bly, MD[a],*

KEYWORDS

- Robotics • Pediatric otolaryngology • Surgical planning

KEY POINTS

- Robotic surgery has been successfully applied to many aspects of pediatric otolaryngology.
- Adoption of robotic technology may be improved with advanced computer-aided surgical planning to compare techniques and approaches.
- Advanced surgical planning includes segmentation, virtual reality, three-dimensional printing, optimization algorithms, intraoperative mirror image overlay, and can incorporate robotic instruments.
- Barriers for integration include specialized pediatric instruments as well as time and expertise needed for advanced surgical planning.

INTRODUCTION

Robotic surgery has been explored in pediatric otolaryngology since 2007.[1] Although its applications have been demonstrated in many different areas of pediatric head and neck surgery, its adoption has been limited to larger centers and its reports limited to feasibility studies. Integration of robotic surgery may improve with advanced preoperative surgical planning and newer, smaller robotic instrumentation. Recent advances in computer-aided surgical planning allow for comparison and implementation of different surgical approaches with varying technology including robotics. The ability to surgically access a specific target is a function of visualization, instrumentation, patient-specific anatomy, and morbidity incurred by gaining the access. The two major components that can be optimized include visualization and instrumentation, both

[a] Department of Otolaryngology–Head and Neck Surgery, Division of Pediatric Otolaryngology, University of Washington, Seattle Children's Hospital, 1959 Northeast Pacific Street, Box 356515, Seattle, WA 98195, USA; [b] Department of Otolaryngology–Head and Neck Surgery, Division of Pediatric Otolaryngology, University of Washington, Seattle Children's Hospital, Seattle, WA, USA
* Corresponding author.
E-mail address: Randall.Bly@seattlechildrens.org

Otolaryngol Clin N Am 53 (2020) 1005–1016
https://doi.org/10.1016/j.otc.2020.07.011
0030-6665/20/© 2020 Elsevier Inc. All rights reserved.

of which are related to surgical robotics. A major opportunity within pediatric robotic head and neck surgery is to perform the same surgical task but with reduced morbidity incurred to the patient.

CURRENT USE OF ROBOTICS IN PEDIATRIC OTOLARYNGOLOGY

Robotic surgery has been used in pediatric surgery since the initial description of transoral robotic surgery (TORS) in laryngeal cleft repair in 2007.[1] In that case series of 5 pediatric patients, the size of the robotic arms was considered to be a limiting factor for application in the pediatric population as 3 cases could not be completed due to lack of visualization and insufficient space to maneuver instruments.

As TORS technology has advanced, its applications in pediatric head and neck surgery have expanded, including in children undergoing surgery for obstructive sleep apnea.[2–4] A retrospective review of 16 patients between ages 5 and 19 years who underwent lingual tonsillectomy via TORS divided the study population into 3 groups in the order of operation and found that the docking times decreased significantly from the first group to the second 2 groups.[4] Operative time and blood loss were not noted to be statistically different among the groups. The investigators attributed their successful completion of all cases to smaller instruments (5 mm instruments, 12 mm endoscope), unmatched exposure of the tongue base musculature, magnification of working area, and visualization of cranial nerve IX. Another study described 9 patients who underwent base of tongue reduction and lingual tonsillectomy via TORS and stated advantages include a three-dimensional (3D) view and more freedom of motion over endoscopic coblation or radiofrequency ablation.[3] There was one postoperative base of tongue bleed that required intraoperative control and was discharged without further complications.

Another case series described use of TORS in 16 children in a variety of oropharyngeal and airway procedures including resection of base of tongue lesions, resection of supraglottic and hypopharyngeal lesions, and repair of laryngeal clefts.[5] This was the first pediatric case series to describe use of TORS in a variety of procedures in children from as young as 14 days to 15 years. Similar to prior reports, wristed-instrument control, 3D visualization, more precise control of the laser, ability to place more sutures in small spaces, and multilayer closure with greater exposure than in standard endoscopic procedures were identified as advantages. Adequate exposure, obtaining surgical access for robotic arms, and need for a bedside surgeon were noted as limitations. Operative and docking time were not reported due to the large variety of cases, and complications were found to be within expected range for the procedures. It was suggested that specialized airway instruments would likely widen pediatric applications.

Since then TORS has been reported in several case reports for use in pediatric airway reconstruction and head and neck resections.[6,7] It has been used for successful resection of supraglottic neurofibroma with parapharyngeal space extension.[7] In this case, surgeons opted for TORS over transoral laser microsurgery (TLM) due to its superior laryngeal and lateral pharyngeal exposure. However, the patient then required resection of residual disease 2 months postoperatively for which they preferred TLM, as they had adequate exposure with a less cumbersome setup and superior tactile feedback.[7] A laryngeal neurofibroma is shown being resected in **Fig. 1** in a 2-year-old via transoral robotic surgery.

These case series suggest that the known advantages of TORS in adults including increased precision, 3D magnification, tremor reduction, motion downscaling, and freedom of motion superior to that of the human hand[4,7] are also advantaged in pediatric head and surgery. However, the same study also notes that when traditional

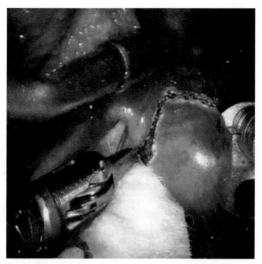

Fig. 1. View of exposure of laryngeal neurofibroma in a 2-year-old resected via TORS.

endoscopic instruments are deemed sufficient during surgical planning, they are preferred due to lack of cumbersome setup and decreased cost.

Most preoperative surgical planning is performed with 2D computed tomography (CT) and MRI combined with the surgeon's experience. Advanced surgical planning can play a role in further adoption of robotic technology, as it could allow for preoperative surgical exploration and comparison of robotic instruments over traditional surgical instruments.

CURRENT ADVANCED SURGICAL PLANNING TOOLS

Preoperative surgical planning provides opportunities for increased patient safety, decreased operative time, and decreased morbidity. Advanced surgical planning refers to the use of technology to enhance the planning process and can include anything from virtual reality to 3D printed models to computer-aided optimization algorithms.

Surgical planning must start with a computer model of the patient-specific anatomy and lesion (**Fig. 2**). In order to use any of the following methods such as virtual reality, hologram visualization, and 3D printed templates, an accurate model must first be created. To do this, typically cross-sectional imagings (CT and MRI) are used either in isolation or merged to create the anatomic model. For certain anatomic regions, this can be straightforward and automatic segmentation can be used to identify bones and vessels with contrast, but many of the smaller structures within the head and neck still require manual segmentation by an expert. Segmenting cartilage, for example, continues to be a challenge using CT alone.[8] This is time consuming and is one of the barriers for using surgical planning. Once a model is created, depending on the application, simply visualizing the approach (eg, virtual endoscopy) may provide enough insight to the surgeon that he or she now has a better understanding of what the surgical task will entail. In other instances, the surgeon needs more than visualization and requires specific templates or other guides to precisely carry out the surgical task. The topics discussed later are some of the available methods to convey the information from the model to the surgeon regarding patient-specific surgery. As this

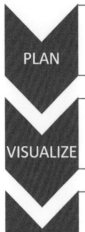

PLAN
- CT/MRI
- Segmentation of critical and relevent structures

VISUALIZE
- 3D modeling/printing
- Virtual endoscopy
- Pre-operative rehearsal

GUIDE
- Virtual reality navigation, heads-up display
- Patient-specific face mask for surgical portals
- 3D printed drill guides

Fig. 2. Stages of advanced surgical planning that can incorporate robotic instrumentation.

process improves, it will be an essential step in adopting new robotic technology to novel surgical approaches.

Virtual Reality

Augmented reality or virtual reality has been well studied in surgical training, and several studies have shown simulation can increase trainee and surgeon confidence.[9] As the patient-specific fidelity and haptic feedback of virtual reality has improved, its use has expanded to preoperative planning. In fact, the benefits of virtual reality surgical rehearsal were shown to improve case selection, selection of surgical tools, and surgical performance in carotid endovascular surgery.[10,11]

With respect to endoscopic skull base surgery, virtual reality can be used to improve surgeon familiarity with important anatomic landmarks with more patient specificity and lower cost than cadaver training. One study created a virtual surgical environment, entitled CardinalSim, and retrospectively reviewed simulation of 10 endoscopic skull base cases.[12] They found excellent correlation in surgical exposure, anatomic features, and location of pathology between the simulation and actual case, suggesting benefits of patient-specific rehearsal before actual surgery. Surgical rehearsal allows surgeons to familiarize themselves with anatomic variations, foresee pitfalls, and adjust operative plans.[12] Several virtual simulators of endoscopic sinus and skull base surgery are available yet their evaluations have been limited to training purposes.[13] However, time and cost needed to manually segment and reconstruct individual patient anatomy from CT scans are major barriers to widespread use in preoperative planning and practice.[13]

In sleep surgery, virtual reality modeled the effects of maxillomandibular advancement.[14,15] Preoperative virtual planning results compared with postsurgical data showed that the simulation reliably predicted facial tissue and anteroposterior airway extension.[14] However, it was not able to accurately predict changes in the lateral velopharyngeal region. Another model guided the surgeon in the extent of maxillomandibular advancement based on goal posterior airway space and tooth-to-lip show in 4 patients.[15] Postoperative posterior airway space and facial aesthetic profile closely matched those predicted by the model.

Virtual reality has also been used to plan and rehearse lateral skull base/otologic surgery.[16–18] Surgical planning via a combination of 3D printing and 3D simulation allowed for avoidance of critical structures in a case study on transcanal endoscopic approach to the petrous apex.[17] Voxelman TempSurg with haptic feedback is a simulation software used for case-specific surgical rehearsal for 24 cadaver temporal bones.[18] Trainee and expert otolaryngologists agreed that knowledge of anatomic variation influenced subsequent surgery on cadaver specimens, particularly the specific boundaries of sigmoid sinus.[18] This study also showed that there was improvement in upload time or time needed to convert a CT scan to a 3D model via segmentation, as surgeons better understood how to use the semiautomatic segmentation process. Surgical planning was rated higher with case-specific data as compared with a generic training model. However, this study still suffered from low fidelity for critical structures such as facial nerve and tegmen.[18] A similar study was conducted in 2 different institutions and also showed that rehearsal increased confidence, which correlated with higher grades on dissection performance.[19]

Despite its complex 3D anatomy, surgical planning for head and neck surgery resection and reconstruction is still mainly done via 2D CTs and MRIs. A recent case series explored the use of virtual reality modeling with patient-specific data before surgery. Surgeons were able to explore the 3D anatomy and practice techniques in cases such as a partial clavicle resection with myocutaneous flap repair and a carotid body tumor. One benefit noted was that the visualization of vascular invasion and intraluminal dimension before surgery—particularly in postradiation cases—could help anticipate operative time and vascular surgery consultation.[20]

Three-Dimensional Printing

3D printing for surgical planning involves the development of a CAD template that is generated from 3D reconstructions from MRI or CT images.[21] Advantages include patient specificity and ability to create single-use models.

3D printed surgical guides have been used in craniofacial surgery to determine the optimal location for internal plates and screws.[20,22,23] Drill and osteotomy guides can be planned and printed in advance to assist the surgeon with regard to optimal orientation, location, and depth. These guides are becoming increasingly accurate and more useful as innovations in transparency and flexibility become available for 3D printing.[24]

In head and neck reconstructive surgery, preoperative simulation with mandibular models were also noted to decrease operative times, as they allowed practice shaping the fibula and fitting it within the mandibular reconstruction plate.[25] Furthermore, cutting guides were 3D printed to allow for cutting and contouring of the fibula bone to fit precisely in segmental mandibular resections defects.[26] Navigation has also been shown to be helpful in planning reconstructions.[27]

A recent systematic review examined the role of 3D printing for the creation of patient-matched surgical guides, templates, and implants in pediatric airway reconstruction.[28] In all cases, preoperative assessment with patient-specific 3D printed models resulted in significant alterations in surgical plans, and expert option was unanimously in favor of using 3D printed models. The use of 3D printed airway models were recommended as a means to reduce complications in complex airway interventions and should be compared with preoperative planning with only 2D and 3D imaging.[28]

NEW DEVELOPMENTS IN ROBOTICS AND ADVANCED SURGICAL PLANNING
Multiobjective Cost Function to Optimize Endoscopic Approach

A multiobjective cost function was recently used to model preoperative planning for skull base surgery.[29] Key skull base structures were segmented using patients' preoperative CT scans. Morbidity costs were assigned to each of the predetermined structures by surgeons, and a weight-based cost function was then used to determine an optimized surgical approach. Resultant pathways were found to be similar to actual approaches performed on patients based on surveys of skull base surgeons when reviewed retrospectively. The algorithm can be expanded to other anatomic regions and potentially be used to optimize approach in many different head and neck surgeries. A major advantage of this method to seek optimized surgical approach is that the boundaries through which instrumentation can function can be defined. As new robotic technology becomes available, the specific surgical pathway through which those instruments need to work can be inputted to identify optimized surgical corridors as a function of lesion location and individual patient anatomy.

A simpler version of this technique can be done without multiobjective cost function optimization, and defines—in great detail—the geometry of the surgical corridor required to perform a specific surgical task (**Fig. 3**).[30] This has been applied for multiple applications to the skull base including the lateral cavernous sinus.[30–32] This permits precise knowledge of the size and shape of surgical corridor, which could enable robotic integration. It could both assess feasibility of current robotic instrumentation but should also be used in the future design of robotic systems.

Mirror Image Overlay

Another method to incorporate surgical planning in guiding the surgeon accurately is the use of mirror image overlay (MIO). This technique can be applied where there is anatomic symmetry. In orbital reconstruction, restoration of the orbital bones to their

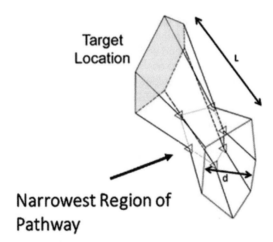

Fig. 3. Mapping of maximal pathway boundaries of potential robotic surgical portal based on the target, entrance, and narrowest region. (*From* Moe KS, Bly RA. Commentary: Comparative Analysis of the Exposure and Surgical Freedom of the Endoscopic Extended Minipterional Craniotomy and the Transorbital Endoscopic Approach to the Anterior and Middle Cranial Fossae. Oper Neurosurg (Hagerstown) 2019;17(2):E47-E49 https://doi.org/10.1093/ons/opy371[published Online First: Epub Date]|.)

correct anatomic position is important to minimize postoperative complications. One advanced surgical planning technique to optimize the orbital bone placement is MIO.[33] This involves duplicating the contralateral (nontraumatized) orbitozygomatic region, reversing (side-to-side) the segment, and superimposing its skeleton onto the fractured, displaced orbit. When combined with intraoperative navigation, MIO can be used to guide a surgical implant into proper anatomic position and has been studied in several cohorts.[33–35]

In another study focused on treating delayed orbitozygomatic fracture with severe enophthalmos, in addition to intraoperative MIO, a model with MIO was 3D printed so that titanium mesh and plates could be prebent on the model.[36] Adequate zygomatic reduction was achieved in 74.3% of the patients with traditional surgery, 85.7% of the cases that used 3D printed models, and 100% of navigation-guided cases.[36] In a larger study, MIO resulted in a significant reduction in postoperative diplopia for complex fractures and reduced the rate of revision surgery from 20% to 4% in 113 orbital fracture repairs.[33]

Flexible Robotic Technology

Flexible robotic technology for endoscopic sinus and skull base surgery has been in development for the past decade[37] but is not yet in clinical use. Ideally, flexible robotic endoscopes would allow for endoscopes to curve around critical structures to reach surgical targets based on patient anatomy. A recent systematic review assessed 11 robotic prototypes for extended skull base surgery and concluded that although there are still technical limitations, clinical feasibility is getting very close.[38] A robotic endoscope holder for anterior skull base surgery was recently introduced, and 30 skull base surgeons were tested on 2 tasks with and without EndoscopeRobot, a robotic endoscope holder.[39] There was a trend toward shorter completion times and increased efficiency in one of the bimanual tasks.

Development of robots for the skull base and the head and neck is being developed on surgical robot platforms such as the RAVEN II including simulation of semiautonomous brain tumor ablation.[40] This research platform robot is important to study because any robot that is cleared by Food and Drug Administration has limitations on its use and cannot be modified.[41] In the research phase, multiple studies have demonstrated both feasibility and have reported the technical limitations. For example, access to the anterior cranial fossa was evaluated on both DaVinci and RAVEN robotic platforms in multiple studies (**Fig. 4**).[42–45] The conclusions were that instrument arms often collided due to the narrow funnel effect of surgical portals too close in proximity. Expanding the surgical portals did improve that, but surgeons were still limited by the ability to instrument at the target location.

BARRIERS TO ADOPTION AND STRATEGIES
Barriers to Robotics in Pediatric Otolaryngology

Barriers to pediatric robotic surgery are similar to those for adult TORS with a few additional limitations. Similar to adult TORS, cost becomes less prohibitive if cases are gathered at a tertiary center.[3] Cumbersome setup and decreased tactile feedback when compared with endoscopic instruments are barriers to adoption.[7] It can be prohibitive in a busy pediatric center with a large variety of cases. As robotic instruments continue to improve, the size of the instruments has become less of a limitation, as one study noted use of TORS in a 14-day-old. However, the same study noted the need for pediatric airway instruments, as many TORS instruments are designed for pharyngeal surgery.[5] Thus far, studies have only been able to show the noninferiority of robotic

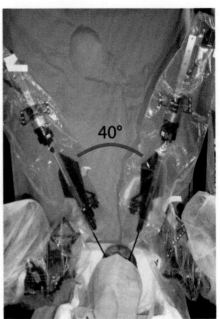

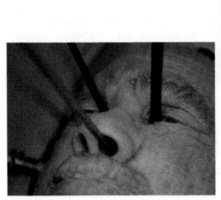

Fig. 4. Multiportal technique with the Raven robot in a cadaver study. (*From* Bly RA, Su D, Lendvay TS, et al. Multiportal robotic access to the anterior cranial fossa: a surgical and engineering feasibility study. Otolaryngol Head Neck Surg 2013;149(6):940-6 https://doi.org/10. 1177/0194599813509587[published Online First: Epub Date]|.)

pediatric surgery. Improvement of the aforementioned limitations may result in the adoption of robotic surgery over endoscopic tools.

Barriers to Preoperative Planning with Virtual Reality

Surgical planning with virtual reality and other visualization methods has been demonstrated to provide insight that can change surgical approach and potentially improve patient outcomes. However, the time of experts needed to create an accurate model continues to be a barrier for widespread adoption as high fidelity simulations require increased time for image rendering as well as manual segmentation.[13] Lower fidelity environments allow for comparison to cadaver surgery and training but do not always provide experts with the soft tissue specifications needed to plan surgery.[18] Virtual reality used for planning of sleep surgery would also incur costs of scanning time and radiation exposure the patient may not otherwise need.[15]

Barriers to Preoperative Planning with Three-Dimensional Printing

3D printing combined with 3D models to plan and print cutting guides and markers are being quickly adopted due to their high clinical utility and increase in surgical efficiency.[20,22,23,28] Cost of printing the model is not usually prohibitive due to significant advances in 3D printing technology. However, commercial programs and expertise are needed to print 3D models with cutting guides, which incurs additional cost. Furthermore, expert surgeons currently determine appropriate cuts, and the margin of resection may change compared with what is predicted on the preoperative imaging. Adding an additional step of modeling may seem unnecessary without more studies showing superiority in patient outcomes compared with the current standard.

SUMMARY

Robotic surgery has been successfully applied to many different areas of pediatric head and neck surgery from sleep surgery to airway reconstruction to resection of pharyngeal masses. Despite some limitations including cumbersome setup and obtaining surgical access for robotic arms, overall studies have shown the feasibility and advantages of the surgical robot in pediatric otolaryngology. However, adoption has been limited, and robotic surgery may be better integrated into practice with advanced preoperative surgical planning, which allows for comparison of different surgical approaches. Computer-aided surgical planning techniques include current technologies of 3D printing and virtual reality as well as new developments of multiobjective cost function for optimization of approach, MIO, and flexible robotics. These promising robotic and advanced surgical planning technologies are more likely to be adopted with future studies noting advantages over current practice. More studies need to be done with actual patient outcomes as well as comparing the different methods.

ACKNOWLEDGMENTS

Vanessa Masco for figure preparation and critical review. The late Dr Eduardo Mendez contributed with involvement in the pediatric case presented in **Fig. 1**.

R.A. Bly is supported through Clinical Scholars Research Program, Seattle Children's Hospital. N. Konuthula is supported through NIH T32 DC000018-33 from the National Institute on Deafness and Other Communication Disorders awarded to the University of Washington Department of Otolaryngology (P.I., Edward Weaver).

DISCLOSURE

Dr N. Konuthula has nothing to disclose. Dr R.A. Bly is co-founder and holds a financial interest of ownership equity with Edus Health, Inc and EigenHealth, Inc. He is Consultant and stock holder, Spiway, LLC.

REFERENCES

1. Rahbar R, Ferrari LR, Borer JG, et al. Robotic surgery in the pediatric airway: application and safety. Arch Otolaryngol Head Neck Surg 2007;133(1):46–50 [discussion: 50].
2. Montevecchi F, Bellini C, Meccariello G, et al. Transoral robotic-assisted tongue base resection in pediatric obstructive sleep apnea syndrome: case presentation, clinical and technical consideration. Eur Arch Otorhinolaryngol 2017; 274(2):1161–6.
3. Thottam PJ, Govil N, Duvvuri U, et al. Transoral robotic surgery for sleep apnea in children: Is it effective? Int J Pediatr Otorhinolaryngol 2015;79(12):2234–7.
4. Leonardis RL, Duvvuri U, Mehta D. Transoral robotic-assisted lingual tonsillectomy in the pediatric population. JAMA Otolaryngol Head Neck Surg 2013; 139(10):1032–6.
5. Zdanski CJ, Austin GK, Walsh JM, et al. Transoral robotic surgery for upper airway pathology in the pediatric population. Laryngoscope 2017;127(1):247–51.
6. Carroll DJ, Byrd JK, Harris GF. The feasibility of pediatric TORS for lingual thyroglossal duct cyst. Int J Pediatr Otorhinolaryngol 2016;88:109–12.
7. Arnold MA, Mortelliti AJ, Marzouk MF. Transoral resection of extensive pediatric supraglottic neurofibroma. Laryngoscope 2018;128(11):2525–8.
8. Saxena RC, Friedman S, Bly RA, et al. Comparison of micro-computed tomography and clinical computed tomography protocols for visualization of nasal

cartilage before surgical planning for rhinoplasty. JAMA Facial Plast Surg 2019; 21(3):237–43.

9. Kashikar TS, Kerwin TF, Moberly AC, et al. A review of simulation applications in temporal bone surgery. Laryngoscope Investig Otolaryngol 2019;4(4):420–4.

10. Willaert W, Aggarwal R, Bicknell C, et al. Patient-specific simulation in carotid artery stenting. J Vasc Surg 2010;52(6):1700–5.

11. Cates CU, Patel AD, Nicholson WJ. Use of virtual reality simulation for mission rehearsal for carotid stenting. JAMA 2007;297(3):265–6.

12. Won TB, Hwang P, Lim JH, et al. Early experience with a patient-specific virtual surgical simulation for rehearsal of endoscopic skull-base surgery. Int Forum Allergy Rhinol 2018;8(1):54–63.

13. Kim DH, Kim Y, Park JS, et al. Virtual reality simulators for endoscopic sinus and skull base surgery: the present and future. Clin Exp Otorhinolaryngol 2019; 12(1):12–7.

14. Frey R, Gabrielova B, Gladilin E. A combined planning approach for improved functional and esthetic outcome of bimaxillary rotation advancement for treatment of obstructive sleep apnea using 3D biomechanical modeling. PLoS One 2018; 13(8):e0199956.

15. Barrera JE. Virtual surgical planning improves surgical outcome measures in obstructive sleep apnea surgery. Laryngoscope 2014;124(5):1259–66.

16. Chan S, Li P, Locketz G, et al. High-fidelity haptic and visual rendering for patient-specific simulation of temporal bone surgery. Comput Assist Surg (Abingdon) 2016;21(1):85–101.

17. Barber SR, Wong K, Kanumuri V, et al. Augmented Reality, Surgical Navigation, and 3D Printing for Transcanal Endoscopic Approach to the Petrous Apex. OTO Open 2018;2(4). 2473974X18804492.

18. Arora A, Swords C, Khemani S, et al. Virtual reality case-specific rehearsal in temporal bone surgery: a preliminary evaluation. Int J Surg 2014;12(2):141–5.

19. Locketz GD, Lui JT, Chan S, et al. Anatomy-Specific Virtual Reality Simulation in Temporal Bone Dissection: Perceived Utility and Impact on Surgeon Confidence. Otolaryngol Head Neck Surg 2017;156(6):1142–9.

20. Li C, Cai Y, Wang W, et al. Combined application of virtual surgery and 3D printing technology in postoperative reconstruction of head and neck cancers. BMC Surg 2019;19(1):182.

21. Kaye R, Goldstein T, Zeltsman D, et al. Three dimensional printing: A review on the utility within medicine and otolaryngology. Int J Pediatr Otorhinolaryngol 2016;89:145–8.

22. Smithers FAE, Cheng K, Jayaram R, et al. Maxillofacial reconstruction using in-house virtual surgical planning. ANZ J Surg 2018;88(9):907–12.

23. Resnick CM. Precise osteotomies for mandibular distraction in infants with Robin sequence using virtual surgical planning. Int J Oral Maxillofac Surg 2018;47(1): 35–43.

24. Kim GB, Lee S, Kim H, et al. Three-dimensional printing: basic principles and applications in medicine and radiology. Korean J Radiol 2016;17(2):182–97.

25. Xu X, Ping FY, Chen J, et al. [Application of CAD/CAM techniques in mandible large-scale defect and reconstruction with vascularized fibular bone graft]. Zhejiang Da Xue Xue Bao Yi Xue Ban 2007;36(5):498–502.

26. Zhang T, Zhang Y, Li YS, et al. [Application of CTA and CAD＼CAM techniques in mandible reconstruction with free fibula flap]. Zhonghua Zheng Xing Wai Ke Za Zhi 2006;22(5):325–7.

27. Harbison RA, Shan XF, Douglas Z, et al. Navigation Guidance During Free Flap Mandibular Reconstruction: A Cadaveric Trial. JAMA Otolaryngol Head Neck Surg 2017;143(3):226–33.
28. Stramiello JA, Saddawi-Konefka R, Ryan J, et al. The role of 3D printing in pediatric airway obstruction: A systematic review. Int J Pediatr Otorhinolaryngol 2020; 132:109923.
29. Aghdasi N, Whipple M, Humphreys IM, et al. Automated surgical approach planning for complex skull base targets: development and validation of a cost function and semantic at-las. Surg Innov 2018;25(5):476–84.
30. Moe KS, Bly RA. Commentary: comparative analysis of the exposure and surgical freedom of the endoscopic extended minipterional craniotomy and the transorbital endoscopic approach to the anterior and middle cranial fossae. Oper Neurosurg (Hagerstown) 2019;17(2):E47–9.
31. Bly RA, Ramakrishna R, Ferreira M, et al. Lateral transorbital neuroendoscopic approach to the lateral cavernous sinus. J Neurol Surg B Skull Base 2014; 75(1):11–7.
32. Noiphithak R, Yanez-Siller JC, Revuelta Barbero JM, et al. Comparative analysis of the exposure and surgical freedom of the endoscopic extended minipterional craniotomy and the transorbital endoscopic approach to the anterior and middle cranial fossae. Oper Neurosurg (Hagerstown) 2019;17(2):174–81.
33. Bly RA, Chang SH, Cudejkova M, et al. Computer-guided orbital reconstruction to improve outcomes. JAMA Facial Plast Surg 2013;15(2):113–20.
34. Gellrich NC, Schramm A, Hammer B, et al. Computer-assisted secondary reconstruction of unilateral posttraumatic orbital deformity. Plast Reconstr Surg 2002; 110(6):1417–29.
35. Schmelzeisen R, Gellrich NC, Schoen R, et al. Navigation-aided reconstruction of medial orbital wall and floor contour in cranio-maxillofacial reconstruction. Injury 2004;35(10):955–62.
36. He D, Li Z, Shi W, et al. Orbitozygomatic fractures with enophthalmos: analysis of 64 cases treated late. J Oral Maxillofac Surg 2012;70(3):562–76.
37. Yoon HS, Oh SM, Jeong JH, et al. Active bending endoscope robot system for navigation through sinus area. IROS'11 - 2011 IEEE/RSJ International Conference on Intelligent Robots and Systems: Celebrating 50 Years of Robotics. San Francisco, September 25-30. 2011. p. 967–72.
38. Bolzoni Villaret A, Doglietto F, Carobbio A, et al. Robotic transnasal endoscopic skull base surgery: systematic review of the literature and report of a novel prototype for a hybrid system (brescia endoscope assistant robotic holder). World Neurosurg 2017;105:875–83.
39. Zappa F, Mattavelli D, Madoglio A, et al. Hybrid robotics for endoscopic skull base surgery: preclinical evaluation and surgeon first impression. World Neurosurg 2020;134:e572–80.
40. Hu D, Gong Y, Hannaford B, et al. Path Planning for Semi-automated Simulated Robotic Neurosurgery. Rep U S 2015;2015:2639–45.
41. Hannaford B, Rosen J, Friedman DW, et al. Raven-II: an open platform for surgical robotics research. IEEE Trans Biomed Eng 2013;60(4):954–9.
42. Lee JY, O'Malley BW Jr, Newman JG, et al. Transoral robotic surgery of the skull base: a cadaver and feasibility study. ORL J Otorhinolaryngol Relat Spec 2010; 72(4):181–7.
43. Kupferman M, Demonte F, Holsinger FC, et al. Transantral robotic access to the pituitary gland. Otolaryngol Head Neck Surg 2009;141(3):413–5.

44. Hanna EY, Holsinger C, DeMonte F, et al. Robotic endoscopic surgery of the skull base: a novel surgical approach. Arch Otolaryngol Head Neck Surg 2007; 133(12):1209–14.

45. Bly RA, Su D, Lendvay TS, et al. Multiportal robotic access to the anterior cranial fossa: a surgical and engineering feasibility study. Otolaryngol Head Neck Surg 2013;149(6):940–6.

The Rise of Upper Airway Stimulation in the Era of Transoral Robotic Surgery for Obstructive Sleep Apnea

Kevin J. Kovatch, MD, Syed Ahmed Ali, MD, Paul T. Hoff, MS, MD*

KEYWORDS

- Obstructive sleep apnea • Hypoglossal nerve stimulation • Upper airway stimulation
- Inspire • Transoral robotic surgery

KEY POINTS

- Upper airway stimulation (UAS) has shown high success rates in carefully selected patients with moderate to severe sleep apnea.
- UAS has shown equivalent or better outcomes with lower morbidity compared with transoral robotic (TORS) base of tongue surgery.
- Studies comparing UAS and TORS directly have shown clear benefit of UAS over TORS in patients meeting UAS criteria; however, many TORS candidates are not UAS candidates under current candidacy criteria.
- Future studies of UAS will further characterize long-term treatment efficacy, adverse event profile, and effect on medical outcomes.

INTRODUCTION/BACKGROUND

Obstructive sleep apnea (OSA) is a chronic sleep disorder characterized by recurrent episodes of upper airway collapse and associated reduction or cessation of airflow with resulting hypoxia. The adverse health effects on both quality of life and medical comorbidities, including cardiac arrhythmia and stroke, are well described.[1,2] First-line treatment of OSA includes medical measures, with continuous positive airway pressure (CPAP) being the gold standard of treatment.[3] Intolerance of CPAP is common and drives many patients to pursue surgical treatment.[4]

The pathophysiology contributing to OSA is multifactorial and includes mechanical airway obstruction from soft tissue and skeletal elements, as well as dynamic collapse related to decreased tone and inadequate reflex airway dilation.[5] Transoral robotic

Department of Otolaryngology Head & Neck Surgery, Michigan Medicine, 1500 East Medical Center Drive, Ann Arbor, MI 48109, USA
* Corresponding author.
E-mail address: phoff@med.umich.edu

Otolaryngol Clin N Am 53 (2020) 1017–1029
https://doi.org/10.1016/j.otc.2020.08.001
0030-6665/20/© 2020 Elsevier Inc. All rights reserved.

multilevel surgery (TORS) was first approved for removal of benign tongue base tissue in 2009 under the Davinci robotic platform; it became increasingly popular over the last decade as a way to address anatomic obstruction from hypertrophied lingual tonsillar tissue that could not be accessed easily or safely by conventional methods.[6] As the understanding of the pathophysiology of OSA has evolved, recent treatments falling into the category of neurostimulation (upper airway stimulation, UAS) have emerged as a dynamic alternative to traditional static soft tissue and skeletal framework surgery. Currently, hypoglossal nerve stimulation (HGNS) is the only UAS device that is Food and Drug Administration (FDA) approved (Inspire, 2014) for the treatment of OSA.[7,8]

TORS is ideally suited for patients with primarily tongue base obstruction from lingual tonsil hypertrophy, although it may be performed in conjunction with other multilevel surgeries when other sites of mechanical obstruction are present[9] (**Fig. 1**). A major benefit of TORS includes improved surgical access, allowing more complete surgical resection of tongue base tissue, which could not otherwise be addressed by traditional surgical methods.

The UAS procedure effectively works at multiple levels of obstructions simultaneously, as targeted nerve stimulation advances the base of tongue to open the retrolingual airway while simultaneously opening the retropalatal space by palatoglossal coupling[10] (**Fig. 2**). UAS is logically an excellent option for patients with tongue base obstruction primarily due to muscular hypertrophy rather than lymphoid tissue hypertrophy. In contrast to static soft tissue and skeletal framework surgery, UAS

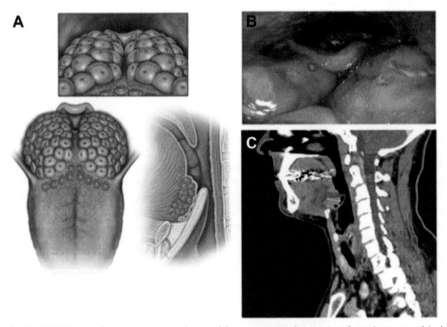

Fig. 1. TORS base of tongue surgery best addresses static obstruction from hypertrophied lingual tonsils. (*A*) Schematic, (*B*) endoscopic, and (*C*) sagittal CT views showing obstruction of the retrolingual space, size 4 lingual tonsils. CT, computed tomography. (*From* Friedman M, Yalamanchali S, Gorelick G, Joseph NJ, Hwang MS. A standardized lingual tonsil grading system: interexaminer agreement. Otolaryngology–head and neck surgery: official journal of American Academy of Otolaryngology-Head and Neck Surgery. 2015;152(4):667-672.)

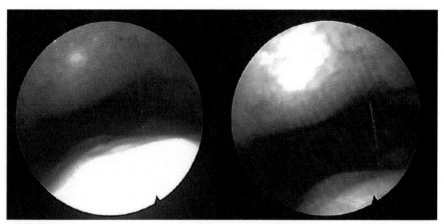

Fig. 2. UAS addresses airway collapse via dynamic airway dilation in phase with respiration. Endoscopic view of hypoglossal nerve stimulation; the base of tongue and palate move together in coordination as a result of palatoglossal coupling.

uniquely addresses the common contributing pathology of low neuromuscular tone by way of dynamic airway dilation during respiration. In its early implementation, highly favorable outcomes in carefully selected patient populations have contributed to the rise of UAS in the current era of sleep medicine.

ASSESSMENT/EVALUATION
Transoral Robotic Surgery

In 2014, TORS was approved for removal of benign base of tongue tissue, rather than specifically for the diagnosis of OSA.[11] Surgical candidates should have significant lymphoid hypertrophy (Friedman lingual tonsil size 3–4), as well as Apnea Hypopnea Index (AHI) less than 60, body mass index (BMI) less than 30, and no evidence of lateral velopharyngeal collapse on drug-induced sleep endoscopy (DISE).[9,11,12] Patients with predominantly muscular tongue hypertrophy should be excluded, as anticipated benefit of muscular resection is low and carries high morbidity. To this point, muscular tongue dissection should be kept to a minimum to prevent dysphagia and foreign body sensation. Swallowing function must be normal and should be routinely assessed preoperatively using a validated questionnaire (eg, MD Anderson Dysphagia Inventory) or formal swallowing evaluation (clinical swallow evaluation or formal swallow study).[13] Feasibility of robotic access must be considered, further excluding patients with retrognathia, or interincisor distance less than 2.5 cm. Patients cannot be on anticoagulation and should have an ASA less than 3.

The surgeon must determine whether lingual tonsil hypertrophy is the entire cause of obstruction or whether there is multilevel collapse of the airway. Thus, patients being considered for TORS should have preoperative DISE. If multilevel obstruction is determined, the surgeon can elect to perform single stage surgery including palate, palatine tonsils, and lingual tonsils. The option to stage the procedure with an interval polysomnogram is also reasonable, with the disadvantage of subjecting the patient to multiple procedures with attendant risk.

To better assess candidacy in patients with OSA, Lin and colleagues[12] developed a scoring system to predict surgical response based on combined measures of BMI, AHI, and DISE findings (**Table 1**). Several measures of success have been reported;

Table 1
Algorithm for transoral robotic surgery candidacy proposed by Lin and colleagues

Clinical	Stratif.	Score
BMI	<30	0
	>30 but <40	1
	>40	2
AHI	<60	0
	>60	1
Lat. VP Collapse	No	0
	Yes	1

Combined Assigned Score		Surgical Response Rate
0		86.7% (13/15)
1		71.4% (5/7)
2		25% (2/8)
3		16.7% (1/6)
4		0.0% (0/3)

Scoring system includes combined measures of BMI, AHI, and DISE pattern of collapse. Surgical response rates highly depend on preoperative score.

Data from Lin HS, Rowley JA, Folbe AJ, Yoo GH, Badr MS, Chen W. Transoral robotic surgery for treatment of obstructive sleep apnea: factors predicting surgical response. *The Laryngoscope.* 2015;125(4):1013-1020.

here, surgical response was defined by greater than 50% reduction in AHI and final AHI less than 15 (mild OSA) with resolution of daytime somnolence (symptomatic improvement).[12,14]

Upper Airway Stimulation

The *Inspire* device was FDA approved in 2014 and is currently the only FDA-approved UAS device available for treatment of OSA. Hypoglossal nerve stimulation is currently approved for adults (age >18 years) with BMI less than 35 and moderate to severe OSA (AHI 15–65, <25% central/mixed apneas)[8] (**Table 2**). Patients must have failed

Table 2
Candidacy criteria for upper airway stimulation

Age	>18
Body mass index	≤35
Polysomnography	AHI 15–65 events per hour <25% central or mixed apneas
DISE	Excludes pattern of concentric collapse at the palate
Contraindications	• Anticipated need for MRI[a] • Some neurologic or psychiatric conditions • Pregnancy

[a] New *Inspire* model is compatible with head and extremity MRI under most conditions.

conservative treatment including CPAP. Patients meeting these criteria and pursuing UAS treatment must have a recent polysomnogram and must undergo DISE to determine the pattern (anteroposterior, lateral, concentric), level (velum, oropharynx, tongue base, epiglottis), and severity of airway collapse.[15] UAS will best address anteroposterior collapse at the tongue base (retroglossal space) and velum (retropalatal space). A pattern of complete circumferential collapse (CCC) is a contraindication to UAS, as patients with this pattern of obstruction on DISE are felt to be poor surgical candidates[16] (**Fig. 3**). Potential candidates for surgery should be evaluated by both the surgeon and sleep medicine physician before undergoing hypoglossal nerve stimulator implantation. Although currently only approved for adults, UAS has been performed in children with hypotonia related to trisomy 21 on a clinical trial basis with encouraging results.[17,18]

SURGICAL TECHNIQUE AND POSTOPERATIVE CARE
Transoral Robotic Surgery

The DaVinci Si robot is the standard platform for the procedure (Xi and SP models are not required). To prepare for robotic access, patients are intubated transnasally, the bed is rotated 180°, and plastic eye shields are placed. The tongue is retracted with a stitch to better expose the lingual tonsils. A tonsil mouth gag with a short tongue blade and integrated suction is used to expose the lingual tonsils. The robot cart is brought into the field and docked. The robotic instruments include a 30-degree camera, monopolar cautery, and Maryland grasper, typically arranged in a tripod configuration (**Fig. 4**). The bedside assistant aids with suction cautery, surgical clips as needed for hemostasis, and retraction.

The lingual tonsil resection is performed sequentially from right to left, and resections of the right and left tonsils are performed separately (**Fig. 5**). Care is taken not to enter the muscular tongue, which avoids postoperative pain, risk to the dorsal branch of the lingual artery, as well as persistent dysphagia and globus sensation. Care should be taken not to demucosalize the lingual surface of epiglottis, and resection of the upper third of epiglottis should be avoided unless there is clear evidence of collapse at this level. If single-stage surgery is performed, it is imperative to leave a bridge of mucosa in the glossotonsillar sulcus between the lingual and palatine

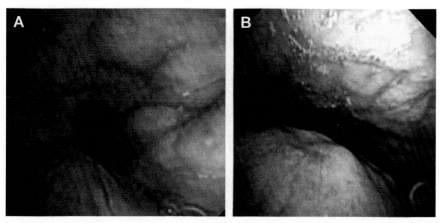

Fig. 3. DISE examination showing (*A*) complete circumferential collapse versus (*B*) anteroposterior collapse at the velum.

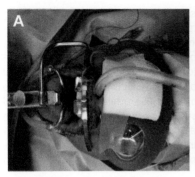
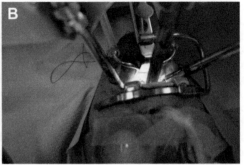

Fig. 4. TORS surgical set up showing (*A*) positioning with mouth gag in place, nasal intubation, and eye shields. (*B*) Robotic arms in tripod configuration including the Maryland retractor and monopolar spatula tip cautery (lateral placement), as well as 30-degree endoscope placed centrally.

tonsillectomy sites in order to prevent circumferential scarring. The volume of resected tissue should be measured and sent to pathology. Measured volume of lymphoid tissue should be greater than 7 to 10 cc; resected volume between 10 and 20 cc has been correlated with improved outcomes as measured by decrease in AHI.[19]

Hypoglossal nerve stimulator

The anatomy and physiology of the hypoglossal nerve allows easy surgical access in the submandibular triangle. Integral to the UAS procedure, the distal branching pattern of the nerve can be leveraged to preferentially stimulate the muscles that protrude and stiffen the tongue. Lateral branches of the hypoglossal nerve innervate the styloglossus and hyoglossus muscles, whereas more medial branches innervate the genioglossus muscle, the geniohyoid muscle (C1 contribution), and intrinsic tongue muscles of the tongue (**Fig. 6**).

The current *Inspire* device has 3 components: a stimulation lead, an implantable pulse generator (IPG), and a breath sensing lead (**Fig. 7**). The stimulating electrode sits around the hypoglossal nerve to deliver mild electrical stimulation in phase with inspiration to maintain multilevel airway patency. The IPG sits in a subcutaneous

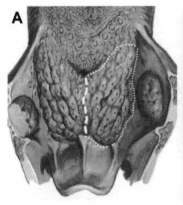
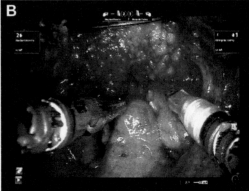

Fig. 5. (*A*) Ideal resection of lingual tonsil tissue (right lingual tonsil outlined) and (*B*) intraoperative view. Resection of the right and left lingual tonsils are performed separately.

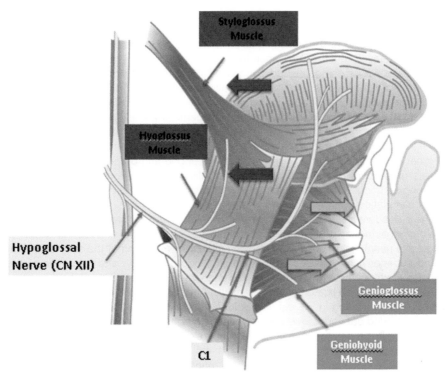

Fig. 6. Distal branching pattern of the hypoglossal nerve. Retractors of the tongue include the styloglossus and hyoglossus. Protrusion muscles of the tongue include the genioglossus and geniohyoid (C1 contribution). The intrinsic muscles of the tongue stiffen the tongue.

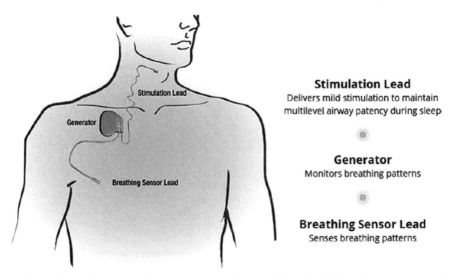

Fig. 7. Inspire UAS device with 3 components: (1) stimulation lead, (2) pulse generator, and (3) breath sensing lead.

pocket overlying the pectoralis fascia and generates the impulses based on input from the sensing lead. The breath sensing lead is placed between the external and internal intercostal muscles at the fourth to sixth rib space and senses breathing patterns, which are relayed to the pulse generator.

For surgical positioning, the bed is turned 180° and a bump is placed under the right chest to allow better access to the chest wall for the breath sensing lead placement. A bite block or other oral retractor is placed to allow placement of the neuromonitoring electrodes: an exclusion lead is placed in the superficial lateral tongue to monitor stimulation of the hyoglossus and styloglossus, and an inclusion lead is placed in the anterior floor of mouth lateral to the frenulum to monitor stimulation of the genioglossus and geniohyoid muscles. The patient is then prepped and draped, including a clear plastic drape over the face to maintain a sterile field while allowing visualization of the tongue. Long-acting paralytics are avoided due to need for neuromonitoring and nerve stimulation during the case.

The procedure includes 3 surgical sites. The first incision is placed 1 to 2 cm below the border of the mandible to the right of midline: dissection to expose the distal hypoglossal nerve includes raising subplatysmal flaps, retraction of the submandibular gland superiorly, retraction of the digastric tendon inferiorly, and retraction of the mylohyoid anteriorly. A ranine vein is often encountered in the vicinity of the hypoglossal nerve and can be ligated or, preferentially, freed and retracted using blunt dissection to avoid bleeding in the surgical field. Meticulous dissection of the hypoglossal nerve is carried out under loupe or microscope magnification, and the nerve is stimulated along its course to identify inclusion and exclusion branches (**Fig. 8**). The stimulation electrode cuff is placed around a 1 cm segment of the hypoglossal nerve, which ideally excludes proximal branches innervating the retractors of the tongue and includes the C1 contribution branch and distal hypoglossal branches that

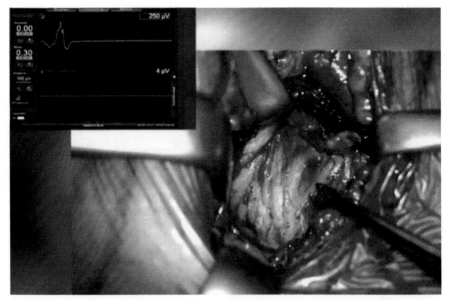

Fig. 8. Intraoperative stimulation of the hypoglossal nerve to determine location of the functional breakpoint. Inset: NIMS monitor output showing inclusion versus exclusion branches.

innervate protrusion and stiffening muscles of the tongue. This location is referred to as the functional breakpoint.

The second incision is made several centimeters below the clavicle centered on the midclavicular line. A subcutaneous pocket superficial to the pectoralis fascia is bluntly dissected to create a pocket for the pulse generator.

The final incision is made at the fourth to sixth rib space, 5 cm lateral to the nipple line. The serratus muscles are retracted to expose the external intercostal muscles, and a window is made in the external intercostal muscles to create a pocket between the internal and external intercostal muscles for placement of the breath sensing lead along a malleable retractor. It is critical that the breath sensing lead be placed in the correct layer and with the correct orientation with the sensing side facing the pleura. Wires from the breath sensing lead and the stimulation lead are then tunneled in a subcutaneous plane to the chest pocket and are connected to the IPG, which is then secured with suture to the pectoralis fascia. Finally, breath sensing and stimulation of the tongue are tested before closing the incisions. A successful test will show gross excursion of the tongue favoring protrusion.

DISCUSSION
Clinical Outcomes

Comparisons of both TORS and UAS with conventional surgery (eg, uvulopalatopharyngoplasty, UPPP) have been made, with each showing benefits over traditional surgical approaches.[11,20] The usage of TORS for management of OSA began with a pilot study by Vicini and colleagues[21] evaluating the utility and feasibility of robotic management of tongue base hypertrophy. Following this innovation, several studies have evaluated and demonstrated the efficacy of TORS tongue base reduction, with a meta-analysis demonstrating impressive success (68%) and cure rates (24%) for patients.[22] Prospective comparison studies to previously established techniques such as radiofrequency tongue base reduction and/or palatoplasty procedures demonstrate potential for improvement in clinical outcomes in those who undergo TORS.[23] In terms of newer technology, TORS is most readily comparable to coblation lingual tonsillectomy, where outcomes are roughly equivalent, and the anticipated TORS benefits including more complete and easier removal for large lingual tonsils are tempered by higher cost, longer hospital stay, and higher morbidity than coblation.[24]

There exists great clinical promise for UAS as well. A landmark study from the Stimulation Therapy for Apnea Reduction (STAR) trial group was published in 2014 evaluating the safety and efficacy of UAS at 12 months. In the original study of 126 patients meeting selection criteria (AHI 15–65, BMI <32, failed CPAP, DISE without CCC), significant improvements were seen in all primary (AHI and oxygen desaturation index [ODI]) and secondary (Epworth sleepiness scale [ESS], functional outcomes of sleep questionnaire [FOSQ], and percentage of sleep with O2 saturation <90%) outcomes.[8] Two-thirds of patients had a successful response, defined as 50% reduction in AHI and AHI score less than 20. Further, responders of this study were randomized to treatment continuation and treatment withdrawal groups, showing significant worsening of AHI and ODI when therapy was withdrawn at 12 months. A 5-year follow-up study was recently published showing that outcomes including AHI, ODI, ESS, FOSQ, and patient-reported snoring, all showed durable responses at 60 months following implantation.[25]

Similar efficacy was demonstrated by early reports from the Adherence and Outcomes of Upper Airway Stimulation for OSA (ADHERE) International Registry, which was designed to study UAS outcomes as the procedure transitioned from trail to clinical practice.[26] The ADHERE registry collects data including demographics, surgical outcomes, complications, quality of life, and other patient-reported outcomes for patients undergoing treatment in the United States and Europe and will prove a powerful tool to study outcomes. Recent results of a cohort of 508 patients from the AHDERE registry notably show significant reductions in AHI (36.3 baseline to 10.2 posttitration, events per hour) and ESS (11.8 baseline to 7.7 posttitration) following implantation, as well as uniformly high percentages of patient satisfaction (94%–96%). Steffen and colleagues[27] observed similarly excellent outcomes for AHI reduction, ESS improvement, and FOSQ improvement in a postmarket study of 60 patients where a BMI cutoff of less than 35 was used.[28] A study by Hofsauer and colleagues also found that in addition to the improved metrics discussed earlier, UAS had significant effects on sleep architecture, with PSG REM time increasing from 9.5% pretreatment to 15.7% posttreatment.

Predictors of success based on AHDERE data included increased age (OR 1.04 for each additional year) and lower BMI (OR 0.91 for each 1 unit BMI increase).[26] Among the STAR trial population, UAS responders had lower VOTE scores on DISE than did UAS nonresponders.[29] Prior studies have shown CCC at the velum to predict poor response to UAS and thus use of this finding as a contraindication to surgery.[16] With regard to other multilevel surgery, UAS has shown higher cure rates (AHI <5) compared with traditional UPPP in patients with moderate to severe OSA intolerant of CPAP.[20] Further, having prior soft tissue or skeletal framework surgery has not been shown to negatively impact UAS outcomes.[26]

These favorable outcomes have prompted consideration of UAS as an alternative to TORS base of tongue reduction.[23,30] As TORS has been used for treatment of OSA since 2009, and UAS was approved for treatment of OSA in 2014, the 2 modalities constitute separate but overlapping eras of treatment. Retrospective cohort comparisons of TORS to UAS have shown consistently superior reduction in AHI and cure rates with UAS when groups are matched to include only the subset of patients who would be potential candidates for both procedures.[30] As we move toward an era of precision medicine and surgery, although, candidacy criteria become increasingly important; when TORS cohorts are evaluated retrospectively for UAS candidacy by the current criteria, dual candidacy has been observed in as low as just 20% of patients.[30] Thus, there is still clearly a role for TORS in a large proportion of patients with tongue base hypertrophy who do not qualify for UAS. When considering a treatment algorithm that includes DISE-directed therapy, this direct comparison of TORS with UAS is a potential area of future study, particularly in the likely event that UAS inclusion criteria broaden.

Serious adverse events following UAS are reported around 2%, most commonly device discomfort requiring surgical revision.[8,26] More commonly, transient changes to tongue sensation, temporary weakness, minor discomfort related to the implanted device, and discomfort during the initial titration period are noted (up to 40% of patients).[7,8] This adverse event profile is distinct from that of TORS, which has longer hospital stay, higher readmission rates, and higher bleeding rates compared with UAS.[11,23]

Considerations/Future Directions

Studies of UAS since FDA approval have reported treatment success rates upward of 80%. Under the current paradigm, criteria for candidacy continue to be highly selective. In light of this, it is unclear why some patients continue to fail treatment, and further studies to determine predictors of treatment success and failure are warranted. This rise of UAS will allow optimization patient outcomes as surgical volume increases and long-term follow up data become available. Treatment effect on medical comorbidities, including cardiovascular outcomes and mortality, will be additional critical areas of future study.

As existing UAS devices continue to evolve and new devices enter the market, the field will likely benefit from increased access, lower cost, and liberalized criteria for candidacy. There are opportunities to improve and optimize multidisciplinary care, training during and after residency, and delivery of care in various practice settings.

SUMMARY

OSA remains a challenging disease process to treat. Given the complexity and unique anatomic profile of each individual patient, the addition of the HGNS to the sleep surgeon's armamentarium has had promising early results. This period is the golden age of sleep surgery, where medical management with CPAP is complemented by cutting edge surgical technology including UAS and TORS to provide sleep physicians with the personalized options that this complex patient population demands.

CLINICS CARE POINTS

1. Candidacy criteria for TORS multilevel surgery include AHI less than 60, BMI less than 30, and DISE finding showing no evidence of lateral velopharyngeal collapse.
2. Candidacy criteria for UAS are selective and include adults (age >18 years) with BMI less than 35, moderate to severe OSA (AHI 15–65), and DISE examination demonstrating absence of complete circumferential collapse.
3. In patients qualifying for both UAS and TORS, studies have shown superior outcomes and lower morbidity in those undergoing UAS.
4. UAS with the HGNS is predominantly being performed in high-volume centers in conjunction with device technicians and sleep medicine physicians to allow for optimal postimplant titration and calibration.

DISCLOSURE

The authors have nothing to disclose.

REFERENCES

1. Gami AS, Pressman G, Caples SM, et al. Association of atrial fibrillation and obstructive sleep apnea. Circulation 2004;110(4):364–7.
2. Wright J, Johns R, Watt I, et al. Health effects of obstructive sleep apnoea and the effectiveness of continuous positive airways pressure: a systematic review of the research evidence. BMJ 1997;314(7084):851–60.
3. McEvoy RD, Antic NA, Heeley E, et al. CPAP for prevention of cardiovascular events in obstructive sleep apnea. N Engl J Med 2016;375(10):919–31.
4. Sawyer AM, Gooneratne NS, Marcus CL, et al. A systematic review of CPAP adherence across age groups: clinical and empiric insights for developing CPAP adherence interventions. Sleep Med Rev 2011;15(6):343–56.
5. Remmers JE, deGroot WJ, Sauerland EK, et al. Pathogenesis of upper airway occlusion during sleep. J Appl Physiol Respir Environ Exerc Physiol 1978;44(6):931–8.
6. Vicini C, Montevecchi F, Campanini A, et al. Clinical outcomes and complications associated with TORS for OSAHS: a benchmark for evaluating an emerging surgical technology in a targeted application for benign disease. ORL J Otorhinolaryngol Relat Spec 2014;76(2):63–9.

7. Yu JL, Thaler ER. Hypoglossal Nerve (Cranial Nerve XII) Stimulation. Otolaryngol Clin North Am 2020;53(1):157–69.
8. Strollo PJ Jr, Soose RJ, Maurer JT, et al. Upper-airway stimulation for obstructive sleep apnea. N Engl J Med 2014;370(2):139–49.
9. Friedman M, Yalamanchali S, Gorelick G, et al. A standardized lingual tonsil grading system: interexaminer agreement. Otolaryngol Head Neck Surg 2015; 152(4):667–72.
10. Heiser C, Edenharter G, Bas M, et al. Palatoglossus coupling in selective upper airway stimulation. Laryngoscope 2017;127(10):E378–83.
11. Hoff PT, D'Agostino MA, Thaler ER. Transoral robotic surgery in benign diseases including obstructive sleep apnea: Safety and feasibility. Laryngoscope 2015; 125(5):1249–53.
12. Lin HS, Rowley JA, Folbe AJ, et al. Transoral robotic surgery for treatment of obstructive sleep apnea: factors predicting surgical response. Laryngoscope 2015;125(4):1013–20.
13. Paker M, Duek I, Awwad F, et al. Long-term swallowing performance following transoral robotic surgery for obstructive sleep apnea. Laryngoscope 2019; 129(2):422–8.
14. Sher AE, Schechtman KB, Piccirillo JF. The efficacy of surgical modifications of the upper airway in adults with obstructive sleep apnea syndrome. Sleep 1996; 19(2):156–77.
15. Vroegop AV, Vanderveken OM, Verbraecken JA. Drug-induced sleep endoscopy: evaluation of a selection tool for treatment modalities for obstructive sleep apnea. Respiration 2020;99(5):451–7.
16. Vanderveken OM, Maurer JT, Hohenhorst W, et al. Evaluation of drug-induced sleep endoscopy as a patient selection tool for implanted upper airway stimulation for obstructive sleep apnea. J Clin Sleep Med 2013;9(5):433–8.
17. Diercks GR, Wentland C, Keamy D, et al. Hypoglossal Nerve Stimulation in Adolescents With Down Syndrome and Obstructive Sleep Apnea. JAMA Otolaryngol Head Neck Surg 2018;144(1):37–42.
18. Caloway CL, Diercks GR, Keamy D, et al. Update on hypoglossal nerve stimulation in children with down syndrome and obstructive sleep apnea. Laryngoscope 2019;130(4):E263–7.
19. Eesa M, Montevecchi F, Hendawy E, et al. Swallowing outcome after TORS for sleep apnea: short- and long-term evaluation. Eur Arch Otorhinolaryngol 2015; 272(6):1537–41.
20. Shah J, Russell JO, Waters T, et al. Uvulopalatopharyngoplasty vs CN XII stimulation for treatment of obstructive sleep apnea: A single institution experience. Am J Otolaryngol 2018;39(3):266–70.
21. Vicini C, Dallan I, Canzi P, et al. Transoral robotic tongue base resection in obstructive sleep apnoea-hypopnoea syndrome: a preliminary report. ORL J Otorhinolaryngol Relat Spec 2010;72(1):22–7.
22. Miller SC, Nguyen SA, Ong AA, et al. Transoral robotic base of tongue reduction for obstructive sleep apnea: A systematic review and meta-analysis. Laryngoscope 2017;127(1):258–65.
23. Huntley C, Topf MC, Christopher V, et al. Comparing upper airway stimulation to transoral robotic base of tongue resection for treatment of obstructive sleep apnea. Laryngoscope 2019;129(4):1010–3.
24. Li HY, Lee LA, Kezirian EJ. Efficacy of coblation endoscopic lingual lightning in multilevel surgery for obstructive sleep apnea. JAMA Otolaryngol Head Neck Surg 2016;142(5):438–43.

25. Woodson BT, Strohl KP, Soose RJ, et al. Upper airway stimulation for obstructive sleep apnea: 5-year outcomes. Otolaryngol Head Neck Surg 2018;159(1): 194–202.
26. Heiser C, Steffen A, Boon M, et al. Post-approval upper airway stimulation predictors of treatment effectiveness in the ADHERE registry. Eur Respir J 2019;53(1): 1801405.
27. Steffen A, Sommer JU, Hofauer B, et al. Outcome after one year of upper airway stimulation for obstructive sleep apnea in a multicenter German post-market study. Laryngoscope 2018;128(2):509–15.
28. Huntley C, Steffen A, Doghramji K, et al. Upper airway stimulation in patients with obstructive sleep apnea and an elevated body mass index: a multi-institutional review. Laryngoscope 2018;128(10):2425–8.
29. Ong AA, Murphey AW, Nguyen SA, et al. Efficacy of upper airway stimulation on collapse patterns observed during drug-induced sedation endoscopy. Otolaryngol Head Neck Surg 2016;154(5):970–7.
30. Yu JL, Mahmoud A, Thaler ER. Transoral robotic surgery versus upper airway stimulation in select obstructive sleep apnea patients. Laryngoscope 2019; 129(1):256–8.

Robotic Thyroidectomy
Past, Future, and Current Perspectives

Emad Kandil, MD, MBA*, Abdallah S. Attia, MD,
Deena Hadedeya, MD, MHS, Areej Shihabi, MD, Ahmad Elnahla, MD

KEYWORDS

- Robotic thyroidectomy • Transaxillary • Transoral • Retroauricular • Facelift

KEY POINTS

- Remote access approaches (RAA) use the axillary approach, the axillary-bilateral breast approach, the bilateral axilla-breast approach, the retroauricular approach, and the transoral approach.
- The installation of the robotic system in surgery overcomes many limitations of the RAA.
- Benefits and the constraints of remote access approaches.

INTRODUCTION

Through the past decades, there was an immense revolution in the surgical approaches for thyroidectomy. In 1997, since Huscher[1] did the first minimally invasive thyroidectomy, this technique and remote access approach (RAA) have gained notoriety. After a year, Paolo Miccoli and colleagues[2] started the minimally invasive video-assisted thyroidectomy in 1998. However, many studies proved its feasibility and safety. It is still questionable whether it can replace the conventional open approach or not.

Remote access approaches (RAA) use the axillary approach, the anterior/breast approach, the axillary-bilateral breast approach, the bilateral axilla-breast approach, the retroauricular approach, and the transoral approach.[3] The introduction of the robotic system in surgery overcomes many limitations of the RAA. Lobe and colleagues[4] performed the first robotic thyroidectomy via a trans-axillary approach in 2005. Since that time, many surgeons have reported their experience with RAA for thyroid surgery. Chung and colleagues[5] published his experience with more than 5000 cases with a comparable rate of complications with the open conventional approach. Others and we reported the most substantial experience in the United States with the transaxillary approach.[6] Duke and colleagues[7] published the first most prominent data on consecutive patients undergoing robotic facelift thyroidectomy (RFT) in 5 North American

Department of Surgery, Tulane University, School of Medicine, New Orleans, LA 70112, USA
* Corresponding author.
E-mail address: ekandil@tulane.edu

academic endocrine surgical practices that were compiled. The study showed that RFT could be offered to selected patients to avoid neck scare. This review details surgical approaches for robotic thyroidectomy: transaxillary, retro auricular, and transoral. In this article, we explain the benefits and the constraints of each approach and future directions of robotic thyroidectomy.

PATIENT SELECTION

Although there are various types of robotic thyroidectomy by far, transaxillary is the most commonly used approach. Moreover, the transoral approach is the most novel described approach. Surgeons must be aware of their skills and should have performed a high-volume of surgery before deciding on which method to use and put into consideration the patient's decision. The American Thyroid Association reported that remote access thyroidectomy might only be performed safely in high-volume centers. They have also highlighted and established strict guidelines for the patient's selection.[8] The indications for thyroidectomy should be the same as for standard surgery. Surgeons should review the following circumstances for patient selection. Factors relating to the patient that should ideally be considered in early experience include (1) lean body habitus (except for the facelift approach) and (2) the absence of excess body fat along the flap trajectory (except for the facelift approach). Factors relating to the thyroid pathology include (1) well-circumscribed nodule less than or equal to 3 cm 2) thyroid lobe less than 7 cm in the largest dimension and 3) underlying thyroid pathology with no evidence of thyroiditis on ultrasound. Factors relating to specific approaches include the fact that the distance between the axilla and the sternal notch should ideally be less than 15 to 17 cm for an axillary approach. Absolute contraindications include: 1) evidence of thyroid cancer with extrathyroidal extension or lymph node involvement; 2) Graves disease; 3) substernal extension; and 4) previous neck surgery; 5) evidence of preoperative recurrent laryngeal nerve palsy.[8,9]

SURGICAL TECHNIQUES

Both the transaxillary and retroauricular approaches are performed in a gasless fashion, whereas the transoral technique requires carbon dioxide (CO_2) gas insufflation. However, Young Min and colleagues[10] reported cases of successful gasless transoral approach and proved its safety and feasibility. Many recommend using intraoperative nerve monitoring (IONM) for robotic thyroidectomy cases.[11] The surgical techniques of these 3 approaches using the da Vinci robots are described later. Despite the chosen approach, there are 3 consistent steps to robotic thyroidectomy: (1) working space creation, (2) docking, and (3) console stages.

THE TRANSAXILLARY APPROACH
Working Space Formation

After general anesthesia is administered, the patient is in the supine position with a slight extension of the neck.[12–14] Neck extension is accomplished by using a large shoulder roll to provide appropriate field exposure.[13] The ipsilateral arm is then stretched and twisted cephalad, fully showing the axilla. It is vital to assess the extent of the patient's arm extension/abduction without implementing additional force to prevent avoidable overextension of the arm, which can lead to accidental brachial plexus injury. Intraoperative nerve monitoring via somatosensory evoked potential (SSEP) has been used to avoid the injury. Ulnar, median, and radial nerves of the arm ipsilateral to the surgical incision were individually stimulated at each nerve's respective location on the wrist. The contralateral arm positioned at the patient's side was stimulated at the median nerve as a positive control. The monitoring of SSEP was initiated preoperatively, recorded during patient positioning, and continued intraoperatively. A warning was relayed to the surgeon if IONM detected an amplitude decrease of greater than or equal to 50% and/or a greater than or equal to 10% increase in signal latency.[15] A 5- to 6-cm curved vertical line is formed just posterior to the anterior axillary fold. This arm is padded and secured, applying a tape. Once the ideal position is reached, the patient's arm, neck, and chest are prepped and draped, exposing the axilla, neck, and upper chest. The incision is created using a 15 blade, and the subcutaneous flap is raised using electrocautery. It is essential to maintain the fascia overlying the pectoralis major muscle to limit postoperative adhesions, which may lead to increased discomfort and pain over the chest area. Once the pectoralis major is exhibited, a careful dissection over the clavicle is performed until the sternocleidomastoid (SCM) muscle is revealed. It is vital to preserving the posterior triangle soft tissue structures to possible avoidable injury to the external jugular vein and an increased risk of postoperative hematoma. Once the SCM is exposed, the dissection proceeds by opening the avascular plane between the clavicular and sternal heads of the SCM. The surgeons must enter this avascular space correctly to avoid possible injury to the major vessels that are lying directly below the route of dissection. Strap muscles are then found. The dissection is then carefully proceeded directly underneath the strap muscles exposing the thyroid gland. The working space is considered to be safe and adequate if sufficient space is created, showing the superior pole of the thyroid and central neck. Once the dissection is completed, Chung retractor or an equivalent retractor is placed holding the subcutaneous flap, anterior SCM, and strap muscles upward to keep the working space exposed. In the case of total thyroidectomy, the contralateral lobe should be completely exposed, and the position of the retractor should be appropriately adjusted to allow safe resection of the contralateral lobe.

Docking Stage

Once the surgeon reaches adequate working space, the robot approaches toward the patient from the opposite side in preparation for the docking of the arms. For the transaxillary procedure, all 4 robotic arms are used. For the right-sided approach, the arm closest to the head of the patient provides the Maryland dissector, followed by the second arm carrying the 30-degree endoscope. On the arm beside the endoscope arm, the ProGrasp forceps is implanted. The arm closest to the patient's feet leads the Harmonic scalpel. The order is shifted when the procedure is approached via the left side. This docking method guarantees that the surgeon operates using the Harmonic scalpel using his right hand, likewise to the open procedures. The Maryland and ProGrasp forceps provide continuous countertraction for safe and precise dissection, following the same surgical concepts used in conventional open surgeries. It is crucial to keep an adequate distance between each robotic arm to avoid clashing between the instruments. The docking stage massively depends on the skills and expertise of the surgeon and his operative team. Even a small variation in the docking position can affect the effectiveness of the console stage, and this statement holds regardless of the robotic thyroidectomy approach.

Console Stage

Once the perfect docking of the robotic arms is accomplished, the surgeon may advance to the console stage. The superior pole is first dissected by determining the superior vessels. This first step is crucial to recognize the superior parathyroid gland and safely make sure to keep it. Once the superior pole is freed, then the attention is directed to the inferior pole. If the central neck dissection (CND) is required, then this is made en bloc before the inferior pole dissection. The recurrent laryngeal nerve (RLN) should be identified inferiorly and dissected superiorly toward Berry's ligament while dissecting the thyroid gland off of the neighboring structures. The isthmus is then divided, which concludes the hemithyroidectomy. The entire CND content and thyroid gland are taken out en bloc. Once the specimen is detached, careful examination of the surgical field is conducted for verifying of hemostasis.

THE RETROAURICULAR APPROACH
Working Space Creation

The patient is placed supine after intubation with general anesthesia with the head turned smoothly to the contralateral side from the approach, showing the posterior auricular sulcus with the posterior area of the neck facing the surgeon. The incision is drawn along the posterior auricular sulcus reaching over the mastoid and inferiorly parallel to the occipital hairline. The patient is prepped and draped, showing the incision line, neck, and the ipsilateral half of the face. Once the cut is made, the subcutaneous retroauricular flap is lifted anteriorly, exposing the parotid tail and the SCM. In our experience, we maintained the flap superficial to the platysma.[6] However, others maintained a subplatysmal flap.[15] Deep dissection beneath the strap muscles is made to identify the thyroid gland. A modified Chung retractor is inserted underneath the strap muscles.

Docking Stage

Once an adequate working space is secured, the robotic system is docked. If the working area allows, it is always preferable to use all 3 robotic divisions (30-degree endoscope with 3 instrument arms) to facilitate the surgery. If the working space is inadequate, the surgeon can still perform the surgery using only 2 instrument arms without the ProGrasp. Operating with 2 instrument arms rather than 3 is technically more challenging. The docking method is similar to the transaxillary approach, where the surgeon's hand controls the Maryland dissector and the right-hand controls the Harmonic scalpel.

Console Stage

The steps of the hemithyroidectomy via the retro auricular approach start with the identification and dissection of the superior pole. The superior pole is smoothly retracted superiorly, and the superior pole vessels are carefully ligated one vessel at a time. During these steps, the surgeon must distinguish the superior parathyroid gland and preserve it. Accurate and gentle dissection is advised to minimize the chance of thermic damage to the parathyroid gland. Once the superior pole is liberated, and the cricothyroid muscle is recognized, the isthmusectomy is then performed, which will assist in the recognition and dissection of the RLN. The nerve is distinguished in the tracheoesophageal groove near the cricothyroid joint, where the nerve accesses the larynx. The IONM probe can be used to confirm the RLN. Once the nerve is correctly recognized and verified via IONM, the rest of the thyroid gland is dissected off of its adjacent soft tissue while keeping the RLN uninjured along its course. With the dissection of the inferior pole, the operation is achieved.

THE TRANSORAL APPROACH
Working Space Creation

After the patient received general anesthesia, the patient's neck should be placed in a slight extension. Three incisions are performed in the gingival-buccal sulcus: one in the midline, about 2 cm up the frenulum labii inferioris and 2 laterally close to the angle of the mouth. The midline incision is marked first. A submental subplatysmal opening is formed to create a tunnel toward the edge of the mandible. Blunt dissection is conducted to raise the platysma of the strap muscles all the way down toward the suprasternal notch. This blunt dissection is aided via injections of saline mixed with epinephrine into the subplatysmal layer. Once a sufficient flap is formed, the endoscope (30 degrees, down-facing) cannula is implanted. CO_2 insufflation (8–10 L/min) is initiated and maintained via the central port. Alike blunt dissection is also made from the 2 lateral incision sites, allowing the introduction of the instrument cannulae into the subplatysmal working area. Vicryl stitches are then applied to help retain the subplatysmal flap superiorly to form a larger working area.

Docking Stage

Once the working space creation is complete, the robotic system is stationed. The cannulae are implanted into the robotic arms, beginning with the central cannula to ensure the position of the endoscope. A Harmonic scalpel and Maryland dissector are embedded into the right and left ports, respectively.

Console Stage

Dissection in the midline raphe is conducted to separate the strap muscles. The strap muscles are cut off the thyroid gland, revealing the lobe of importance. The pyramidal lobe is cut off the thyroid cartilage, followed by isthmusectomy is delivered. Once the thyroid lobe is released from the trachea medially, the superior pole is marked. Careful dissection of the superior lobe is made ligating one vessel at a time. The superior parathyroid gland is distinguished and protected. The thyroid lobe is retracted inferiorly to aid the identification of the RLN at its entry point into the larynx. Once the RLN is identified and carefully protected, Berry's ligament is identified. The dissection is then carried out, inferiorly protecting the inferior parathyroid gland. Once the inferior lobe is liberated off of its surrounding soft tissue, hemithyroidectomy is complete.

ADVANTAGES AND DISADVANTAGES

In this review, the authors discuss different types of remote access thyroidectomy; each of them has its advantages and disadvantages, given all the steps to perform those types of thyroidectomy. Knowing the benefits and limitations of each approach will help the surgeon make the best recommendations for each patient.

The transaxillary approach was invented primarily by doing 2 separate incisions, one in the axillary crease and the other on the anterior chest. Recently, just using one incision through the axillary crease, surgeons can perform thyroidectomy safely. The main advantages of the transaxillary approach are to ease the console stage, facilitate the detection of the recurrent laryngeal nerve, more access to do central and lateral neck dissection, and well-established literature showing its safety and feasibility. Not only that, but it is also the only approach that does not disrupt the area between the superficial neck muscles, which in turn aims for more favorable swallowing outcomes compared with other plans.[12,16–18] One of the main disadvantages of the transaxillary method is the possible risk of brachial plexus injury,[19–22] which can be avoided with proper arm positioning and extrapadded support. In our early experience, 137 robotic transaxillary surgeries using SSEP monitoring were performed on 123 patients. Seven patients (5.1%) developed significant changes, with an average SSEP amplitude reduction of 73% ± 12% recorded at the signals' nadir. Immediate arm repositioning resulted in the recovery of signals and complete return to baseline parameters in 14.3 ± 9.2 minutes.[23] Also, others reported no brachial plexus injury with a high-volume surgeon,[1] high volume hemorrhage, and damage to the esophagus are other reported complications however these events are rare and deceased when surgeons became used to the lateral approach.[6,24,25] But these complications are rare and deceased when the surgeons became used to the lateral approach. We routinely perform monitoring for the median and ulnar nerves using somatosensory evoked potentials (SSEP) (Biotronic, Ann Arbor, MI, USA) to avoid neuropraxia. However, many other robotic surgeons did not use SSEP and were able to prevent this severe complication by careful positioning of the arm. Patients could experience anterior chest paresthesia over the clavicular area with nonavoided injury to the sensory nerves of the cervical plexus chain. These nerves are encountered as the subplatysmal flap is elevated off the clavicle toward the SCM and needs to be sacrificed to create a safe working space. For most of the cases, this paresthesia is temporary, but it was reported as permanent in rare tiny cases. Therefore, this complication should be discussed with the patient while obtaining informed consent.[26]

Terris first described the advantage of a retroauricular approach over the transaxillary one,[19,27] contemplating that the significantly reduced field of dissection in the transaxillary method, when compared with the retroauricular approach, is associated with faster recovery and decreased postoperative distress.[27] He also describes the retroauricular technique to be more comfortable than the transaxillary method when working on obese patients.[27] This statement seems to be verified by the American Thyroid Association, as its last statement on robotic surgery states that remote-access surgery should be carried out in patients with normal body weight without extra body fat except for the retroauricular approach.[8] The retroauricular approach also reduced the risk of damage to the vessels, the esophagus, or the anterior chest nerves because these structures are hard to be dodged during the working space creation. Some disadvantages are integral to this approach: injury to greater auricular and marginal mandibular nerves.[24,25,27] These adverse events are usually temporary and fully resolve within a few months following surgery. But these possible adverse events should be discussed in detail for informed consent before surgery.

The transoral approach described by Kim and colleagues can cause a mental nerve injury as they come out from the mental foramina radiating its branches to the lip which has been by overcame by adjusting the sites of incisions.[28] This has since been overcome by adjusting the sites of incisions to avoid damage to the mental nerves as they come out from the mental foramina radiating its branches to the lip. This approach's main benefits are the completely unseen intraoral scars, excellent access, display of the bilateral thyroid lobes for total thyroidectomy, and a reported lower adverse events profile compared with other remote-access procedures. The transoral technique offers the unique superiority of reaching the thyroid gland from a natural opening, and its midline access provides excellent exposure to the whole thyroid gland, making this the most harmless approach to perform a total thyroidectomy when compared with other approaches.

The main limitations of this technique are the necessity for postoperative antibiotics and incapability to do lateral neck dissections. There were no reports of postoperative infections following transoral robotic thyroidectomy; however, postoperative antibiotics are supplied for all patients due to the possible risk of infection. The transoral thyroidectomy is not acknowledged as a clean procedure, unlike its traditional open equivalent. Recent studies on transoral approaches reported shorter hospital stay than bilateral axillo-breast approach robotic thyroidectomy.[29] Another potential downside of this approach is the incapability to control substantial hemorrhage through the intraoral incision in case of accidental great vessel injury. If such hemorrhage were to happen, then an anterior neck incision would be performed to control the bleeding. The most significant weakness of the transoral approach is the incapability to do lateral neck dissections. This challenge may never be overcome, given the anatomic limitations, and may indicate the usage of 2 approaches when performing neck dissections on patients with extended lateral neck disease. Lateral neck dissections are performed via remote-access approaches (RAA) frequently around the world, except the United States. In a study by Adam and colleagues[30] they reported there were no differences in hospital length of stay between robotic and conventional thyroidectomy groups even when the patient underwent neck dissection. Also, there was a nonsignificant trend toward a higher odds of positive surgical margins with robotic thyroidectomy. However, according to the American Thyroid Association statements, the presence of lateral neck disease is currently a contraindication to remote-access thyroid,[10] yet the transoral approach is vital for the surgeons to consider it while operating on obese patients, which is essential for the population of North America.[31]

All RAA shared one disadvantage, which is the high cost in comparison to the conventional transcervical approach. Cabot and colleagues[29] reported that the transaxillary robotic thyroidectomy approach was compared based on medical costs in the United States. A higher total cost for the transaxillary approaches was reported compared with the conventional technique ($13,087 vs $9028).[32] Broome and colleagues[33] mentioned the increase in cost as $3127 as higher than the conventional approach. Equivalence in cost for both procedures was noted, once the total operative time was decreased in the robotic approach to 111 minutes.[29] Although the cost is higher with RAA, it is of great value for patients who are motivated to avoid a visible neck scar. Multiple studies showed that cosmesis is a primary concern, especially for women; neck scars can cause disfigurement and significant stress, which would affect the patients psychologically and may impair their quality of life.[34–36]

SUMMARY

RAA is safe for a specific type of patient. It should be performed by experienced specialized surgeons in centers with high patients' volume. Yet, it did not completely replace the conventional approach, due to a high degree of training that is required before practice, high expenses that should be paid to perform a single operation, and the highly integrated teamwork that should be considered. Furthermore, studies and investigation should be considered regarding RAA, especially after proving its efficacy in reducing the risk of complications with an expert surgeon.

DISCLOSURE

The authors have nothing to disclose.

CLINICS CARE POINTS

- Offer remote access approach to eligible patients only.
- Remote access approach should be only performed by high-volume, well trained surgeons.
- Adequate training should be provided ahead of initiating their practice

REFERENCES

1. Hüscher CS, Chiodini S, Napolitano C, et al. Endoscopic right thyroid lobectomy. Surg Endosc 1997;11(8):877.
2. Miccoli P, Berti P, Conte M, et al. Minimally invasive surgery for thyroid small nodules: preliminary report. J Endocrinol Invest 1999;22(11):849–51.
3. Miccoli P, Bendinelli C, Vignali E, et al. Endoscopic parathyroidectomy: report of an initial experience. Surgery 1998;124(6):1077–80. https://doi.org/10.1067/msy. 1998.92006. Available at:.
4. Lobe TE, Wright SK, Irish MS. Novel uses of surgical robotics in head and neck surgery. J Laparoendosc Adv Surg Tech 2005;15(6):647–52.
5. Lee J, Chung WY. Robotic thyroidectomy and neck dissection: past, present, and future. Cancer J 2013;19(2):151–61.
6. Kandil EH, Noureldine SI, Yao L, et al. Robotic transaxillary thyroidectomy: an examination of the first one hundred cases. J Am Coll Surg 2012;214(4):556–8.
7. Duke WS, Holsinger FC, Kandil E, et al. Remote access robotic facelift thyroidectomy: a multi-institutional experience. World J Surg 2017;41(1):116–21.
8. Berber E, Bernet V, Fahey TJ, et al. American thyroid association statement on remote-access thyroid surgery. Thyroid 2016;26(3):331–7.
9. Dionigi G, Lavazza M, Wu CW, et al. Transoral thyroidectomy: why is it needed? Gland Surg 2017;6(3):272–6.
10. Park YM, Kim DH, Moon YM, et al. Gasless transoral robotic thyroidectomy using the DaVinci SP system: Feasibility, safety, and operative technique. Oral Oncol 2019;95:136–42. https://doi.org/10.1016/j.oraloncology.2019.06.003. Available at:.
11. Al-Qurayshi Z, Randolph GW, Alshehri M, et al. Analysis of variations in the use of intraoperative nerve monitoring in thyroid surgery. JAMA Otolaryngol Head Neck Surg 2016;142(6):584–9.
12. Lee J, Chung WY. Robotic surgery for thyroid disease. Eur Thyroid J 2013;2(2): 93–101.
13. Holsinger FC, Chung WY. Robotic thyroidectomy. Otolaryngol Clin North Am 2014;47(3):373–8.
14. Kang S-W, Lee SC, Lee SH, et al. Robotic thyroid surgery using a gasless, transaxillary approach and the da Vinci S system: the operative outcomes of 338 consecutive patients. Surgery 2009;146(6):1048–55. https://doi.org/10.1016/j. surg.2009.09.007. Available at:.
15. Holsinger FC, Terris DJ, Kuppersmith RB. Robotic thyroidectomy: operative technique using a transaxillary endoscopic approach without CO2 insufflation. Otolaryngol Clin North Am 2010;43(2):381–8, ix-x.
16. Lee J, Nah KY, Kim RM, et al. Differences in postoperative outcomes, function, and cosmesis: open versus robotic thyroidectomy. Surg Endosc 2010;24(12): 3186–94.
17. Son SK, Kim JH, Bae JS, et al. Surgical safety and oncologic effectiveness in robotic versus conventional open thyroidectomy in thyroid cancer: a systematic review and meta-analysis. Ann Surg Oncol 2015;22(9):3022–32.
18. Axente DD, Silaghi H, Silaghi CA, et al. Operative outcomes of robot-assisted transaxillary thyroid surgery for benign thyroid disease: early experience in 50 patients. Langenbeck's Arch Surg 2013;398(6):887–94.
19. Terris DJ, Singer MC, Seybt MW. Robotic facelift thyroidectomy: patient selection and technical considerations. Surg Laparosc Endosc Percutan Tech 2011;21(4): 237–42.

20. Ban EJ, Yoo JY, Kim WW, et al. Surgical complications after robotic thyroidectomy for thyroid carcinoma: a single center experience with 3,000 patients. Surg Endosc 2014;28(9):2555–63.
21. Kuppersmith RB, Holsinger FC. Robotic thyroid surgery: an initial experience with North American patients. Laryngoscope 2011;121(3):521–6.
22. Landry CS, Grubbs EG, Warneke CL, et al. Robot-assisted transaxillary thyroid surgery in the United States: is it comparable to open thyroid lobectomy? Ann Surg Oncol 2012;19(4):1269–74.
23. Huang S, Garstka ME, Murcy MA, et al. Somatosensory evoked potential: preventing brachial plexus injury in transaxillary robotic surgery. Laryngoscope 2019;129(11):2663–8.
24. Sung ES, Ji YB, Song CM, et al. Robotic thyroidectomy: comparison of a postauricular facelift approach with a gasless unilateral axillary approach. Otolaryngol Head Neck Surg 2016;154(6):997–1004.
25. Byeon HK, Kim DH, Chang JW, et al. Comprehensive application of robotic retroauricular thyroidectomy: the evolution of robotic thyroidectomy. Laryngoscope 2016;126(8):1952–7.
26. Terris DJ, Singer MC. Qualitative and quantitative differences between 2 robotic thyroidectomy techniques. Otolaryngol Neck Surg 2012;147(1):20–5.
27. Terris DJ, Singer MC, Seybt MW. Robotic facelift thyroidectomy: II. Clinical feasibility and safety. Laryngoscope 2011;121(8):1636–41.
28. Choo JM, You JY, Kim HY. Transoral robotic thyroidectomy: the overview and suggestions for future research in new minimally invasive thyroid surgery. J Minim Invasive Surg 2019;22(1):5–10.
29. Cabot JC, Lee CR, Brunaud L, et al. Robotic and endoscopic transaxillary thyroidectomies may be cost prohibitive when compared to standard cervical thyroidectomy: a cost analysis. Surgery 2012;152(6):1016–24.
30. Abdelgadir Adam M, Speicher P, Pura J, et al. Robotic thyroidectomy for cancer in the us: patterns of use and short-term outcomes. Ann Surg Oncol 2014;21(12): 3859–64.
31. Lee HY, You JY, Woo SU, et al. Transoral periosteal thyroidectomy: cadaver to human. Surg Endosc 2015;29(4):898–904.
32. Chabrillac* E, Zerdoud S, Graff-Cailleaud SF P, et al. Report of a track seeding of thyroid papillary carcinoma during robotassisted transaxillary thyroidectomy. J Thyroid Disord Ther 2017;6. Available at: https://www.longdom.org/open-access/report-of-a-track-seeding-of-thyroid-papillary-carcinoma-during-robotassisted-transaxillary-thyroidectomy-2167-7948-1000218.pdf.
33. Broome JT, Pomeroy S, Solorzano CC. Expense of robotic thyroidectomy: a cost analysis at a single institution. Arch Surg 2012;147(12):1102–6.
34. Kandil E, Hammad AY, Walvekar RR, et al. Robotic thyroidectomy versus nonrobotic approaches: a meta-analysis examining surgical outcomes. Surg Innov 2016;23(3):317–25.
35. Tae K, Ji YB, Song CM, et al. Robotic and endoscopic thyroid surgery: evolution and advances. Clin Exp Otorhinolaryngol 2019;12(1):1–11.
36. Ji YB, Song CM, Bang HS, et al. Long-term cosmetic outcomes after robotic/ endoscopic thyroidectomy by a gasless unilateral axillo-breast or axillary approach. J Laparoendosc Adv Surg Tech 2014;24(4):248–53.

Robotic Neck Dissection

Neal Rajan Godse, MD[a], Toby Shen Zhu, BS[b],
Umamaheswar Duvvuri, MD, PhD[a,c],*

KEYWORDS

- Neck dissection • Head and neck cancer • Robot-assisted surgery • Robotics

KEY POINTS

- Neck dissection is a key surgical tool in the management of nodal disease in head and neck squamous cell carcinoma.
- Robot-assisted neck dissections have been procedurally well validated and appear to have oncologic and perioperative outcomes similar to open neck dissection.
- Robot-assisted neck dissections have the potential for improved cosmesis compared with open neck dissections, which is increasingly important in the younger, human papilloma virus–related disease cohort.
- Increased operative times and cost are important factors that currently limit the universal adoption of robot-assisted neck dissections.
- Further work and research are required to establish long-term outcomes and to increase experience with this novel surgical approach.

INTRODUCTION

Head and neck squamous cell carcinoma (HNSCC) is a family of malignancies that arise from epithelial tissues of the head and neck. Primary tumors arise in the upper aerodigestive tract, most commonly from carcinogenic exposures (eg, tobacco smoke and alcohol) or in response to infection by the oncogenic human papilloma virus. Local metastasis begins with involvement of the cervical lymphatics and then may proceed to distant metastases. Management of HNSCC involves surgery, chemotherapy, and radiation, depending on patient and tumor characteristics. The surgical neck dissection is a key component of surgical management of HNSCC and involves the systematic removal of cervical lymphatics for diagnostic and therapeutic purposes. Typically, neck dissections are performed with open approaches,

[a] Department of Otolaryngology, University of Pittsburgh, 203 Lothrop Street, Suite 500, Pittsburgh, PA 15213, USA; [b] University of Pittsburgh, School of Medicine, 401 Scaife Hall, 3550 Terrace Street, Pittsburgh, PA 15261, USA; [c] Department of Veterans Affairs, Pittsburgh Health System, University Drive C, Pittsburgh, PA 15240, USA
* Corresponding author. University of Pittsburgh, 203 Lothrop Street, Suite 500, Pittsburgh, PA 15213.
E-mail address: duvvuriu@upmc.edu

allowing for direct visualization of the key neurovascular structures in the neck. More recently, however, some surgeons have begun exploring the use of surgical robotic platforms to perform minimally invasive neck dissections via incisions that spare the visible, anterior neck. Resultant research has been focused on understanding the pros and cons of these novel approaches.

HISTORY

The neck dissection as an operation has a rich history that begins in the early nineteenth century. Early surgeons, including Warren and Chelius, recognized cancer could spread to the local cervical lymphatics and the poor prognosis it portended and attempted surgical removal of individually affected nodes.[1] In the absence of anesthesia, aseptic technique, and a biological understanding of the disease process, these surgeries often carried significant morbidity and mortality with no survival benefit to the patient.

In the mid to late nineteenth century, Billroth, von Langenbeck, Volkmann, and Kocher described a variety of extirpative surgeries combined with some form of neck dissection.[2] These neck dissections involved removal of surrounding normal structures, not just single-node excisions. Sir Henry Butlin built on these techniques and incorporated Halstedian principles of surgical oncology, ultimately publishing a large series of patients who underwent surgeries for tongue cancer with neck dissections. He used the classic Y-shaped Kocher incision and removed the cervical lymphatics along with the internal jugular vein (IJV), sternocleidomastoid (SCM) muscles, and submandibular gland. Butlin recognized nodal involvement in tongue cancer was common and that lymph nodes could be removed prior to being clinically involved, thus creating the concept of an elective neck dissection. By employing this strategy, Butlin improved 3-year survival of patients with tongue cancer from 29% (n = 44, no elective neck dissection) to 42% (n = 70, elective neck dissection).[2,3]

In 1905, George Crile[4] published an article that described a systematic, radical en bloc neck dissection performed 121 times in 105 patients. Crile[5] went on to publish an expanded series of 132 surgeries in 1906 with 3-year follow-up. The publications included 12 meticulously illustrated figures that demonstrated the key anatomy. In the Crile radical neck dissection, the IJV, SCM, submandibular gland, tail of parotid, and often the spinal accessory nerve (SAN) all were resected routinely as part of the tissue block. In these landmark articles, Crile discussed the inferiority of subradical surgery and advocated for elective neck dissection in the clinically negative neck. The outcomes and techniques that Crile proposed in his original articles were so widely adopted that he now is credited as the father of the neck dissection.

The neck dissection continued to evolve in the twentieth century. Osvaldo Suarez proposed the functional neck dissection based on the anatomic understanding that the cervical lymphatics were contained within fascial sheaths that may allow other key structures in the neck to be spared.[6,7] Bocca observed the Suarez neck dissection and, along with Pignataro, went on to publish a series of 843 patients in the English literature who underwent the functional neck dissection as well as long-term outcomes.[8] In the late twentieth century, patterns of cervical metastases were identified, allowing surgeons to perform level-specific neck dissections based on the location of the primary tumor.[9] Thus the modern era of the neck dissection came about in which a customized neck dissection (eg, risk-stratified primary site–specific neck dissections, elective neck dissections for the clinically negative neck, and selective neck dissections that spare the SCM, IJV, SAN, and so forth) could be used based on the clinical scenario to maximize oncologic control and minimize surgical morbidity and mortality.

It is in this environment, rich in history, innovation, and discovery, that the concept of a robot-assisted neck dissection is introduced.

DISCUSSION

Robot-assisted surgery has become adopted in a variety of surgical fields due to the minimally invasive nature and ability to access difficult anatomy, visualize small structures in superb detail, and reduce physiologic tremor. Transoral robotic surgery commonly is used in otolaryngology for cancers of the oropharynx and supraglottis due to issues with access and visualization with more traditional approaches. As the use of robotic platforms in otolaryngology has increased, the potential for other applications in the head and neck have been proposed. Early work focused on robot-assisted transaxillary approaches for thyroidectomy with the potential advantage of no visible cervical incision.[10] As these surgeries were shown to be feasible and became widely practiced, particularly in Asia, the possibility of a robot-assisted neck dissection in cases of HNSCC was explored.[11] Potential benefits included improved cosmesis and reduced postoperative lymphedema. In the current state, robot-assisted neck dissections typically are performed using the da Vinci Surgical System (Intuitive, Sunnyvale, California) via a modified face lift/postauricular incision due to ease of access to the lymphatic packet of the neck while minimizing centrally located, visible incisions.

In this procedure, an incision is made first directly under the lobule of the ear and then carried postauricularly to approximately the middle of the ear and then inferiorly to the hairline. Subplatysmal flaps are raised medially to the anterior border of the SCM muscle. The great auricular nerve can be used to judge the depth of the subplatysmal flap laterally in the neck (**Fig. 1**). After the initial dissection, a Chung retractor is used to suspend the subplatysmal flap superiorly. The da Vinci surgical robot then is docked in the surgical field (**Fig. 2**). A 5-mm Maryland dissector and 5-mm Harmonic scalpel are used for deeper dissection. The structures within the deep cervical fascia are dissected, taking care to identify and preserve the SAN, IJV, and hypoglossal nerve (**Fig. 3**), while removing the lymphatic packet (**Fig. 4**). With the specimen removed, the wound bed is examined for hemostasis, the robot is removed, and the wound is closed over a suction drain (**Fig. 5**).

Oncologic control is of utmost importance for any proposed surgical intervention in HNSCC—as such, assessing the oncologic outcomes of robotic neck dissection versus open neck dissection is critical. Sukato and colleagues[12] looked at 11 published studies on robotic neck dissections and found that the total lateral lymph node yield, pathologic nodal yield, and 6-month locoregional recurrence rates were not statistically significant between open and robotic approaches. Because robotic neck dissection is a relatively new procedure, long-term control and survival rates have yet to be determined. Furthermore, they found that rates of common perioperative complications (eg, hematoma, chyle leaks, Horner syndrome, marginal mandibular nerve weakness, seroma, and wound infection) and length of stay in the hospital were similar between open and robotic approaches. Although more work needs to be done to establish long-term outcomes, it appears that the oncologic and perioperative outcomes of robotic neck dissection are comparable to those of open neck dissections.

The major advantage of a robotic operation is its minimally invasive approach. In a traditional open surgery, an incision is made in the anterior neck for adequate exposure of the entirety of the lymphatic packet but leaves a visible scar. By contrast, the modified facelift incision used for a robotic neck dissection is well disguised in

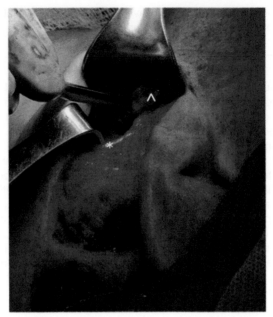

Fig. 1. Initial approach. A modified facelift incision is created and subplatysmal flaps are raised using open techniques. The great auricular nerve (*) is used to guide the depth of the flap laterally. Gross nodal disease is encountered in the level II lymphatics (^).

the postauricular tissue and in the hairline. As human papilloma virus–related disease reveals itself in a younger patient population, cosmesis increasingly is becoming a major concern. Although subjective, studies done by Sukato and colleagues[12] and Albergotti and colleagues[13] reported increased cosmesis (as determined by the surgeon) and patient satisfaction after robotic surgery.

Another advantage is the distance between the incision and the operative bed, especially as this relates to adjuvant radiation therapy. In patients considered high

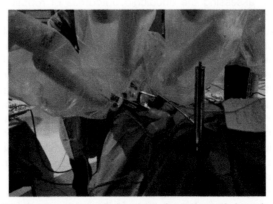

Fig. 2. Robotic setup. The head is turned toward the right and the robot arms (Maryland dissector and Harmonic scalpel) are inserted directly into the left neck. A Chung retractor is used to suspend the subplatysmal flap (*).

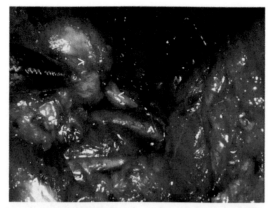

Fig. 3. Intraoperative image of left neck from a superior view with the robotic system. The accessory nerve (*), IJV (ˆ), and hypoglossal nerve (<) have been dissected and preserved while raising the lymphatic packet (>).

risk for locoregional recurrence (eg, locally advanced T3/T4 disease, positive resection margins, extranodal extension, 2 or more pathologically positive lymph nodes, perineural invasion, and lymphovascular space invasion), adjuvant chemotherapy and radiation therapy often are used to improve oncologic control. Numerous complications can occur from radiating a relatively new operative site, including wound infection, incisional dehiscence and breakdown,[14] pharyngocutaneous fistula, and carotid rupture. The risk of developing these complications often necessitates a delay between the conclusion of surgery and the initiation of radiation to allow for postoperative wound healing to occur. With an incision that is positioned away from the operative bed and out of the field of irradiation, there potentially is a reduced risk of these wound healing complications.

Although robot-assisted neck dissections have advantages, there also are pertinent disadvantages that would discourage its use. One key issue in robotic surgery is the prolonged operation time. Although operational times for each surgery vary drastically

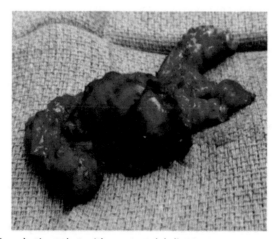

Fig. 4. Resected lymphatic packet with gross nodal disease.

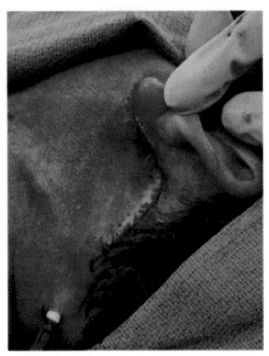

Fig. 5. Final wound closure. The incision is closed over a suction drain hidden in the postauricular tissue and hair line.

depending on degree of disease and experience of the surgeon with robotic procedures, on average robotic neck dissections can take an hour longer (189 minutes vs 254 minutes[12]) or twice as long (110 minutes vs 234 minutes[13,15]) compared with traditional open neck dissections. This prolonged operative time is attributed to preparation of the robot and the learning curve associated with use of a novel technology. Increased operative and anesthesia times also could increase the rates of perioperative complications. Over time, however, the operational time for robotic neck dissections is expected to decrease with experience but may not ever reach or be faster than open neck dissections due to the inherent delays with using an additional technology.

Another important consideration is cost—current robotic systems are highly advanced and expensive systems and, as such, robotic surgeries are more expensive than traditional approaches. Factors that affect cost include the direct cost of the equipment, maintenance costs, and costs associated with increased times in the operating room. The details of cost analysis, including hospital costs, insurance costs, and costs charged to the patient, are beyond the scope of this article but must be considered at an institutional and systems level when studying how feasible it is to routinely adopt robotic surgeries.

There are advantages and disadvantages to both open and robotic neck dissections in the treatment of HNSCC and there are different indications for the use of either technique. A proposed algorithm of how to choose between robotic and open neck dissection is presented in **Fig. 6**. The authors believe the most important indication for performing a robotic neck dissection is if cosmesis is a primary concern, such as in the case of a younger patient or potentially in a patient with extensive wound healing

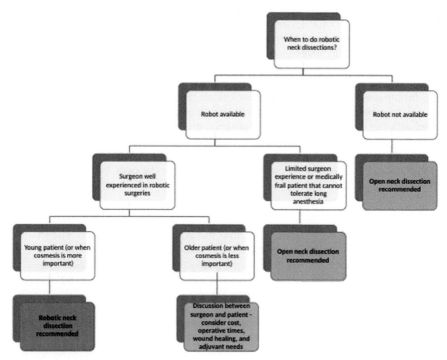

Fig. 6. Proposed algorithm of when to employ robotic neck dissection. Key considerations are surgeon experience, equipment availability, cosmetic needs, wound healing issues, medical comorbidities, and patient preference.

issues that require adjuvant radiation. Open surgery is indicated as the gold standard procedure and is indicated particularly when cost or experience eliminate the possibility of robotic surgery. As always, a careful discussion must be had on a patient-by-patient basis to evaluate whether a robotic neck dissection is the appropriate surgical therapy in a given scenario.

SUMMARY

From the days of Crile's radical neck dissections to the modern, minimally invasive robotic surgeries, there have been drastic advancements in the treatment of HNSCC. Early radical neck dissections removed many important structures in the patient's neck; elective and functional neck dissections refined the process and spared patients significant postoperative morbidity; and, finally, site-specific risk stratified selective neck dissections further refined the process while maintaining oncologic outcomes. Each new discovery improved some aspect of patient care but took time to become disseminated and adopted by the community of head and neck surgeons. In the modern age, robotic and minimally invasive surgery have been popularized among clinicians, and patient demand for improved cosmesis has increased. It still is imperative, however, to systematically examine the advantages and disadvantages of adopting robotic and minimally invasive techniques in the management of nodal disease of the neck in order to deliver evidence-based recommendations to patients.

Current literature suggests that perioperative outcomes and oncologic control are comparable between robotic and the gold standard open neck dissection, although long-term survival outcomes still need further research. The main advantage of robotic surgery is its minimally invasive approach, offering improved cosmesis by avoiding scarring of the anterior neck. There also may be important implications of having an incision distant from the operative bed when it comes to wound healing and the need for adjuvant radiation. Robotic neck dissections are associated, however, with a longer operative time, due to the physical setup of the robot and learning curve associated with the new technique, and increased costs. Both of these are expected to decrease with experience and technological advancements. Careful considerations of surgical experience, cost, patient disease status, and patient values are imperative in the decision to use robotic cervical lymphadenectomy over the traditional open procedure.

CLINICS CARE POINTS

- Robot-assisted neck dissections offer the possibility of minimally invasive approaches to the cervical lymphatics with potentially improved cosmesis
- When equipment and experience are available, robot-assisted neck dissection should be offered to young patients with cosmetic concerns and potentially in patients with wound healing issues.
- Robot-assisted neck dissection should not be used in situations when equipment, support personnel, or surgeon experience is lacking; in these scenarios, the open neck dissection should be employed.
- More research and experience are required to assess long-term oncologic outcomes and to assess whether cost and operative times decrease.

DISCLOSURE

The authors have nothing to disclose.

REFERENCES

1. Rinaldo A, Ferlito A, Silver CE. Early history of neck dissection. Eur Arch Otorhinolaryngol 2008;265(12):1535–8.
2. Ferlito A, Johnson JT, Rinaldo A, et al. European surgeons were the first to perform neck dissection. Laryngoscope 2007;117(5):797–802.
3. Uttley AR, Mcgurk M. Sir Henry Trentham Butlin: the father of British head and neck surgery. Br J Oral Maxillofac Surg 2000;38(2):114–20.
4. Crile GW. On the surgical treatment of cancer of the head and neck. With a summary of one hundred and twenty-one operations performed upon one hundred and five patients. Trans South Surg Gynecol Assoc 1905;18:108–27.
5. Crile G. Excision of cancer of the head and neck. With special reference to the plan of dissection based on one hundred and thirty-two operations. JAMA 1906;47:1780–6.
6. Suarez O. El problema de las metastasis linfaticas y alejadas del cancer de laringe e hipofaringe. Rev Otorrinolaringol 1963;23:83–99.
7. Ferlito A, Rinaldo A. Osvaldo Suárez: often-forgotten father of functional neck dissection (in the non-Spanish-speaking literature). Laryngoscope 2004;114(7):1177–8.
8. Bocca E, Pignataro O, Oldini C, et al. Functional neck dissection: an evaluation and review of 843 cases. Laryngoscope 1984;94(7):942–5.

9. Shah JP. Patterns of cervical lymph node metastasis from squamous carcinomas of the upper aerodigestive tract. Am J Surg 1990;160(4):405–9.
10. Kang SW, Jeong JJ, Yun JS, et al. Robot-assisted endoscopic surgery for thyroid cancer: experience with the first 100 patients. Surg Endosc 2009;23(11): 2399–406.
11. Kim WS, Lee HS, Kang SM, et al. Feasibility of robot-assisted neck dissections via a transaxillary and retroauricular ("TARA") approach in head and neck cancer: preliminary results. Ann Surg Oncol 2012;19(3):1009–17.
12. Sukato DC, Ballard DP, Abramowitz JM, et al. Robotic versus conventional neck dissection: A systematic review and meta-analysis. Laryngoscope 2019;129(7): 1587–96.
13. Albergotti WG, Byrd JK, Almeida JRD, et al. Robot-assisted level II-IV neck dissection through a modified facelift incision: initial North American experience. Int J Med Robot 2014;10(4):391–6.
14. Payne WG, Naidu DK, Wheeler CK, et al. Wound healing in patients with cancer. Eplasty 2008;8:e9.
15. Albergotti WG, Byrd JK, Nance M, et al. Robot-assisted neck dissection through a modified facelift incision. Ann Otol Rhinol Laryngol 2016;125(2):123–9.

Robotic Management of Salivary Glands

Jennifer E. Douglas, MD[a], Christopher Z. Wen, BA[b], Christopher H. Rassekh, MD[a],*

KEYWORDS

- Transoral robotic surgery • Robotic surgery • Salivary gland disease • Sialadenitis
- Salivary gland tumors • Parapharyngeal space • Minor salivary glands • Sialolithiasis

KEY POINTS

- Robotic surgery for salivary gland diseases can be performed transorally or transcervically.
- Transoral robotic surgery is primarily indicated for neoplasms of the oropharynx, including minor salivary gland tumors of the pharynx, base of tongue, and palate.
- Transoral robotic surgery can be combined with other approaches for resection of nasopharyngeal salivary gland malignancies.
- Transoral robotic surgery is helpful for inflammatory diseases of the submandibular gland and sublingual gland such as sialoliths and ranula.
- Transoral robotic surgery and retroauricular robotic surgery are alternatives to conventional transcervical approaches for removal of the submandibular gland.

INTRODUCTION

There are several ways to use robotics in the management of salivary gland disease. These include transoral robotic surgical resection of benign and malignant minor salivary gland tumors in the oropharynx, which are performed with classic operations such as radical tonsillectomy and base of tongue resections. Transoral approach and excision of parapharyngeal space minor salivary gland tumors have been employed successfully also. Transoral robotic surgery (TORS)-assisted submandibular gland excision and TORS-assisted combined approaches for submandibular stones are presented. Finally, unusual applications such as nasopharyngectomy, soft palate resection and reconstruction, sublingual gland excision, and resection of congenital anomalies such as salivary duct remnants in the oropharynx represent innovations that are also of interest (**Table 1**). Although the use of the robot for some of these indications is technically off label, this is explained to patients who agree to its use.

[a] Department of Otorhinolaryngology–Head and Neck Surgery, University of Pennsylvania Health System, 5th Floor Silverstein Building, 3400 Spruce Street, Philadelphia, PA 19104, USA; [b] Perelman School of Medicine, University of Pennsylvania, 3400 Civic Center Boulevard, Building 421, Philadelphia, PA 19104, USA
* Corresponding author.
E-mail address: Christopher.Rassekh@pennmedicine.upenn.edu

Otolaryngol Clin N Am 53 (2020) 1051–1064
https://doi.org/10.1016/j.otc.2020.07.013
0030-6665/20/© 2020 Elsevier Inc. All rights reserved.

Table 1
Robotic salivary gland surgery overview

		Indication			
	Pharyngeal Minor Salivary Gland Neoplasms	**Parapharyngeal Space (PPS) Neoplasms**	**Submandibular Gland (SMG) Pathology**	**Other TORS**	**Retroauricular Robotic Surgery**
Frequency of use at our institution	Most common	TORS posterior hemiglossectomy	TORS PPS space resection	TORS-Sialo		
	More common	TORS radical tonsillectomy		TORS SMG excision		
	Less common	TORS palatectomy with local flap reconstruction			Sublingual gland excision	
	Rare	TORS-assisted Nasopharyngectomy	TORS PPS resection combined with open approach		Congenital salivary fistula	
	Not performed					SMG excision

DISCUSSION
Transoral Robotic Surgical Resection of the Base of Tongue (Posterior Hemiglossectomy)

Background
Transoral robotic surgery was initially developed for the surgical management of squamous cell carcinoma (SCC) of the base of tongue (BOT) and tonsil.[1,2] Based on its significant success with this pathology and subsites, the technology was quickly extended to additional pathology and subsites, as will be discussed here. Early on, it was most easily extended to additional BOT neoplasms (**Fig. 1**). To study the efficacy of TORS for non-SCC pathology at the base of tongue, Schoppy and colleagues reviewed 20 patients managed with endoscopic approaches, either TORS or transoral laser microsurgery (TLM). Eighty percent of cases were minor salivary gland tumors, the most common of which was adenoid cystic carcinoma.[3] Notably, 75% of cases were BOT neoplasms, 10 of which underwent TORS followed by adjuvant radiation therapy. Only 1 of 20 patients had recurrence and underwent salvage TORS with good outcome. One patient underwent elective bilateral neck dissection because of pathology showing myoepithelial carcinoma.

Procedure
Exposure of the BOT is achieved using the Feyh-Kastenbauer retractor. A 5 mm spatula-tip cautery is used, with the goal of achieving grossly negative margins. Intraoperative frozen sections are performed to confirm adequacy of resection.[3] Based on patient factors (eg, body mass index [BMI] and medical comorbidities) and extent of resection, tracheostomy and feeding tube placement can be considered

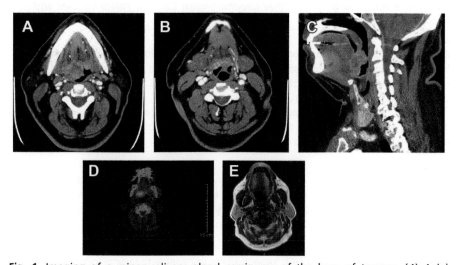

Fig. 1. Imaging of a minor salivary gland carcinoma of the base of tongue. (*A*) Axial computed tomography (CT) scan with contrast demonstrating right BOT mass. (*B*) Axial CT scan also shows multiple pathologic ipsilateral nodes. (*C*) Sagittal CT showing that tumor has both exophytic and submucosal components. (*D*) Positron emission tomography (PET) scan showing avidity (biopsy showed high-grade mucoepidermoid carcinoma). The patient underwent TORS, neck dissection, and postoperative radiation. (*E*) MRI 8 years after TORS showing no recurrence at the primary site but a new contralateral deep lobe parotid tumor that was not felt to be amenable to TORS. It was resected with a parotidectomy approach and was found to be a low-grade hyalinizing clear cell carcinoma.

intraoperatively at the discretion of the treating surgeon. In contrast to the primary indication for TORS posterior hemiglossectomy, chemoradiation is much less effective, so that surgery is almost always preferred for salivary pathology.

Advantages
Benefits of the TORS approach for minor salivary gland neoplasms of the BOT are those that have been described in the literature as general advantages of robotic surgery. These include enhanced magnification, 3-dimensional optics affording greatly improved visualization, improved manual dexterity, and the ability to better utilize a bedside assistant allowing for 4-handed surgery in tandem with the surgeon at the console. The assistant provides feedback to the console surgeon and helps with retraction, suction, and clipping of vessels. These all enhance the adequacy of resection and reduce the risk of hemorrhage. By avoiding large open approaches for access such as mandibulotomy, lingual-mandibular release, and suprahyoid pharyngotomy, tracheotomy can usually be avoided. Additionally, there can be a decreased rate of need for prolonged enteral access, and better short- and long-term swallowing outcomes can be achieved.

Disadvantages
As with TORS for SCC, the risk of post-TORS hemorrhage in the management of minor salivary gland neoplasms of the BOT remains the most significant risk. This is estimated at approximately 10% based on a variety of studies.[4] This risk can be minimized by performing neck dissection before the resection with ligation of the facial, lingual, and superior laryngeal arteries.[5] In some cases, a large resection of the tongue base is required, which necessitates a free flap reconstruction.

Transoral Robotic Surgery for Other Oropharyngeal Cancers, Palate Cancers and Reconstruction

Background
Although the BOT is the predominant oropharyngeal site for minor salivary gland malignancies, tumors of the tonsil and glossotonsillar sulcus also occur. These tumors may require a radical tonsillectomy in addition to a TORS BOT resection.[3] The most common site for minor salivary glands is the hard palate, but many of these tumors may involve the soft palate and other oropharyngeal and nasopharyngeal sites also. The soft palate represents an anatomically difficult location to access, making it ripe for the application of TORS to enable visualization.

Procedure
Basic patient positioning is as described previously with exposure typically achieved with a modified Crow Davis mouth gag A 70° endoscope with a 45° angled monopolar cautery is set-up on the robot. Bipolar cautery is additionally available, which provides optimized hemostasis in the right circumstances.

Advantages
The advantages of TORS for BOT resection are applicable to radical tonsillectomy and palate resection also. In addition, robotically assisted elevation of the buccinators myomucosal flap and buccal fat pad flap enhances visualization and 4-handed surgery for the reconstruction. These procedures can be hybrid (partially nonrobotic) in nature.

Disadvantages
Although there is a theoretic risk of velopalatal insufficiency with soft palate resection, there is no clear evidence showing an increased risk with TORS-assisted soft palate

resection. One can argue that this surgery can be done without robot; however, this has been argued for many of the indications, and the authors believe that TORS adds value for all of these resections, as it does for the BOT.

Transoral Robotic Surgery Approach to the Parapharyngeal Space for Salivary Gland Tumors

Background

The parapharyngeal space is divided anatomically into the pre- and poststyloid parapharyngeal space (PPS) based on the relative location to the styloid process. Salivary gland tumors arise in the prestyloid parapharyngeal space, which contains the deep lobe of the parotid gland and minor salivary glands. Most (70%–80%) of parapharyngeal space masses are benign, most commonly pleomorphic adenoma (**Figs. 2** and **3**).[6,7] Because of this, it is important to perform preoperative work-up with fine needle aspiration, as transoral resection is relatively contraindicated in malignancy. In addition, tumors that minimally involve the deep lobe of parotid gland may be resectable transorally, but those that approach or traverse the stylomandibular tunnel require an alternate approach externally.

A retrospective review and systematic review both previously confirmed the safety and feasibility of TORS for PPS tumors. TORS is primarily indicated for benign tumors of the PPS as previously mentioned, but if malignancy is identified at the time of final pathology, radiation or additional surgery is not precluded.[8,9] O'Malley and colleagues performed a prospective study of well-defined PPS tumors. Ten patients were enrolled, with TORS completed in 9 of 10 patients.[10] There were no significant complications, and in patients with pleomorphic adenomas, local control was 100%.

Procedure

Technical details are reviewed elsewhere, with an approach similar to that of a radical tonsillectomy, with division of the medial pterygoid and blunt dissection.[11]

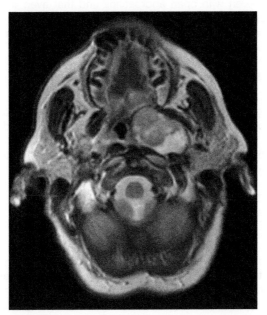

Fig. 2. T2-weighted axial MRI of a prestyloid parapharyngeal space pleomorphic adenoma that underwent TORS with good results.

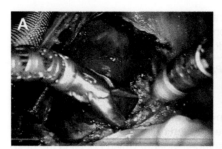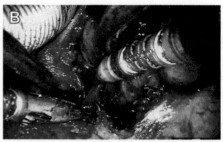

Fig. 3. TORS approach to the parapharyngeal space for a benign tumor. (*A*) Approach and exposure of prestyloid PPS tumor with division of medial pterygoid muscle to improve access. (*B*) 4-handed dissection of prestyloid PPS tumor.

Advantages

Advantages of the TORS approach for PPS tumors include enhanced visualization, avoidance of an external scar, reduced operative time, and the possibility of 4-handed surgery, all while offering comparable return to oral intake times.[10,12] A major advantage of this approach is avoidance of major external approaches such as described for oropharyngeal cancer and parotidectomy or other approaches that require dissection or retraction of the facial nerve. In addition, the risk of first-bite syndrome has been found to be virtually nonexistent, whereas it is a rather frequent occurrence in external approaches.[13]

Disadvantages

The use of the robot increases the cost and technical skill required for the procedure. There is also concern for the risk of tumor spillage, particularly with pathology such as pleomorphic adenoma. However, the open approach literature suggests that tumor rupture can occur even with open approaches and that even with tumor capsule rupture, the risk of recurrence is low.[11] With transoral approaches, there is risk of pharyngeal dehiscence, although this can be avoided by meticulous closure with horizontal mattress sutures.

Transoral Robotic Surgery-Assisted Resection of Nasopharyngeal Salivary Gland Tumors

Traditional approaches to the nasopharynx and infratemporal fossa overlap with those used for the parapharyngeal space.[14,15] TORS has been employed for nasopharyngeal malignancy combined with endoscopic endonasal or transpalatal approaches.[14,16] The robot provides an additional level of visualization and dexterity as it does for many TORS applications.[16,17]

Transoral Robotic Surgery Approach to the Parapharyngeal Space for Submandibular Gland Excision

Background

Transoral excision of the SMG via the PPS was first demonstrated in 2005 by Terris and colleagues[18] and has been reviewed in various publications since, but has never been widely adopted because of the technical difficulty of a predominantly anterior transoral approach.[19] Kauffman and colleagues[20] performed a retrospective review of 9 patients over 10 years, showing its application for the management of chronic sialadenitis (n = 6) and benign cystic lesions (n = 3). There are isolated case reports of TORS SMG excision,[19,21,22] and in their institution, the authors have been working on refining the technical details of a TORS parapharyngeal space approach to make transoral SMG excision safer.

Procedure

The procedure is the most challenging of all TORS procedures in the authors' experience. However, their technical refinements have resulted in successful removal of benign neoplasms and selected glands with chronic sialadenitis. The technique involves a combination of the Crow Davis mouth gag and Jennings mouth gag with tongue retractor and cheek retractor using dual side arms (**Fig. 4**). The dissection is done inside out, so steps that are generally carried out late in the transcervical SMG excision are done earlier. For example, identification and mobilization of the lingual nerve is done immediately after making an incision that is much like that used for PPS tumors but extending further onto the floor of the mouth. The mylohyoid muscle and digastric muscle are identified, and it is critical to ligate the facial vessels. The duct may be used as a handle. The operation is often a hybrid procedure with some of the dissection done under direct vision with loupe magnification. A third assistant may provide upward pressure on the gland to deliver it into the oral cavity. Care is taken to avoid damage to the tumor capsule, as the operation is most commonly performed for pleomorphic adenoma.

Advantages

Transoral removal of the SMG avoids the visible scar inherent with the transcervical approach and also minimizes risk to the marginal mandibular nerve. If required, the transcervical approach can always be employed should transoral resection fail.

Disadvantages

A TORS transoral approach requires a more challenging and complex dissection that leads to longer operative times and increased risk of tumor rupture, vascular complications like critical hemorrhage, and lingual nerve injury. It also requires the patient to

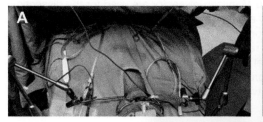
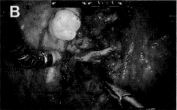
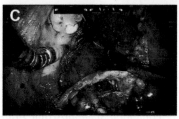

Fig. 4. TORS approach for submandibular gland excision. (*A*) Set-up for TORS SMG excision with Jennings mouth gag and dual side arms; the gland excision is often started with the Crow Davis mouth gag to get the parapharyngeal space exposure first. The same set-up as is shown is used for TORS-Sialendoscopy (*B*) TORS SMG excision-using duct as handle and showing lingual nerve. (*C*) Exposure of very large SMG pleomorphic adenoma with blunt dissection from mylohyoid after division of SMG ganglion.

be on a modified diet. Because of these significant disadvantages, it is generally suitable for patients with keloid potential or those who want to avoid a visible scar. Additionally, because of the operative difficulty, this operation should only be done by centers with extraordinarily high volume of TORS experience with standard modules and ideally in centers that have successfully incorporated TORS PPS resection into their practice. It should also be avoided when gland excision is caused by sialolithiasis, as such cases usually have severe chronic inflammation that makes the procedure dangerous.

Transoral Robotic Surgery Resection of Sublingual Gland for Ranula

Background
Ranulas are salivary gland-associated pseudocysts, typically arising from the sublingual gland (SLG), which are either congenital or acquired in the setting of intraoral trauma.[23] Simple ranulas may require minimal intervention, whereas plunging ranulas involving the musculature of the floor of the mouth may need a more comprehensive resection. At a minimum, removal of the associated salivary gland is necessary for adequate resection. For SLG-associated ranulas, management is typically with standard transoral excision. However, the authors have employed TORS combined with sialendoscopy, which allows improved visualization of the lingual nerve and can be used for cases where the submandibular duct is also abnormal.[24] This minimizes risk of injury to the surrounding neurovasculature and maximizes resection to limit risk of recurrence.[19,24,25] The 2 case reports in the literature detail the approach.[24,25]

Procedure
The procedure is done with the same incision as without the robot, but the magnification improves visualization of the lingual nerve and the extent of the SLG. The authors use a Jennings mouth gag for this operation. Sialendoscopy of the submandibular duct can be used to visualize the sublingual and submandibular ducts and facilitate leaving a stent to aid in localization and limit risk of duct injury. The zero-degree robotic endoscope, monopolar cautery, and Maryland dissector are used for the dissection. An incision is made over the mass, and blunt dissection through the floor of mouth is performed, ensuring safe dissection of the lingual nerve. After identifying sublingual gland, ranula, and the portion of the ranula that extends beyond the sublingual space, the ranula and associated sublingual gland are excised. Postexcision sialendoscopy can be performed to ensure the submandibular duct is intact and entry of the sublingual duct is adequately ligated. The wound is closed with simple interrupted 3-0 Vicryl sutures.

Advantages
Advantages for the technique for SLG resection in cases of ranula are similar to that of TORS used in the oropharynx as previously discussed.

Disadvantage
The primary disadvantage is the complexity of set-up and cost. As such, this technique should be used in very select cases.

Transoral Robotic Surgery Combined Sialendoscopic Approaches to the Submandibular Hilum for Sialoliths

Background
Combining sialoendoscopic approaches with open approaches has shown great success in sialolith removal without the need for gland excision.[26] The combined transoral approach for SMG sialoliths avoids the external scar of traditional sialoadenectomy,

but 2% of cases still have postoperative lingual nerve damage.[27] This risk is higher with larger stones, which occur primarily at the hilum, where Wharton's duct is in close proximity to the lingual nerve.[28] The use of a TORS combined sialendoscopic approach to better protect the lingual nerve has been reported to reduce the risk of permanent lingual nerve injury and have a high gland preservation rate.[29,30]

Procedure

The patient is anesthetized and intubated with a nasotracheal tube, and the sialolith is localized with either palpation (large stones) or sialendoscopy and transillumination (nonpalpable or multiple stones). A Jennings mouth gag is used, and a tongue retractor/cheek retractor combination is used to remove the tongue from the surgical field and stabilize the head. The robot is docked, and low-setting monopolar cautery is used to make a mucosal incision over the stone. Blunt dissection is performed until the lingual nerve is identified, retracted, and protected. Wharton duct can then be found in a triangle between the lingual nerve, mylohyoid, and sublingual gland. Depending on the location of the sialolith, excision of part of or all of the sublingual gland may be necessary to visualize the relationship between the duct and nerve. After confirming the location of the sialolith, an incision is made in the duct, and the sialolith can be delivered (**Fig. 5**).[23] Sialendoscopy is performed after TORS to irrigate the duct, visualize patency, and ensure absence of retained sialoliths. The floor of mouth is then closed with 3-0 or 4-0 Vicryl sutures.

Advantages

The TORS combined sialendoscopic approach allows for safer dissection of the lingual nerve in a multitude of ways. The stereoscopic 3-dimensional magnified view and 6-handed surgical approach allow for finer motions, smaller incisions, and decreased tissue manipulation.[29,30] Decreasing crowding around the already small working space of the posterior floor of the mouth improves ease of access to the surgeon and assistants.[29] Finally, the flexibility this approach offers allows the surgeon to utilize a combination of the direct approach, endoscopic approach, and robotic approach for complex sialolithotomies. In this way, the benefits of TORS assistance allow for easy cases to be performed more quickly and difficult cases to be performed more safely.

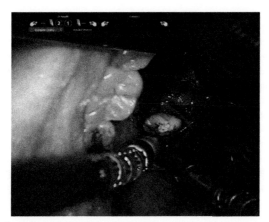

Fig. 5. TORS-sialo for left hilar SMG sialolith with stone shown in the opened duct in the triangle with sublingual gland anteriorly, mylohyoid laterally, and lingual nerve medially.

Disadvantages

Similar to other robotic procedures, a TORS-assisted sialendoscopic approach has increased cost but may not have increased operation duration.[31] Razavi and colleagues[30] reported a decreased operating time (67 vs 90 minutes) when compared with a nonrobotic combined approach, and operative times decreased with increased case experience. Furthermore, difficult cases are longer whether the robot is used or not.

Transoral Robotic Surgery Resection of Congenital Cervical Salivary Duct Fistulas

Congenital cervical salivary duct fistulas (CCSDF) are a rare cause of drainage from the anterolateral neck due primarily to heterotopic salivary gland tissue.[32] Because of the risk of malignancy, definitive treatment is complete excision of the fistula and surrounding salivary tissue.[33] Although uncomplicated cases are unlikely to benefit from robotic assistance, cases that present with tonsillar or posterior oropharyngeal involvement may.[32,34] The authors previously published the report of a patient who presented with asymptomatic bilateral CCSDFs with a tract extending to the posterior oropharynx. TORS direct pharyngolaryngoscopy was able to visualize the tract and demonstrate that the internal opening was not patent to the external opening. The external approach could not access the entire tract, as it narrowed significantly at the level of the digastric muscle. The final centimeters of dissection were completed with TORS and the entire tract delivered transorally. Given the narrow parapharyngeal space, a tonsillectomy would have been otherwise required had TORS not been used.[34] Those rare cases where the SMG is the origin of CCSDF drainage may also benefit from TORS assistance.[30,31,35]

RETROAURICULAR ROBOTIC SMG EXCISION
Retroauricular Approach

Background

The robot-assisted retroauricular approach to SMG excision was developed to avoid the cervical scars that result from a transcervical approach endoscopic-assisted retroauricular approach.[36] Although primarily developed in South Korea,[37,38] this approach has also been reported in India.[39] Robot-assisted approaches have similar safety and efficacy as endoscopic and transcervical approaches in small prospective studies.[40]

Procedure

The procedure begins with either a modified facelift incision or a retroauricular incision that extends posteriorly along the hairline.[41] The subplatysmal flap is raised anteriorly toward the midline about 10 cm, with care to identify and protect the great auricular nerve and external jugular vein.[31,41] A self-retaining retractor maintains the flap to create a working space.[41] The sternocleidomastoid muscle is retracted to reveal the SMG, and dissection begins at the lower border near the posterior belly of the digastric muscle.[31,39,41] Dissection proceeds in a subcapsular fashion with either Harmonic shears or monopolar cautery.[41] The facial artery is identified and ligated with clips or the Harmonic shears.[41] After retracting the mylohyoid and with traction on the SMG, the lingual nerve can be separated from the SMG ganglion, and Wharton duct can be divided.[31,40,41] The SMG can be released from the digastric and mylohyoid muscles and excised after ensuring the integrity of the hypoglossal nerve.[39,41]

Advantages

The primary advantage of this approach is the improved cosmesis.[37–40,42,43] In addition, the wider, 3-dimensional surgical field and improved instrument articulation allow for finer surgical control and easy access to the superior and medial aspects of the SMG just inferior to the mandible, which are otherwise difficult to access with straight endoscopes.[37,42,43]

Disadvantages

As previously noted, similar concerns exist about cost and increased operative time, although this decreases with increased surgeon experience.[40,44] One study did note a greater incidence of transient marginal mandibular nerve paresis in the robot-assisted approach, which could be due in part to the large skin flap of the retroauricular approach.[40]

Transhairline Approach

A separate South Korean group advocates for a transhairline approach as an alternative to the retroauricular approach.[45] The procedural steps are similar, apart from a smaller (sub 5vcm) incision with the transhairline incision that can be hidden at the hairline.[45,46] This maximizes postoperative cosmesis and provides a favorable option for some patients. Without the postauricular limb, the resulting skin flap is much smaller, further limiting the working space but decreasing the risk of flap necrosis or injury to the auricular branches of sensory nerves.[46] If the working space is ultimately too limited, such as for patients with adhesion caused by chronic inflammation, the transhairline approach can easily be converted to the retroauricular approach.[46]

SUMMARY

TORS-assisted combined approaches allow for advanced approaches to multiple sites within the head and neck for management of inflammatory and neoplastic salivary gland disease. In addition to enhanced visualization and ease of dissection, robotic approaches enable improved surgeon posture, which likely decreases the likelihood of a work-related musculoskeletal disorder and may contribute to a longer active surgical career.[31] The authors put forth that the robot be considered as a helpful adjunct to the management of salivary gland disease in high-volume centers with experienced head and neck surgeons.

CLINICS CARE POINTS

TORS has proven benefits for oropharyngeal cancer. The lessons learned from management of oropharyngeal cancer can be applied to salivary gland diseases of the nasopharynx, parapharyngeal space, and the floor of mouth.

TORS allows for minimally invasive surgery to be performed safely. Alternate approaches such as retroauricular approach for submandibular gland excision can be done robotically also. Although some may say that robotic surgery is not needed, for salivary gland indications, the have chosen to be innovators and early adopters akin to the paradigm shift following the application of TORS for oropharyngeal carcinoma[1,47]

ACKNOWLEDGMENTS

The authors would like to acknowledge the vision and leadership of Dr .Gregory S. Weinstein and Dr. Bert W. O'Malley, Jr. who are the inventors of TORS and who supported the development of salivary gland applications within the authors' department.

DISCLOSURE

Dr C.H. Rassekh has a contract with Cook Medical, which provided support for the 5th International Salivary Gland Congress including funds for a faculty dinner program.

REFERENCES

1. Weinstein GS, O'Malley BW, Cohen MA, et al. Transoral robotic surgery for advanced oropharyngeal carcinoma. Arch Otolaryngol Head Neck Surg 2010; 136(11):1079–85.
2. Weinstein GS, O'Malley BW, Magnuson JS, et al. Transoral robotic surgery: a multicenter study to assess feasibility, safety, and surgical margins. Laryngoscope 2012;122(8):1701–7.
3. Schoppy DW, Kupferman ME, Hessel AC, et al. Transoral endoscopic head and neck surgery (eHNS) for minor salivary gland tumors of the oropharynx. Cancers Head Neck 2017;2:5.
4. Chia SH, Gross ND, Richmon JD. Surgeon experience and complications with transoral robotic surgery (TORS). Otolaryngol Head Neck Surg 2013;149(6): 885–92.
5. Hay A, Migliacci J, Karassawa Zanoni D, et al. Haemorrhage following transoral robotic surgery. Clin Otolaryngol 2018;43(2):638–44.
6. Carrau RL, Myers EN, Johnson JT. Management of tumors arising in the parapharyngeal space. Laryngoscope 1990;100(6):583–9.
7. Hughes KV, Olsen KD, McCaffrey TV. Parapharyngeal space neoplasms. Head Neck 1995;17(2):124–30.
8. De Virgilio A, Costantino A, Mercante G, et al. Trans-oral robotic surgery in the management of parapharyngeal space tumors: a systematic review. Oral Oncol 2020;103:104581.
9. Samoy K, Lerut B, Dick C, et al. Transoral robotic surgery for parapharyngeal lesions: a case series of four benign tumours. B-ENT 2015;(Suppl 24):55–9.
10. O'Malley BW, Quon H, Leonhardt FD, et al. Transoral robotic surgery for parapharyngeal space tumors. ORL J Otorhinolaryngol Relat Spec 2010;72(6):332–6.
11. Rassekh CH, Weinstein GS, Loevner LA, et al. Transoral robotic surgery for prestyloid parapharyngeal space masses. Oper Tech Otolaryngol Head Neck Surg 2013;24(2):99–105.
12. Chan JY, Tsang RK, Eisele DW, et al. Transoral robotic surgery of the parapharyngeal space: a case series and systematic review. Head Neck 2015;37(2): 293–8.
13. Linkov G, Morris LGT, Shah JP, et al. First bite syndrome: incidence, risk factors, treatment, and outcomes. Laryngoscope 2012;122(8):1773–8.
14. Carrau RL, Prevedello DM, de Lara D, et al. Combined transoral robotic surgery and endoscopic endonasal approach for the resection of extensive malignancies of the skull base. Head Neck 2013;35(11):E351–8.
15. Bradley PJ. Infratemporal fossa surgical approaches to primary/recurrent malignancies of salivary origin: paradigm surgical shift, patient selection, and oncologic outcomes. Curr Opin Otolaryngol 2020;28:79–89.
16. Henry LE, Haugen TW, Rassekh CH, et al. A novel transpalatal-transoral robotic surgery approach to clival chordomas extending into the nasopharynx. Head Neck 2019;41(8):E133–40.
17. Yin Tsang RK, Ho WK, Wei WI. Combined transnasal endoscopic and transoral robotic resection of recurrent nasopharyngeal carcinoma. Head Neck 2012; 34(8):1190–3.

18. Terris DJ, Haus BM, Gourin CG, et al. Endo-robotic resection of the submandibular gland in a cadaver model. Head Neck 2005;27(11):946–51.
19. Liang LM, Lin XZ, Shao XJ, et al. [Trans-oral robotic submandibular gland removal]. Zhonghua Kou Qiang Yi Xue Za Zhi 2019;54(4):263–5.
20. Kauffman RM, Netterville JL, Burkey BB. Transoral excision of the submandibular gland: techniques and results of nine cases. Laryngoscope 2009;119(3):502–7.
21. Lin XZ, Liang LM, Shao XJ, et al. Trans-oral robotic surgery of submandibular gland removal with preservation of sublingual gland and Wharton's duct. J Craniofac Surg 2019;30(1):237–8.
22. Prosser JD, Bush CM, Solares CA, et al. Trans-oral robotic submandibular gland removal. J Robot Surg 2013;7(1):87–90.
23. Mueller DT, Callanan VP. Congenital malformations of the oral cavity. Otolaryngol Clin North Am 2007;40(1):141–60, vii.
24. Carey RM, Hodnett BL, Rassekh CH, et al. Transoral robotic surgery with sialendoscopy for a plunging ranula. ORL J Otorhinolaryngol Relat Spec 2017;79(6):306–13.
25. Walvekar RR, Peters G, Hardy E, et al. Robotic-assisted transoral removal of a bilateral floor of mouth ranulas. World J Surg Oncol 2011;9:78.
26. Atienza G, López-Cedrún JL. Management of obstructive salivary disorders by sialendoscopy: a systematic review. Br J Oral Maxillofac Surg 2015;53(6):507–19.
27. Zenk J, Constantinidis J, Al-Kadah B, et al. Transoral removal of submandibular stones. Arch Otolaryngol Head Neck Surg 2001;127(4):432–6.
28. Capaccio P, Bottero A, Pompilio M, et al. Conservative transoral removal of hilar submandibular salivary calculi. Laryngoscope 2005;115(4):750–2.
29. Walvekar RR, Tyler PD, Tammareddi N, et al. Robotic-assisted transoral removal of a submandibular megalith. Laryngoscope 2011;121(3):534–7.
30. Razavi C, Pascheles C, Samara G, et al. Robot-assisted sialolithotomy with sialendoscopy for the management of large submandibular gland stones. Laryngoscope 2016;126(2):345–51.
31. Marzouk MF. Robot-assisted glandular surgery. Atlas Oral Maxillofac Surg Clin North Am 2018;26(2):153–7.
32. Ogawa K, Kondoh K, Kanaya K, et al. Bilateral cervical fistulas from heterotopic salivary gland tissues. ORL J Otorhinolaryngol Relat Spec 2014;76(6):336–41.
33. Lassaletta-Atienza L, López-Ríos F, Martín G, et al. Salivary gland heterotopia in the lower neck: a report of five cases. Int J Pediatr Otorhinolaryngol 1998;43(2):153–61.
34. Rassekh CH, Kazahaya K, Livolsi VA, et al. Transoral robotic surgery–assisted excision of a congenital cervical salivary duct fistula presenting as a branchial cleft fistula. Head Neck 2016;38(2):E49–53.
35. Morii M, Hebiguchi T, Watanabe R, et al. [Congenital cervical salivary fistula from the submandibular gland]. J Jpn Soc Pediatr Surg 2017;53(7):1316–9.
36. Song CM, Jung YH, Sung MW, et al. Endoscopic resection of the submandibular gland via a hairline incision: a new surgical approach. Laryngoscope 2010;120(5):970–4.
37. De Virgilio A, Park YM, Kim W, et al. Robotic sialoadenectomy of the submandibular gland via a modified face-lift approach. Int J Oral Maxillofac Surg 2012;41(11):1325–9.
38. Lee HS, Park DY, Hwang CS, et al. Feasibility of robot-assisted submandibular gland resection via retroauricular approach: Preliminary results. Laryngoscope 2013;123(2):369–73.

39. Nagpal K, Naruka SS, Rana N, et al. Robot-assisted submandibular gland excision via retroauricular approach in a patient with known keloid formation tendency – a case report. Acta Sci Otolaryngol 2020;2(4):7–9.
40. Singh RP, Sung ES, Song CM, et al. Robot-assisted excision of the submandibular gland by a postauricular facelift approach: comparison with the conventional transcervical approach. Br J Oral Maxillofac Surg 2017;55(10):1030–4.
41. Byeon HK, Koh YW. The new era of robotic neck surgery: the universal application of the retroauricular approach. J Surg Oncol 2015;112(7):707–16.
42. Park YM, Byeon HK, Chung HP, et al. Robotic resection of benign neck masses via a retroauricular approach. J Laparoendosc Adv Surg 2013;23(7):578–83.
43. Lee HS, Kim D, Lee SY, et al. Robot-assisted versus endoscopic submandibular gland resection via retroauricular approach: a prospective nonrandomized study. Br J Oral Maxillofac Surg 2014;52(2):179–84.
44. Yang TL, Ko JY, Lou PJ, et al. Gland-preserving robotic surgery for benign submandibular gland tumours: a comparison between robotic and open techniques. Br J Oral Maxillofac Surg 2014;52(5):420–4.
45. Yang TL, Li H, Holsinger FC, et al. Submandibular gland resection via the trans-hairline approach: a preclinical study of a novel flexible single-port surgical system and the surgical experiences of standard multiarm robotic surgical systems. Head Neck 2019;41(7):2231–8.
46. Yang TL. Robotic surgery for submandibular gland resection through a trans-hairline approach: The first human series and comparison with applicable approaches. Head Neck 2018;40(4):793–800.
47. Moore GA. Crossing the chasm: marketing and selling disruptive products to mainstream customers. 3rd edition. New York: Harper Business, an imprint of HarperCollins Publishers; 2014.

Robotic Ear Surgery

Katherine E. Riojas, BS[a], Robert F. Labadie, MD, PhD[b],*

KEYWORDS

- Surgical robots • Minimally invasive • Stapes • Cochlear implant

KEY POINTS

- Three classifications of surgical robots in ear surgery are discussed: collaborative (eg, passive parallel robot to guide drilling), teleoperated (eg, the daVinci surgical system), or autonomous (eg, bone-mounted robot performing mastoidectomy).
- Current clinical trials include minimally invasive drilling approaches to the cochlea with both collaborative guides and autonomous robots as well as stapes surgery and cochlear implant electrode array insertion using a teleoperated system.
- Within otology/neurotology, while autonomous robots may have the potential for higher impact (eg, drilling translabyrinthine approaches to the internal auditory canal), collaborative or teleoperated manipulators are likely to be clinically translated first, given less disruption to current surgical workflow and less rigorous regulatory criteria.
- Market forces will largely determine when adoption of robots as standard of clinical practice within otology will occur.

INTRODUCTION

Surgical robots are of considerable interest to clinicians and patients for their perceived benefit in more accurately targeting structures and more effectively accomplishing surgical tasks, often in a minimally invasive fashion while overcoming human limitations (eg, inherent tremor, limited tactile feedback, and technique variability). In this article aimed at covering the current state of the art regarding robotic ear surgery, the authors first begin by defining 3 classes of robotic devices in ear surgery to be used. These definitions are largely based on the surgeon-device-patient interaction with "end effector" defined as the surgical instrument that is contacting the patient.

- *Collaborative Robot/Guide.* The surgeon's hands directly actuate the end effector. The robot/guide passively (eg,[1]) or actively (eg,[2]) constrains and potentially augments surgical motion.

---

[a] Department of Mechanical Engineering, Vanderbilt University, 101 Olin Hall, 2400 Highland Avenue, Nashville, TN 37212, USA; [b] Department of Otolaryngology, Vanderbilt University Medical Center, 10450 Medical Center East, South Tower, Nashville, TN 37232-8605, USA
* Corresponding author.
E-mail address: robert.labadie@vumc.org

Otolaryngol Clin N Am 53 (2020) 1065–1075
https://doi.org/10.1016/j.otc.2020.07.014
0030-6665/20/© 2020 Elsevier Inc. All rights reserved.
oto.theclinics.com

- *Teleoperated Robot.* The surgeon remotely controls the end effector during the surgery (ie, surgeon motions map to end effector motion with potential modification [ie, tremor reduction, scaling]; eg,[3]).
- *Autonomous Robot.* The end effector interacts with the patient independently, whereas the surgeon supervises (eg,[4]). Note, the surgeon initiates the interaction (perhaps with a button push/hold) and closely monitors progression with intervention, if necessary.

Also pertinent to understanding the current and future state of the art is some appreciation of regulatory oversight that may help to explain why autonomous robots—which are standard of care in most high-volume manufacturing facilities (eg, car assembly) where they are considered safer and more efficient than human operators—have yet to be widely introduced into our surgical armamentarium while teleoperated systems, such as Intuitive's da Vinci surgical system (Intuitive Surgical Inc., Sunnyvale, CA) have been introduced.

With respect to ear surgery, surgical robotic devices have the potential to give surgeons superhuman abilities by augmenting their existing training. One specific example of when this augmentation would be clinically useful is during cochlear implant (CI) electrode array insertion. Past studies[5,6] have demonstrated that human surgeon perception is on the same order of magnitude as severe intracochlear trauma. A logical extension of these findings is that subtle intracochlear trauma cannot be appreciated by human surgeons, yet CI companies instruct surgeons to stop electrode array insertion when increased force is perceived, which seems to not be humanly possible. Perhaps as important as development of robotic technology is recognition by surgeons that the technology is necessary. This example is but one of the broad potential applications in this field that is discussed in the following section. In this article, the authors focus on clinical applications of the devices defined in the classes mentioned earlier. Interested readers may also find further details on many of the technologies discussed later in the cited references as well as in other review articles on this topic.[7,8] For each defined class of surgical robot, the authors first describe the general landscape of that robot in ear surgery and then discuss known clinical implementations with regulatory approval.

APPLICATIONS
Collaborative Surgical Robot/Guides

The authors begin the discussion with perhaps the simplest approach to robotic assistance in ear surgery—the collaborative robot/guide. One example of this type of device is a template or frame that aligns a tool/implant to a patient-specific trajectory and the surgeon then carries out the remaining surgical tasks. Such technology has been in use in neurosurgery since the 1970s, first with rigid N-frames[9] and then articulated arm robots[10] and now includes 2 Food and Drug Administration (FDA)-cleared and clinically used models—the Neuromate (Renishaw, Inc.) and the Rosa (MedTech, Inc.)—which are used for minimally invasive intracranial biopsy, deep brain stimulator placement, and ablative therapy for intractable epilepsy. Extension of such collaborative guides to target the cochlea for minimally invasive access to the cochlea has been reported by numerous groups including setting the trajectory with a patient-customized microstereotactic frame[11] (details on clinical implementation discussed later) or setting the trajectory with a passive parallel robot.[1,12]

Another type of collaborative robot is one that constrains surgical motion to establish so-called no-fly zones to prevent surgeons from damaging healthy tissue. This type of robot allows the surgeon to freely move the drill but uses active braking with motors[2] (**Fig. 1**) or passive braking[13] to enforce safety boundaries. Both the patient and robot are tracked using an infrared image guidance system (IGS). When a boundary is approached—boundaries are set during preoperative planning—the system sends an audible signal followed by braking to prevent the drill from violating the boundary. These types of robots could have utility during training and/ or in complex cases where unusual anatomy may be encountered.

Several groups have worked on variations of collaborative "micromanipulators" modified for ear surgery to overcome inherent physiologic tremor and improve repeatable positioning. The Steady Hand Robot from Johns Hopkins University[14] is a robot designed to reduce hand tremor and has undergone preclinical testing for stapes surgery and is being commercialized by Galen Robotics, Inc. (Baltimore, MD). This robot has also been used for improved cochlear implant insertions with the implementation of no-fly zones.[15] The Micron is another micromanipulator modified for stapes footplate surgery, with past studies showing 50% reduction in hand tremor.[16]

Clinical implementation

Labadie and colleagues[11] reported in 9 patients the ability to use a customized microstereotactic frame to access the cochlea via a narrow tunnel drilled from the surface of the mastoid through the facial recess. Their initial cohort included a patient with a heat-induced facial nerve paresis, which resolved to a House-Brackmann II/VI. Because of regulatory changes at the United States FDA via the 2012 Safety and Innovation Act, their work was halted, whereas technological improvements and obtainment of an Investigational Device Exemption was sought. They reported reinitiation of clinical trials in a recent case report under review. The same group has also clinically used the customized microstereotactic frame approach to drain a petrous apex lesion via both the subacurate and infralabyrinthine approaches.[17]

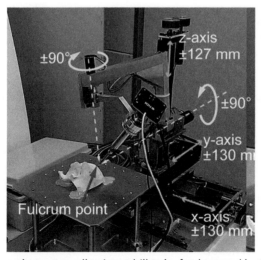

Fig. 1. Collaborative robot system allowing a drill to be freely moved by the surgeon within a specified workspace but restricted from violating preset boundaries (eg, tegmen, sigmoid sinus, facial nerve, labyrinthine, and external auditory canal). (*From* Auris Nasus Larynx, 43(2), Lim H, Matsumoto N, Cho B, et al. "Semi-manual mastoidectomy assisted by human-robot collaborative control - A temporal bone replica study", pages 161-165, © (2015) Elsevier Ireland Ltd, with permission from Elsevier.)

Teleoperated Surgical Robots

Teleoperated surgical robots have relatively broad clinical use with Intuitive's da Vinci, perhaps the most recognized example. The da Vinci system has found widespread use in urology with more limited applications in otolaryngology where it has been used for tumor resection without the need to split the jaw for access.[3] The use of the da Vinci surgical system for ear surgery, while proposed and even demonstrated in cadaver models, does not seem to offer immediate cost-effective value or advantages over traditional techniques.[18] Although the da Vinci surgical system is not designed for ear surgery, the concept of a teleoperated robot for ear surgery has high yield, as many of the interventions ear surgeons perform are at or near the threshold of human abilities including stapes surgery, CI electrode array insertion, and cochleostomy drilling. Efforts describing teleoperated systems specifically designed for ear surgery include the system developed by Zhang and colleagues[19] for insertion of steerable CI electrode arrays. Yasin and colleagues[20] developed a teleoperated robot with a dexterous gripper demonstrating increased reachability and precision capabilities in the middle ear space. A teleoperated system that seems to be close to clinical implementation is from Technische Universität München and the Department of Otolaryngology from the University Hospital of Leipzig in Munich where they have built a teleoperated micromanipulator[21] that includes a 3 degree-of-freedom (DOF) manipulator controlled via a joystick similar to what is used in laboratories for control of micropipettes injecting into and/or extracting from individual cells. They have performed a clinical study showing decreased learning curve for stapedotomy.[22] The regulatory status of this project regarding clinical use is uncertain as of this writing.

Clinical implementation

To the best knowledge of the authors, the only teleoperated robot approved by a regulatory body for ear surgery is the RobOtol developed at Pierre and Marie Curie University in Paris, France and now offered commercially within the European Union by Collin Ltd (Bagnuex, France) with CE mark approval.[23] RobOtol (**Fig. 2**) consists of a platform placed on the opposite side of the patient as the surgeon (eg, where a scrub technician would typically stand) and has up to two effector arms (eg, endoscope and/or surgical instrument) that may be positioned by the surgeon using either a mouse and/or stylet interface. Motions can be scaled to accomplish gross versus microscopic motions. Initial clinical familiarity on simple procedures (eg, myringotomy and tube placement), is recommended before undertaking more challenging cases (eg, stapes surgery). A paper describing initial clinical use as an endoscope holder or microinstrument holder is under review as of this writing. Another potential[24] application of the RobOtol would be pairing with a force feedback control drill end effector allowing drilling of a stapedotomy or cochleostomy with minimal trauma to internal endosteum. Such technology was developed at Birmingham University in the United Kingdom,[25] and efficacy was dramatically demonstrated by drilling a hole in an uncooked egg without violating the membranous lining.[26]

Autonomous Surgical Robots

Autonomous robots are the types of robots that most people envision when they think of robots. Many would be surprised to learn that these autonomous robots have been used in surgical interventions for decades with first reports dating back to the mid-1980s when a neurosurgeon used an articulated robot arm to biopsy intracranial lesions.[10]

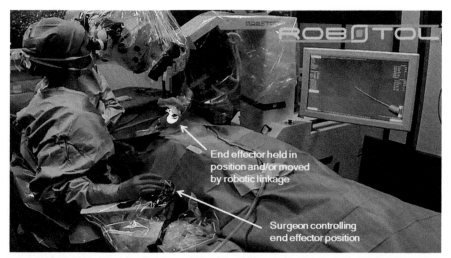

Fig. 2. Teleoperated RobOtol system. The surgeon sits opposite the robot that can hold an endoscope and/or an end effector, which is controlled via mouse and/or stylus. In this photograph, the surgeon is visualizing via the microscope and is moving an end effector (visible on the computer screen) with a mouse.

One area of otologic surgery where autonomous robots may bring value includes those robots that, in a semi- or fully automated fashion, drill the mastoid. Different groups have demonstrated drilling a minimally invasive tunnel to the cochlea with an autonomous robot either using an industrial arm robot with image guidance[27,28] or using a custom-built image-guided robotic system[4] (more later on clinical implementation of this robot). Autonomous robots can also be used to drill more of the mastoid than just a tunnel to the cochlea—they can perform a full mastoidectomy independently. For robotic mastoidectomy, the position of the robotically positioned drill tip relative to the patient's anatomy must be known. Position feedback can be provided by image guidance (eg, infrared tracking) or by rigidly linking the robot to the skull, creating a single rigid body from which drill tip calculations relative to anatomy can be made. First demonstration of image-guided, autonomous robotic mastoidectomy drilling was reported by Danilchenko and colleagues.[29] They modified an industrial-grade robot arm to hold a high-speed surgical drill. The robot, drill, and skull were tracked using an infrared image-guidance system. Although the system accomplished the task at hand, the need for line of sight of the tracked fiducial markers was made more difficult by the bone dust and irrigation that accumulated on the infrared markers. Another tracking system that does not require line of site is an electromagnetic tracking system, but this option does not currently support a level of tracking accuracy sufficient for this task. The need for line of sight tracking can be avoided by rigidly linking a robot to a patient's skull, and at least 2 groups have pursued this technique. Dillon and colleagues[30] developed a lightweight, 5 DOF (x, y, z, and rotation about 2 of these axes) robot (**Fig. 3**), which they used to drill translabyrinthine approaches to the internal auditory canal (IAC) in cadavers. The hypothesized advantage of this robot is that it performs the tedious bulk dissection of bone leaving a rim of bone over vital structures (eg, facial nerve, opening to the IAC) to be manually removed by a highly skilled, human surgeon. Similar work was done by Couldwell and colleagues[31] using a 5 DOF computer numeric control machine rigidly affixed to a cadaver by means of a Mayfield head holder.

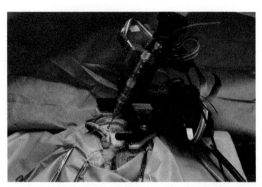

Fig. 3. Bone-affixed 5 DOF autonomous robot drilling translabyrinthine approach to IAC.

Autonomous robots also have great potential in insertion of CI electrode arrays. If a CI trajectory is specified, electrode array insertion can be largely reduced to linear advancement of the array along that trajectory especially for straight (a.k.a., lateral-wall) arrays. Such placement occurs at the limits of human perception with intracochlear trauma during insertion—including tip fold-over and translocation from scala tympani to scala vestibuli—occurring relatively frequently. For precurved (a.k.a., perimodiolar) electrode arrays, a second motion is necessary to stop stylet motion during insertion. These insertion motions can be automated by highly precise actuators such as those described[32] that consists of a linear advancement coupled with a stylet stop. Comparison of a modified version of this tool to manual, human insertion showed that although a human—at their best—may outperform the robot, the robotic insertion tool consistently and repeatably achieved very low insertion forces[33] likely to be associated with less intracochlear trauma and improved audiological outcomes[34] as compared with the human operator. The latest automated insertion tool from the RobOtol developers can be coupled to the RobOtol and has demonstrated smoother insertion force profiles compared with manual insertions.[37] Another automated linear tool that is nonmagnetic has been developed to be incorporated into a magnetic steering system meant to provide atraumatic insertion of magnet-tipped CI arrays.[36] Building on the aforementioned work of Zhang and colleagues[19] have developed a multi-DOF automated insertion solution using a parallel robot design that can be teleoperated or autonomous. This robot was initially designed and tested[35] and was the first robot to incorporate control feedback during CI insertion.[38] Perhaps the most unique of the CI electrode array insertion robots is one proposed to be surgically implanted in the mastoid, allowing slow insertion over hours or days and/or advancement of a hybrid CI electrode array if, over time, the patient's hearing were to further degrade.[39]

Clinical implementation

Caversaccio and colleagues[4] have clinical trials underway for their HEARO robot (**Fig. 4**), which has certification mark (CE) approval being offered by Cascination AG (Bern, Switzerland). Their approach uses a custom-built multiarticulated arm robot with image guidance to guide drilling from the surface of the mastoid through the facial recess during which the drill functions as a facial nerve stimulator with concurrent monitoring. Initially performed at University Hospital in Bern, Switzerland, they have now extended their study to Antwerp University in Belgium. The modularity of the

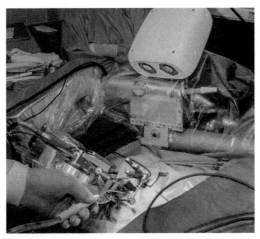

Fig. 4. HEARO system showing the IGS system (*white box* houses infrared tracking cameras) monitoring the robotic arm relative to the patient. The human hand is holding suction-irrigation clearing away debris so that humans can visualize the interaction between the end effector and the patient. (*From* PLoS One. 2019; 14(8): e0220543. Published online 2019 Aug 2. https://doi.org/10.1371/journal.pone.0220543.)

system allows for future expansion to include force-feedback drilling preserving endosteum (eg,[25]) and robotic CI electrode array insertion.

DISCUSSION

From an engineering standpoint, robotic interventions are obvious solutions to interventions that require high precision and border on the limits of human abilities. In the world of industrial manufacturing (eg, car assembly), robots are *preferred* over human operators, given the improved accuracy and reliability (ie, although robots occasionally need servicing, they can work 24 hours a day, 7 days a week, and do not have to deal with human stresses that can degrade operation). Why, then, have robots not been equally embraced within surgical realms, especially otology, where their utility doing high-precision work seems obvious? The answer to this question is complex but involves both inertia of existing behavior and uncertainty regarding regulatory approval processes.

Regarding inertia of existing behavior, ear surgery requires high manual dexterity skill levels that are acquired during lengthy training. Entry into the field is relatively exclusive with compensation and status commensurate with the training involved. This exclusivity may lead to conscious and/or unconscious bias in adopting technology that could lessen the exclusivity of these skill sets and allow less-experienced surgeons to be able to perform complex procedures without the need for lengthy, income-delaying training. This resistance to adoption of technology has been seen in other labor markets (eg, elevator operators who were obviated by the development of the automated elevator) and is typically overcome by economic incentives.

Regarding regulatory approval in the United States, highly automated systems, for example, autonomous surgical robots, are heavily regulated by the FDA. Although autonomous surgical robots have the potential for high impact in otology, such robots are highly disruptive to current surgical techniques and workflow, which can lead to delayed clinical adoption. A further barrier to their clinical implementation is stringent regulatory controls that are often prohibitively expensive to pursue especially by academic research teams. FDA compliance is achieved either by Premarket Notification 510(k) process in which a manufacturer can claim substantial equivalence to a device on the market before 1976 to be FDA-cleared or Premarket Approval (PMA) to be FDA approved. The 510(k) process is a much quicker and cheaper pathway for medical devices to reach clinical realization, and—not surprisingly—the pathway most often pursued especially in high-risk devices.[40] In contrast, the PMA pathway is much more costly, primarily due to the need for clinical testing. Relevant to surgical robots, the prototypical teleoperated manipulator, the da Vinci surgical system, was FDA cleared via the 510(k) pathway with a predicate device difficult to trace but likely either a manual retractor and/or and endoscope holder.[41] It is likely that autonomous otologic robots will require the much more costly PMA.

SUMMARY

Ultimately, as with most new behaviors within health care, innovations are adopted either because they have dramatic improvement in outcomes and/or because they provide similar results at a much-reduced cost compared with the current standard. Regarding robots for otologic interventions, otology is a relatively small field with good clinical outcomes. Clinical adoption of an otologic robot will require extensive investment by industry to obtain regulatory approval, intensive marketing to hospital administrators regarding increased through-put and/or decreased cost, and buy-in from highly trained otologists/neurotologists who may resist adoption of the technology. However, as is typical in capitalist economies such as the United States, over time, market forces largely dictate behaviors and are driven by often unforeseen occurrences (eg, the introduction of the Internet and electronic medical records). As of this writing, the world is dealing with the COVID19 pandemic that may push the adoption of otologic robots, allowing human surgeons to stay safely afar from potentially infectious debris.

CLINICS CARE POINTS

- Surgical robots have exciting potential in ear surgery but are not yet the standard of care.
- Most promising initial applications include cochlear implant and stapes surgery.
- Robots will only become standard of care if most of the ear surgeons deem them useful and/or necessary and if substantial regulatory hurdles are overcome.

DISCLOSURE

R.F. Labadie is a consultant for Advanced Bionics and Spiral Therapeutics. Funding Source Addition Grant received from National Science Foundation Graduate Research Fellowship DGE-1445197/1937963.

REFERENCES

1. Kratchman LB, Blachon GS, Withrow TJ, et al. Design of a bone-attached parallel robot for percutaneous cochlear implantation. IEEE Trans Biomed Eng 2011; 58(10 PART 1):2904–10.
2. Lim H, Matsumoto N, Cho B, et al. Semi-manual mastoidectomy assisted by human-robot collaborative control - A temporal bone replica study. Auris Nasus Larynx 2016;43(2):161–5.

3. Weinstein GS, O'Malley BW, Magnuson JS, et al. Transoral robotic surgery: A multicenter study to assess feasibility, safety, and surgical margins. Laryngoscope 2012;122(8):1701–7.

4. Caversaccio M, Wimmerid W, Ansoid J, et al. Robotic middle ear access for cochlear implantation: First in man. PLoS One 2019. https://doi.org/10.1371/journal.pone.0220543.

5. Kratchman LB, Schuster D, Dietrich MS, et al. Force perception thresholds in cochlear implantation surgery. Audiol Neurotol 2016;21(4):244–9.

6. Schuster D, Kratchman LB, Labadie RF. Characterization of intracochlear rupture forces in fresh human cadaveric cochleae. Otol Neurotol 2015;36(4):657–61.

7. Robot-based otological surgery- ClinicalKey. Available at: https://www.clinicalkey.com/#!/content/book/3-s2.0-B9782294760129000112. Accessed October 31, 2019.

8. O'Toole Bom Braga G, Schneider D, Weber S, et al. Computer assistance, image guidance, and robotics in otologic surgery. Thieme. doi:10.7892/BORIS.134224.

9. Brown RA. A stereotactic head frame for use with CT body scanners. Invest Radiol 1979;14(4):300–4.

10. Kwoh YS, Hou J, Jonckheere EA, et al. A robot with improved absolute positioning accuracy for CT guided stereotactic brain surgery. IEEE Trans Biomed Eng 1988;35(2):153–60.

11. Labadie RF, Balachandran R, Noble JH, et al. Minimally invasive image-guided cochlear implantation surgery: First report of clinical implementation. Laryngoscope 2014;124(8):1915–22.

12. Kobler JP, Nuelle K, Lexow GJ, et al. Configuration optimization and experimental accuracy evaluation of a bone-attached, parallel robot for skull surgery. Int J Comput Assist Radiol Surg 2016;11(3):421–36.

13. Yoo MH, Lee HS, Yang CJ, et al. A cadaver study of mastoidectomy using an image-guided human-robot collaborative control system. Laryngoscope Investig Otolaryngol 2017;2(5):208–14.

14. Taylor R, Jensen P, Whitcomb L, et al. A steady-hand robotic system for microsurgical augmentation. In: Lecture notes in computer science (including subseries lecture notes in artificial intelligence and lecture notes in bioinformatics), vol. 1679. Springer Verlag; 1999. p. 1031–41. https://doi.org/10.1007/10704282_112.

15. Wilkening P, Chien W, Gonenc B, et al. Evaluation of virtual fixtures for robot-assisted cochlear implant insertion. In: Proceedings of the IEEE RAS and EMBS International Conference on Biomedical Robotics and Biomechatronics. IEEE Computer Society. 2014. p. 332–8. 12-15 August, 2014, Sao Paulo, Brazil. https://doi.org/10.1109/biorob.2014.6913798.

16. Montes Grande G, Knisely AJ, Becker BC, et al. Handheld micromanipulator for robot-assisted stapes footplate surgery. In: Proceedings of the Annual International Conference of the IEEE Engineering in Medicine and Biology Society, EMBS. Vol. 2012. NIH Public Access. 2012. p. 1422–5. 28 August-1 September, 2012, San Diego, CA, USA. https://doi.org/10.1109/EMBC.2012.6346206.

17. Balachandran R, Tsai BS, Ramachandra T, et al. Minimally invasive image-guided access for drainage of Petrous apex lesions: A case report. Otol Neurotol 2014; 35(4):649–55.

18. Liu WP, Azizian M, Sorger J, et al. Cadaveric feasibility study of da Vinci Si-assisted cochlear implant with augmented visual navigation for otologic surgery. JAMA Otolaryngol Head Neck Surg 2014;140(3):208–14.

19. Zhang J, Wei W, Ding J, et al. Inroads toward robot-assisted cochlear implant surgery using steerable electrode arrays. Otol Neurotol 2010;31(8):1199–206.

20. Yasin R, O'Connell BP, Yu H, et al. Steerable robot-assisted micromanipulation in the middle ear. Otol Neurotol 2017;38(2):290–5.
21. Strauß G, Maier T, Krinninger M, et al. Clinical use of a micromanipulator: First experience in middle ear and temporal bone surgery. HNO 2012;60(9):807–13.
22. Maier T, Strauss G, Scholz M, et al. A new evaluation and training system for micro-telemanipulation at the middle ear. In: Proceedings of the Annual International Conference of the IEEE Engineering in Medicine and Biology Society, EMBS. 2012. p. 932–5. 28 August-1 September, 2012, San Diego, CA, USA. https://doi.org/10.1109/EMBC.2012.6346085.
23. Nguyen Y, Bernardeschi D, Sterkers O. Potential of robot-based surgery for otosclerosis surgery. Otolaryngol Clin North Am 2018;51(2):475–85.
24. Vittoria S, Lahlou G, Torres R, et al. Robot-based assistance in middle ear surgery and cochlear implantation: first clinical report. European Archives of Oto-rhino-laryngology: Official Journal of the European Federation of Oto-rhino-laryngological Societies (EUFOS): 2020.
25. Coulson CJ, Zoka Assadi M, Taylor RP, et al. A smart micro-drill for cochleostomy formation: A comparison of cochlear disturbances with manual drilling and a human trial. Cochlear Implants Int 2013;14(2):98–106.
26. Brett P, Du X, Zoka-Assadi M, et al. Feasibility study of a hand guided robotic drill for cochleostomy. BioMed research international: 2014.
27. Majdani O, Rau TS, Baron S, et al. A robot-guided minimally invasive approach for cochlear implant surgery: Preliminary results of a temporal bone study. Int J Comput Assist Radiol Surg 2009;4(5):475–86.
28. Baron S, Eilers H, Munske B, et al. Percutaneous inner-ear access via an image-guided industrial robot system. Proc Inst Mech Eng H J Eng Med 2010;224(5): 633–49.
29. Danilchenko A, Balachandran R, Toennies JL, et al. Robotic mastoidectomy. Otol Neurotol 2011;32(1):11–6.
30. Dillon NP, Balachandran R, Siebold MA, et al. Cadaveric testing of robot-assisted access to the internal auditory canal for vestibular schwannoma removal. Otol Neurotol 2017;38(3):441–7.
31. Couldwell WT, MacDonald JD, Thomas CL, et al. Computer-aided design/computer-aided manufacturing skull base drill. Neurosurg Focus 2017;42(5). https://doi.org/10.3171/2017.2.FOCUS16561.
32. Hussong A, Rau T, Eilers H, et al. Conception and design of an automated insertion tool for cochlear implants. In: 2008 30th Annual International Conference of the IEEE Engineering in Medicine and Biology Society. Vol. 2008. IEEE. 2008. p. 5593–6. 20-25 August, 2008, Vancouver, BC, Canada. https://doi.org/10.1109/IEMBS.2008.4650482
33. Majdani O, Schurzig D, Hussong A, et al. Force measurement of insertion of cochlear implant electrode arrays in vitro: comparison of surgeon to automated insertion tool. Acta Otolaryngol 2010;130(1):31–6.
34. Carlson ML, Driscoll CLW, Gifford RH, et al. Implications of minimizing trauma during conventional cochlear implantation. Otol Neurotol 2011;32(6):962–8.
35. Nguyen Y, Kazmitcheff G, De Seta D, et al. Definition of metrics to evaluate cochlear array insertion forces performed with forceps, insertion tool, or motorized tool in temporal bone specimens. Biomed Res Int 2014;2014. https://doi.org/10.1155/2014/532570.
36. Bruns TL, Riojas KE, Ropella DS, et al. Magnetically steered robotic insertion of cochlear-implant electrode arrays: system integration and first-in-cadaver results. IEEE Robot Autom Lett 2020;5(2):2240–7.

37. Pile J, Simaan N. Modeling, design, and evaluation of a parallel robot for cochlear implant surgery. IEEE ASME Trans Mechatron 2014;19(6):1746–55.
38. Pile J, Wanna GB, Simaan N. Robot-assisted perception augmentation for online detection of insertion failure during cochlear implant surgery. Robotica 2017; 35(7):1598–615.
39. Kaufmann CR, Henslee AM, Claussen A, et al. Evaluation of insertion forces and cochlea trauma following robotics-assisted cochlear implant electrode array insertion. Otol Neurotol 2020;1. https://doi.org/10.1097/mao.0000000000002608.
40. Zuckerman DM, Brown P, Nissen SE. Medical device recalls and the FDA approval process. Arch Intern Med 2011;171(11):1006–11.
41. Lefkovich C. The use of predicates in FDA regulation of medical devices: a case study of robotic surgical devices. 2018. . Available at: https://scholarworks.rit.edu/theses/9895. Accessed April 13, 2020.

Robotic Skull Base Surgery

Mitchell Heuermann, MD[a], Alex P. Michael, MD[b],
Dana L. Crosby, MD, MPH[a],*

KEYWORDS

- Skull base • Sinonasal • Robotic surgery • Robotic skull base
- Transoral robotic surgery

KEY POINTS

- Robotic surgery has made an important impact in head and neck surgery, although its use in skull base surgery has been limited.
- Current approaches to the anterior and central skull base remain fundamentally limited by robotic systems that were never designed to navigate the intricate, delicate anatomy of the skull base.
- New robotic technology is in development to address the current technical limitations of existing robotic systems.
- Cost, safety, and clinical outcomes need to be factored into the indications for usage of robotics in skull base surgery.

INTRODUCTION

Robotic surgery has had a significant impact on multiple surgical specialties and has gained wide usage since the introduction of the da Vinci robotic system (Intuitive Surgical, Sunnyvale, CA) in the early 2000s.[1] Head and neck surgeons have adopted it for use in transoral robotic surgery (TORS) of the oropharynx, hypopharynx,[2] and approaches have also been described for laryngectomy,[3,4] parapharyngeal space tumors,[5] thyroidectomy,[6,7] and neck dissections.[8] Compared with open procedures, TORS procedures promote less-invasive surgical approaches, better visualization of critical structures,[9] and faster operating times.[10] TORS has also been shown to result in better postoperative swallow function,[11] faster recovery, higher rate of margin negativity, and shorter hospital stays[12] than open procedures. Similarly, robotic thyroid procedures have shown improved postoperative pain, swallow, and cosmesis.[6,7]

Despite early success in other areas of the head and neck, the use of robotics in the anterior and central skull base has been limited to date. Several surgical robots have been repurposed for use in skull base surgery, but none are currently marketed or

[a] Department of Otolaryngology–Head and Neck Surgery, SIU School of Medicine, 720 North Bond Street, Springfield, IL 62702, USA; [b] Division of Neurosurgery, Neuroscience Institute, SIU School of Medicine, PO Box 19638, Springfield, IL 62794-9638, USA
* Corresponding author.
E-mail address: dcrosby53@siumed.edu

Otolaryngol Clin N Am 53 (2020) 1077–1089
https://doi.org/10.1016/j.otc.2020.07.015
0030-6665/20/© 2020 Elsevier Inc. All rights reserved.

oto.theclinics.com

designed specifically for the skull base. This has imposed limitations, largely because of the discrepancy between the size and maneuverability of current robotic instruments and the small confines of the anterior skull base. Nevertheless, several approaches have been investigated in cadaveric and human studies that use current robotic technology. These include pure transoral, transnasal, transantral, and transcervical approaches, and combinations thereof. This article reviews the currently available surgical robot technologies and their role in anterior and middle skull base surgery.

CURRENT ROBOTIC TECHNOLOGY
Surgical Robots

The da Vinci robot has become the prototypical and most widely used surgical robot to date. It was first approved for use in 2000 and acquired Food and Drug Administration approval for otolaryngologic surgery in 2009.[13] It has undergone several iterations since its inception (**Table 1**), and is currently controlled by a separate surgeon console that integrates the movement of four rigid arms, three for active instrumentation and one to hold and maneuver the endoscope. Its most recent iteration, the da Vinci SP, notably allows instrumentation through a single 25-mm port as opposed to independent placement of the arms with previous iterations.

To solve the flexibility issues that the da Vinci system faced, the Flex System (Medrobotics, Raynham, MA) was developed and Food and Drug Administration–approved in 2017 for "access to the oropharynx, hypopharynx, and larynx."[19] It features two 3-mm flexible instruments on both sides of a flexible endoscope, all of which are capable of three-dimensional movement (**Fig. 1**). The endoscope is controlled robotically, whereas the instruments are controlled manually. Unlike the da Vinci system, the Flex System does have limited haptic feedback, but only displays images in two dimensions.[19] Despite the size reduction, this system is still too large to perform traditional endonasal surgery.

Given the size and functionality limitations of existing surgical robots, experimental systems are in development. The SmartArm (Department of Mechanical Engineering, The University of Tokyo, Tokyo, Japan) was designed specifically for endonasal surgery, particularly suturing at the skull base (**Fig. 2**). This system features haptic feedback, 3-mm flexible working tools with 9° of freedom, and a 4-mm endoscope.[20] Wurm and colleagues[21] developed a fully automated robot, featuring an endoscope, drill capable of speeds up to 40,000 RPM, and two ports for irrigation and suction, all within a single 5-mm arm (**Fig. 3**).[22] A novel robotic system being developed by Vanderbilt University features four robotic arms based on a series of tiny concentric tubes, which allow for greater maneuverability along a nonlinear course, making them better suited for pure endonasal surgery (**Fig. 4**).[23–26] This system features arms measuring 2.32 mm in greatest diameter and instruments measuring up to 1.75 mm in diameter, although at present does not support haptic feedback or wristed instruments.[25] It has even been suggested that the concentric tube arms could be custom made for each patient based on their anatomy.[27]

Surgically Assistive Robots

Surgically assistive robots, although not effectors of the surgery itself, aid the surgeon in one or more aspects of the procedure. In the context of skull base surgery, this is usually in the form of an instrument holder or surgically assistive devices. These include the ROVOT-m (Synaptive Medical Corporation, Toronto, Canada),[28] Endoscope Robot (Medineering Surgical Robots, Munich, Germany),[29–31] SoloAssist

Table 1
The da Vinci system in its various iterations, including year of release, number of arms (including instrumentation and camera), and changes compared with prior iterations

Iteration	Released	Arms	Improvements Over Prior Iteration
Standard	2000	3	4th arm added in 2002[14]
S	2006	4	Improved range of motion; improved docking[15]
Si	2009	4	Higher definition camera; second teaching console; single-site surgery using curved trocars[16]
Xi	2014	4	Slimmer, boom-mounted arms; improved maneuverability and reach; integration with operating tables[17]
X	2017	4	Lower purchase cost; no boom-mounting or operating table integration[17]
SP	2018	4	All instruments operate through single 25-mm port[18]

Data from Refs.[14–18]

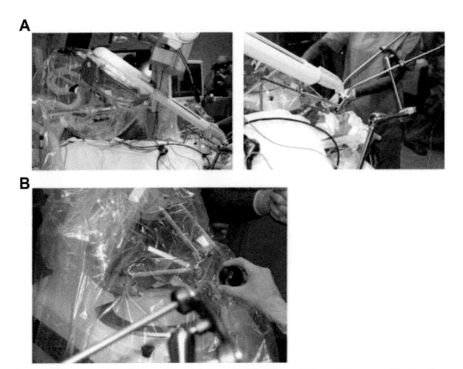

Fig. 1. (*A*) Setup and docking using an integrated flexible robotic endoscope with two flexible instrument arms. (*B*) Control arm for the flexible endoscope. (*Adapted from* Mandapathil M, Duvvuri U, Güldner C, et al. Transoral surgery for oropharyngeal tumors using the Medrobotics® Flex® System – a case report. Int J Surg Case Rep. 2015;10:173-175; with permission.)

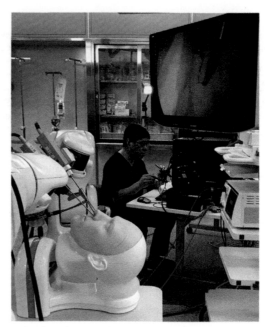

Fig. 2. Setup of a novel robot designed for pure transnasal skull base work. (*From* Marinho MM, Harada K, Morita A, et al. SmartArm: Integration and validation of a versatile surgical robotic system for constrained workspaces. Int J Med Robotics Comput Assist Surg. January 2020:e2053; with permission.)

endoscope holder (AKTORmed Robotic Surgery, Barbing, Germany),[32] the now defunct voice-operated or eye movement–operated AESOP system,[33,34] and other experimental assistive robotic systems.[35] Similarly, the iArmS system automatically follows and supports the surgeon's arm during microdissection helping reduce fatigue and enabling more accurate, fluid motion for long-duration cases.[36]

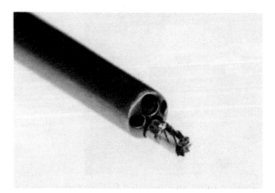

Fig. 3. An example of an integrated robot arm, comprising a drill, endoscope, and two ports for irrigation and suction. (*From* Wurm J, Bumm K, Steinhart H, et al. Entwicklung eines aktiven Robotersystems für die multimodale Chirurgie der Nasennebenhöhlen. HNO. 2005;53(5):446-454; with permission.)

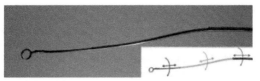

Fig. 4. A representative arm of a concentric tube robot. *Inset image* details the axes of motion for each tube for a three-tube system. (*From* Swaney P, Gilbert H, Webster R, et al. Endonasal Skull Base Tumor Removal Using Concentric Tube Continuum Robots: A Phantom Study. J Neurol Surg B Skull Base. 2014;76(02):145-149; with permission.)

CURRENT SURGICAL APPROACHES

Until recently, most robotic head and neck surgery was limited to use of the da Vinci system. Given the limitations inherent to this system when used for skull base surgery, most studies to date have focused on alternative routes of access for rigid-arm robotic systems.

MULTIORIFICE APPROACHES

The slow adoption of surgical robotics to pure transnasal skull base surgery is likely from smaller diameter of the nostril compared with other natural orifices and design limitation of the da Vinci system that prevent physical interference with the camera and the surgical arms. As such, transnasal access using the da Vinci robot has been limited to a single working endoscopic port while other natural or artificial orifices are used.

Combined Transantral-Transnasal

The feasibility of using surgical robots to access the anterior skull base was first shown in 2007 in a series of four cadaveric specimens.[37] Access was based on bilateral Caldwell-Luc maxillary antrostomies, middle meatal maxillary antrostomies, and posterior septectomy, with placement of the da Vinci arms transantrally and the endoscope transnasally (**Fig. 5**). The authors were then able to surgically access the cribriform plate, planum sphenoidale, sella turcica, and parasellar regions. This approach has been further replicated in other cadaver studies for access to the nasopharynx,[38] sella and cavernous sinus,[39] and infratemporal fossa.[40] To date, there are no reports in the literature using any of these techniques in live patients.

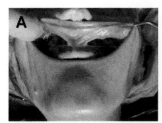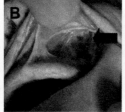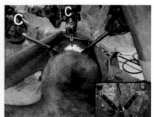

Fig. 5. An example of the transantral approach. (*A*) Bilateral vestibular incisions to expose the anteroinferior maxilla. (*B*) Infraorbital nerve (*black arrow*) relative to surgical field. (*C*) Setup of two robotic instrument arms through maxillary antrostomies and the endoscope transnasally. (*From* Kupferman ME, Hanna E. Robotic Surgery of the Skull Base. Otolaryngol Clin North Am. 2014;47(3):415-423; with permission.)

Combined Transoral-Transnasal

One of the major limitations of pure transoral approaches is the lack of drilling equipment for currently available robotic systems. As such, traditional endonasal instrumentation is often needed to help traverse the bony skull base. This approach has been described in cadaver[41,42] and in live patients for access to the nasopharynx[43,44] and clivus.[42]

Combined Transcervical Approaches

To overcome access limitations of traditional TORS for nasopharyngeal procedures, a group from the University of Pennsylvania described a modified approach (C-TORS) in a cadaver model, in which robotic instrumentation trocars are placed transcervically posterior to the submandibular gland (**Fig. 6**). These terminate in the lateral hypopharynx, and allow access to the nasopharynx, clivus, sphenoid, sella, and anterior fossa.[45,46] Dallan and colleagues[47] described a similar success in a cadaver model with endonasal visualization rather than transoral. McCool and colleagues[48] described a modified approach in a cadaver using two transoral ports and one suprahyoid port for improved access to the infratemporal fossa.

SINGLE-ORIFICE APPROACHES
Transoral

Early pure transoral approaches (**Fig. 7**) to the skull base with the four-arm da Vinci system used a midline or lateral soft palate split for improved access. These have been described in cadaver studies,[49,50] and in several live patients with nasopharyngeal[43,51,52] and infratemporal fossa[53] tumors. By gaining exposure through the hard palate, Ozer and colleagues[54] were able to access the skull base from crista galli to C1. Although splitting the palate dramatically improves surgical access, it carries with it the risk of oronasal fistula formation and scar contracture leading to velopharyngeal insufficiency.[18]

With the reduction in size of the da Vinci arms from 8 mm to 5 mm, cadaver studies have shown the feasibility of nonpalate split transoral approaches to the

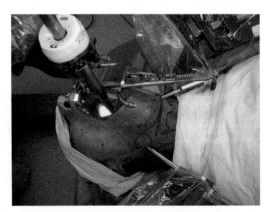

Fig. 6. An example setup of C-TORS, with the two working robotic arms placed transcervically just posterior to the submandibular glands (*outlined*), and the endoscope placed transorally. (*From* O'Malley BW, Weinstein GS. Robotic Anterior and Midline Skull Base Surgery: Preclinical Investigations. Int J Radiat Oncol Biol Phys. 2007;69(2):S125-S128; with permission.)

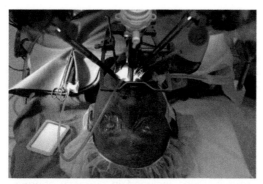

Fig. 7. Setup for a pure transoral approach using one 30° endoscope and two wristed instrument arms. (*From* Newman JG, Kuppersmith RB, O'Malley BW. Robotics and Telesurgery in Otolaryngology. Otolaryngol Clin North Am. 2011;44(6):1317-1331; with permission.)

nasopharynx,[55] sella,[56] infratemporal fossa, and clivus.[46] With the development of the da Vinci SP model, access to the nasopharynx was explored by Tsang and Holsinger with excellent exposure.[18] Nonpalate split approaches have been validated in live patients for access to the infratemporal fossa,[45] sella,[57] and clivus.[58] Access to the nasopharynx using the Flex System has also been demonstrated in cadaver studies,[59,60] although there exist no published studies of its use in live patients.

Transnasal

The transnasal endoscopic approach is currently the preferred method of accessing the anterior skull base, clivus, sella, and parasellar regions. Given the size of currently available robotic systems, published studies on pure transnasal robotic approaches have been comparatively few, limited to a single cadaver study using the Flex System. This approach, however, required partial midface degloving, partial nasal septectomy, and partial removal of the maxillary frontal processes for complete visualization.[61] Nevertheless, this approach allowed access to all paranasal sinuses and wide access to the anterior skull base, sella, clivus, and posterior cranial fossa.

Supraorbital

Hong and colleagues[62] explored the possibility of access to the anterior skull base from above using a supraorbital keyhole craniotomy in a cadaver model, and found adequate exposure and maneuverability for work in the anterior skull base, including suturing. Marcus and colleagues,[63] however, reported conflicting results when a 25-mm keyhole was made and concluded that robotic access was not safe with the da Vinci system because of the bulk of the instruments and camera.

BENEFITS

Compared with endoscopy, robotic-assisted skull base surgery with the da Vinci affords enhanced three-dimensional visualization. This alone may enable improved surgical precision. The da Vinci endowrist allows greater flexibility than what is achieved by the human hand leading to better maneuverability around angled bony structures. Similarly, the enhanced fine motor control of the Da Vinci robotic arms makes suture repair of the dura possible.[36] Robotic surgery can eliminate the issues commonly encountered in traditional four-hand transnasal endoscopic surgery, such as fatigue and tremor. The narrow surgical corridors encountered in endoscopic skull base approaches leads to frequent conflicts between instruments and endoscopes. This may be lessened with alternative robotic approaches with wristed instrumentation. Additionally, the ergonomically designed surgeon's console integrates control of all of the robotic arms, offering the surgeon complete control of the camera and three working instruments. Finally, the newer da Vinci models have the option of using dual consoles, which allows seamless transfer of functions to a second surgeon or allow instruction of a student.[64,65]

LIMITATIONS

Major limitations for incorporation of robotics into skull base surgery still exist. One main drawback is lack of instruments designed for delicate skull base procedures.[64,66] Specifically, the instrumentations included in currently approved devices do not include a drill for skull base bone work.[67] Furthermore, the adoption of surgical robotics to pure transnasal surgery has been limited by the smaller diameter of the nostril compared with other natural orifices, and design limitations of the da Vinci system, which require the surgical arms to be aligned at a minimum of 20° to each other to avoid physical interference with themselves and the camera.[68] Because of these design limitations, a direct approach via a transnasal route is currently impossible. Additionally, the currently available robots do not support integration with image-guidance systems. Lack of haptic feedback for da Vinci instrument contact can prove dangerous, especially when working with delicate structure of the skull base, although this may be offset by exceptional three-dimensional optics afforded by the robot.[64,69] Emerging robotic technologies, such as concentric tube robots, may solve many of these limitations. A cost comparison analysis of robotic head and neck surgery to traditional approaches has not yet been performed, although literature from other specialties generally agree that the cost of robotic surgery is higher because of surgical supply and operating room costs.[70,71] Whether these costs carry with them reduced complication rates, shorter recovery, and improved oncologic control remains to be seen. Furthermore, as with all new technology, there is a significant learning curve especially for surgeons who are otherwise not familiar with robotic technology.[10,72] Adequate training and proficiency before clinical use is paramount to success.

FUTURE DIRECTIONS

With new robotic technologies in development, it is important to develop systems that are safe, versatile, durable, and that provide advantage over traditional surgical approaches. To this end, an ideal robot for use in skull base surgery would be entirely endonasal; be compatible with image guidance; move intuitively with the surgeon's movements; use a self-cleaning endoscope; and allow simultaneous use of multiple instruments that are small, flexible, durable, easily exchangeable, and capable of haptic feedback.[73,74] Clinical trials to date have been limited,[75] but are of paramount importance to show that robotic procedures can be done safely and provide measurable improvement in patient outcomes and quality of life to justify their increased costs. Robotic surgery brings with it the possibility of long-distance telesurgery, although implementation of this has been limited in otolaryngology.[76,77]

SUMMARY

Although TORS has made an important impact in head and neck surgery, robotic skull base surgery is comparatively in its infancy. Although successful access to the anterior skull base has been shown through several approaches, these approaches remain fundamentally limited by systems that were never designed to navigate the intricate, delicate anatomy of the skull base. These limitations are likely to be overcome in the future with the development of specifically designed robotic systems, although cost, safety, and patient outcomes all need to be factored into the indications for their use.

CLINICS CARE POINTS

- No currently available surgical system is approved for use in the skull base
- Several experimental approaches to the skull base with existing surgical robots have been described but are generally not considered to be the current standard of care
- Effective robotic surgery at the anterior and central skull base will likely require new robotic systems or dramatic changes in existing systems
- Novel robotic systems are currently being developed specifically for use in the skull base

DISCLOSURE

The authors have nothing to disclose.

REFERENCES

1. Lane T. A short history of robotic surgery. Ann R Coll Surg Engl 2018; 100(6_sup):5–7.
2. Dias FL, Walder F, Leonhardt FD. The role of transoral robotic surgery in the management of oropharyngeal cancer. Curr Opin Oncol 2017;29(3):166–71.
3. Mendelsohn AH, Remacle M. Transoral robotic surgery for laryngeal cancer. Curr Opin Otolaryngol Head Neck Surg 2015;23(2):148–52.
4. Dowthwaite S, Nichols AC, Yoo J, et al. Transoral robotic total laryngectomy: report of 3 cases. Head Neck 2013;35(11):E338–42.
5. O'Malley BW, Quon H, Leonhardt FD, et al. Transoral robotic surgery for parapharyngeal space tumors. ORL J Otorhinolaryngol Relat Spec 2010;72(6):332–6.
6. Lee J, Nah KY, Kim RM, et al. Differences in postoperative outcomes, function, and cosmesis: open versus robotic thyroidectomy. Surg Endosc 2010;24(12): 3186–94.
7. Kang S-W, Jeong JJ, Yun J-S, et al. Robot-assisted endoscopic surgery for thyroid cancer: experience with the first 100 patients. Surg Endosc 2009;23(11): 2399–406.
8. Lee HS, Kim WS, Hong HJ, et al. Robot-assisted supraomohyoid neck dissection via a modified face-lift or retroauricular approach in early-stage cN0 squamous cell carcinoma of the oral cavity: a comparative study with conventional technique. Ann Surg Oncol 2012;19(12):3871–8.
9. O'Malley BW, Weinstein GS, Snyder W, et al. Transoral robotic surgery (TORS) for base of tongue neoplasms. Laryngoscope 2006;116(8):1465–72.
10. Lawson G, Matar N, Remacle M, et al. Transoral robotic surgery for the management of head and neck tumors: learning curve. Eur Arch Otorhinolaryngol 2011; 268(12):1795–801.
11. Hutcheson KA, Holsinger FC, Kupferman ME, et al. Functional outcomes after TORS for oropharyngeal cancer: a systematic review. Eur Arch Otorhinolaryngol 2015;272(2):463–71.

12. Lee SY, Park YM, Byeon HK, et al. Comparison of oncologic and functional outcomes after transoral robotic lateral oropharyngectomy versus conventional surgery for T1 to T3 tonsillar cancer. Head Neck 2014;36(8):1138–45.
13. U.S. Food and Drug Administration (FDA). Center for Devices and Radiological Health (CDRH). Notice to Intuitive Surgical, Inc. K090993. Trade/Device Name: da Vinci, da Vinci S and da Vinci Si Surgical System and EndoWrist SP Instruments, and Accessories. Silver Spring (MD): FDA. December 9AD. May 31, 2018.
14. Shah J, Vyas A, Vyas D. The history of robotics in surgical specialties. Am J Robot Surg 2014;1(1):12–20.
15. Shah K, Abaza R. Comparison of intraoperative outcomes using the new and old generation da Vinci robot for robot-assisted laparoscopic prostatectomy. BJU Int 2011;108(10):1642–5.
16. Intuitive Surgical, Inc. da Vinci Si/Si-e. da Vinci Surgery Community. 2020.
17. Azizian M, Liu M, Khalaji I, et al. The da Vinci Surgical System. In: Abedin-Nasab MH, editor. Handbook of robotic and image-guided surgery. Elsevier; 2020. p. 39–55.
18. Tsang RK, Holsinger FC. Transoral endoscopic nasopharyngectomy with a flexible next-generation robotic surgical system: robotic nasopharyngectomy with a flexible robot. Laryngoscope 2016;126(10):2257–62.
19. U.S. Food and Drug Administration (FDA), Center for Devices and Radiological Health (CDRH). Notice to Medrobotics Corporation. K170453. Trade/device Name: Medrobotics Flex robotic system. Silver Spring (MD): FDA; 2017.
20. Marinho MM, Harada K, Morita A, et al. SmartArm: integration and validation of a versatile surgical robotic system for constrained workspaces. Int J Med Robot 2020;16:e2053.
21. Wurm J, Bumm K, Steinhart H, et al. Entwicklung eines aktiven Robotersystems für die multimodale Chirurgie der Nasennebenhöhlen. HNO 2005;53(5):446–54.
22. Bumm K, Wurm J, Rachinger J, et al. An automated robotic approach with redundant navigation for minimal invasive extended transsphenoidal skull base surgery. Minim Invasive Neurosurg 2005;48(3):159–64.
23. Swaney P, Gilbert H, Webster R, et al. Endonasal skull base tumor removal using concentric tube continuum robots: a phantom study. J Neurol Surg B Skull Base 2014;76(02):145–9.
24. Swaney PJ, Croom JM, Burgner J, et al. Design of a quadramanual robot for single-nostril skull base surgery. In: ASME Dynamic Systems and Control Conference. Meeting held at October 17–19, 2012. Florida, USA: Fort Lauterdale; 2012. p. 387–93.
25. Burgner J, Rucker DC, Gilbert HB, et al. A telerobotic system for transnasal surgery. IEEE ASME Trans Mechatron 2014;19(3):996–1006.
26. Gilbert H, Hendrick R, Remirez A, et al. A robot for transnasal surgery featuring needle-sized tentacle-like arms. Expert Rev Med Devices 2014;11(1):5–7.
27. Morimoto TK, Greer JD, Hsieh MH, et al. Surgeon design interface for patient-specific concentric tube robots. In: 2016 6th IEEE International Conference on Biomedical Robotics and Biomechatronics (BioRob). Meeting held at June 26–29. Singapore: University Town; 2016. p. 41–8.
28. Kassam AB, Rovin RA, Walia S, et al. The operating room of the future versus the future of the operating room. Otolaryngol Clin North Am 2017;50(3):655–71.
29. Zappa F, Mattavelli D, Madoglio A, et al. Hybrid robotics for endoscopic skull base surgery: preclinical evaluation and surgeon first impression. World Neurosurg 2019;134:e572–80.

30. Mattheis S, Schlüter A, Stähr K, et al. First use of a new robotic endoscope guiding system in endoscopic orbital decompression. Ear Nose Throat J 2019. https://doi.org/10.1177/0145561319885803.
31. Friedrich DT, Sommer F, Scheithauer MO, et al. An innovate robotic endoscope guidance system for transnasal sinus and skull base surgery: proof of concept. J Neurol Surg B Skull Base 2017;78(6):466–72.
32. Kristin J, Kolmer A, Kraus P, et al. Development of a new endoscope holder for head and neck surgery: from the technical design concept to implementation. Eur Arch Otorhinolaryngol 2015;272(5):1239–44.
33. Nathan C-AO, Chakradeo V, Malhotra K, et al. The voice-controlled robotic assist scope holder AESOP for the endoscopic approach to the sella. Skull Base 2006; 16(3):123–31.
34. Ali SM, Reisner LA, King B, et al. Eye gaze tracking for endoscopic camera positioning: an application of a hardware/software interface developed to automate Aesop. Stud Health Technol Inform 2008;132:4–7.
35. Bolzoni Villaret A, Doglietto F, Carobbio A, et al. Robotic transnasal endoscopic skull base surgery: systematic review of the literature and report of a novel prototype for a hybrid system (Brescia endoscope assistant robotic holder). World Neurosurg 2017;105:875–83.
36. Ogiwara T, Goto T, Nagm A, et al. Endoscopic endonasal transsphenoidal surgery using the iArmS operation support robot: initial experience in 43 patients. Neurosurg Focus 2017;42(5):E10.
37. Hanna EY, Holsinger C, DeMonte F, et al. Robotic endoscopic surgery of the skull base: a novel surgical approach. Arch Otolaryngol Head Neck Surg 2007; 133(12):1209–14.
38. Cho H-J, Kang JW, Min HJ, et al. Robotic nasopharyngectomy via combined endonasal and transantral port: a preliminary cadaveric study: robotic nasopharyngectomy. Laryngoscope 2015;125(8):1839–43.
39. Kupferman M, DeMonte F, Holsinger FC, et al. Transantral robotic access to the pituitary gland. Otolaryngol Head Neck Surg 2009;141(3):413–5.
40. Blanco RGF, Boahene K. Robotic-assisted skull base surgery: preclinical study. J Laparoendosc Adv Surg Tech A 2013;23(9):776–82.
41. Tsang RKY, Ho WK, Wei WI. Combined transnasal endoscopic and transoral robotic resection of recurrent nasopharyngeal carcinoma. Head Neck 2011;34(8): 1190–3.
42. Carrau RL, Prevedello DM, de Lara D, et al. Combined transoral robotic surgery and endoscopic endonasal approach for the resection of extensive malignancies of the skull base: combined TORS and EEA for resection of extensive malignancies of skull base. Head Neck 2013;35(11):E351–8.
43. Tsang RK, To VS, Ho AC, et al. Early results of robotic assisted nasopharyngectomy for recurrent nasopharyngeal carcinoma: early results of robotic nasopharyngectomy. Head Neck 2015;37(6):788–93.
44. Sreenath SB, Rawal RB, Zanation AM. The combined endonasal and transoral approach for the management of skull base and nasopharyngeal pathology: a case series. Neurosurg Focus 2014;37(4):E2.
45. O'Malley BW, Weinstein GS. Robotic anterior and midline skull base surgery: preclinical investigations. Int J Radiat Oncol Biol Phys 2007;69(2):S125–8.
46. Lee JYK, O'Malley BW Jr, Newman JG, et al. Transoral robotic surgery of the skull base: a cadaver and feasibility study. ORL J Otorhinolaryngol Relat Spec 2010; 72(4):181–7.

47. Dallan I, Castelnuovo P, Seccia V, et al. Combined transnasal transcervical robotic dissection of posterior skull base: feasibility in a cadaveric model. Rhinology 2012;50(2):165–70.

48. McCool RR, Warren FM, Wiggins RH, et al. Robotic surgery of the infratemporal fossa utilizing novel suprahyoid port. Laryngoscope 2010;120(9):1738–43.

49. Ozer E, Waltonen J. Transoral robotic nasopharyngectomy: a novel approach for nasopharyngeal lesions. Laryngoscope 2008;118(9):1613–6.

50. Fernandez-Nogueras FJJ, Katati MJ, Arraez Sanchez MA, et al. Transoral robotic surgery of the central skull base: preclinical investigations. Eur Arch Otorhinolaryngol 2014;271(6):1759–63.

51. Wei WI, Ho W-K. Transoral robotic resection of recurrent nasopharyngeal carcinoma. Laryngoscope 2010;120(10):2011–4.

52. Tsang RKY, Ho W-K, Wei WI, et al. Transoral robotic assisted nasopharyngectomy via a lateral palatal flap approach. Laryngoscope 2013;123(9):2180–3.

53. Kim GG, Zanation AM. Transoral robotic surgery to resect skull base tumors via transpalatal and lateral pharyngeal approaches. Laryngoscope 2012;122(7): 1575–8.

54. Ozer E, Durmus K, Carrau RL, et al. Applications of transoral, transcervical, transnasal, and transpalatal corridors for robotic surgery of the skull base: robotic approaches to the skull base. Laryngoscope 2013;123(9):2176–9.

55. Harichane A, Chauvet D, Hans S. Nasopharynx access by minimally invasive transoral robotic surgery: anatomical study. J Robot Surg 2018;12(4):687–92.

56. Chauvet D, Missistrano A, Hivelin M, et al. Transoral robotic-assisted skull base surgery to approach the sella turcica: cadaveric study. Neurosurg Rev 2014; 37(4):609–17.

57. Chauvet D, Hans S, Missistrano A, et al. Transoral robotic surgery for sellar tumors: first clinical study. J Neurosurg 2017;127(4):941–8.

58. Henry LE, Haugen TW, Rassekh CH, et al. A novel transpalatal-transoral robotic surgery approach to clival chordomas extending into the nasopharynx. Head Neck 2019;41(8):E133–40.

59. Richmon JD. Transoral palate-sparing nasopharyngectomy with the Flex System: preclinical study: transoral palate-sparing Nasopharyngectomy. Laryngoscope 2015;125(2):318–22.

60. Schuler PJ, Hoffmann TK, Duvvuri U, et al. Demonstration of nasopharyngeal surgery with a single port operator-controlled flexible endoscope system: flexible nasopharyngeal surgery. Head Neck 2016;38(3):370–4.

61. Schuler PJ, Scheithauer M, Rotter N, et al. A single-port operator-controlled flexible endoscope system for endoscopic skull base surgery. HNO 2015;63(3): 189–94.

62. Hong W-C, Tsai J-C, Chang SD, et al. Robotic skull base surgery via supraorbital keyhole approach: a cadaveric study. Neurosurgery 2013;72:A33–8.

63. Marcus HJ, Hughes-Hallett A, Cundy TP, et al. da Vinci robot-assisted keyhole neurosurgery: a cadaver study on feasibility and safety. Neurosurg Rev 2015; 38(2):367–71.

64. Newman JG, Kuppersmith RB, O'Malley BW. Robotics and telesurgery in otolaryngology. Otolaryngol Clin North Am 2011;44(6):1317–31.

65. Smith AL, Scott EM, Krivak TC, et al. Dual-console robotic surgery: a new teaching paradigm. J Robot Surg 2013;7(2):113–8.

66. Chauvet D, Hans S. Transoral robotic surgery applied to the skull base. In: Assaad F, Wassmann H, Khodor M, editors. Pituitary diseases. IntechOpen; 2019.

67. Kupferman ME, Hanna E. Robotic surgery of the skull base. Otolaryngol Clin North Am 2014;47(3):415–23.
68. Bly RA, Su D, Lendvay TS, et al. Multiportal robotic access to the anterior cranial fossa: a surgical and engineering feasibility study. Otolaryngol Head Neck Surg 2013;149(6):940–6.
69. Friedrich DT, Dürselen L, Mayer B, et al. Features of haptic and tactile feedback in TORS: a comparison of available surgical systems. J Robot Surg 2018;12(1): 103–8.
70. Bolenz C, Gupta A, Hotze T, et al. Cost comparison of robotic, laparoscopic, and open radical prostatectomy for prostate cancer. Eur Urol 2010;57(3):453–8.
71. Breitenstein S, Nocito A, Puhan M, et al. Robotic-assisted versus laparoscopic cholecystectomy: outcome and cost analyses of a case-matched control study. Ann Surg 2008;247(6):987–93.
72. White HN, Frederick J, Zimmerman T, et al. Learning curve for transoral robotic surgery: a 4-year analysis. JAMA Otolaryngol Head Neck Surg 2013;139(6): 564–7.
73. Schneider JS, Burgner J, Webster RJ III, et al. Robotic surgery for the sinuses and skull base: what are the possibilities and what are the obstacles? Curr Opin Otolaryngol Head Neck Surg 2013;21(1):11–6.
74. Eichhorn KWG, Bootz F. Clinical requirements and possible applications of robot assisted endoscopy in skull base and sinus surgery. In: Pamir MN, Seifert V, Kiris T, editors. Intraoperative imaging, vol. 109. Vienna: Springer Vienna; 2011. p. 237–40.
75. Fondation Ophtalmologique Adolphe de Rothschild. Da Vinci Transoral Robotic-assisted Surgery of Pituitary Gland (ROBOPHYSE). ClinicalTrials.gov Identifier: NCT02743442.
76. Klapan I, Vranješ Ž, Rišavi R, et al. Computer-assisted surgery and computer-assisted telesurgery in otorhinolaryngology. Ear Nose Throat J 2006;85(5): 318–21.
77. Wirz R, Torres LG, Swaney PJ, et al. An experimental feasibility study on robotic endonasal telesurgery. Neurosurgery 2015;76(4):479–84.

Transoral Robotic Surgery for Residual and Recurrent Oropharyngeal Cancers

Vinidh Paleri, MS, FRCS[a,b,]*, John Hardman, MSc, MRCS[a,c],
Grainne Brady, MRes, MRCSLT[d], Ajith George, FRCS[e,f],
Cyrus Kerawala, FDSRCS, FRCS[a,g]

KEYWORDS

- Recurrence • Cancer • Robotics • Surgery • Head and neck

KEY POINTS

- Transoral robotic surgery (TORS) for residual, recurrent tumors and new primaries in radiation-exposed fields is becoming increasingly adopted as more centers gain access to robotic systems and as favorable outcome data emerge.
- Achieving clear resection margins can be technically challenging in these cases and a TORS program should be considered only by experienced and appropriately trained surgeons.
- Transoral reconstruction additionally may be required and presents its own technical complexities.
- Successful functional outcomes are achievable but require a well-resourced and motivated team to manage patients' expectations and to support them through a potentially prolonged period of rehabilitation.

INTRODUCTION

The most widely used treatment of the management of residual, recurrent, and new primary radiation-exposed (ReRuNeR) oropharyngeal cancer (OPC) is open surgery, with or without reconstruction.[1–4] Open surgery is prolonged, involves significant disruption to normal anatomy to gain access to the tumor (mandibulotomy, floor of mouth dissection, and lingual release), almost always needs reconstruction, and increases recovery time. Additionally, the irradiated bone can be beset with healing

[a] Head and Neck Unit, The Royal Marsden NHS Foundation Trust, Fulham Road, London SW3 6JJ, UK; [b] The Institute of Cancer Research, Brompton Road, London SW3 6JJ, UK; [c] North London, UK; [d] Department of Speech, Language and Swallowing, The Royal Marsden NHS Foundation Trust, Fulham Road, London SW3 6JJ, UK; [e] University Hospitals North Midlands, North Staffordshire, England; [f] Keele University Medical School, Staffordshire, UK; [g] University of Winchester, Winchester, UK
* Corresponding author.
E-mail address: vinidh.paleri@rmh.nhs.uk
Twitter: @VinPaleri (V.P.)

Otolaryngol Clin N Am 53 (2020) 1091–1108
https://doi.org/10.1016/j.otc.2020.07.016   oto.theclinics.com
0030-6665/20/© 2020 Elsevier Inc. All rights reserved.

issues in nearly half of patients.[5] A transoral robotic surgery (TORS) approach abrogates these disadvantages. The superior ability to maneuver instruments in a confined space and perform an en bloc resection makes TORS-based approaches a viable option for ReRuNeR OPCs.

Salvage surgery continues to be the most effective treatment modality in ReRuNeR OPCs, as demonstrated in the systematic review by Jayaram and colleagues.[2] Recent studies show that the difference in survival can be as much as 50%,[6] with salvage surgery reducing the risk of death from residual cancers by half.[7] In the human papillomavirus (HPV)-positive squamous cell carcinoma population, recurrence at the primary site is uncommon and seen in only 5% to 7% of patients after intensity-modulated radiation therapy,[8,9] because most index tumors are of early stage with excellent response rates to primary surgery or nonsurgical treatments.[10] HPV-negative squamous cancers are more likely to recur at the primary site, but higher rates of comorbidities in this group may reduce their tolerance of any postoperative aspiration. As such, a smaller proportion of the HPV-negative, compared with HPV-positive, patients may be suitable for salvage surgery. All things considered, patients with ReRuNeR cancers may not be offered salvage surgery, given the significant morbidity of open surgery, resource utilization, and the wide perception of relatively poor outcome.

Significant expertise in TORS has been accrued since its use has been described in the management of treatment-naïve cancers in early years of this century. The experience with TORS for recurrent cancer has been described in single centers and also has been the subject of a systematic review and meta-analysis by the authors' group.[11] The oncological and functional outcomes of TORS for recurrent cancer are supportive and, in carefully selected patients, transoral resection is an acceptable procedure to perform with satisfactory functional outcomes.

This article aims to offer readers the principles of case selection, decision making, tips on robotic surgical resection of these cancers, principles of reconstruction, rehabilitation, and future trends for using TORS in the management of ReRuNeR OPCs. Although the clinical and technical aspects and functional outcomes are based on the authors' experience, the oncological outcome data discussed are based on the systematic review and meta-analysis published recently by the authors' group.[11]

ASSESSMENT OF RESIDUAL, RECURRENT, AND NEW PRIMARY RADIATION-EXPOSED OROPHARYNGEAL CANCERS FOR TRANSORAL ROBOTIC SURGERY

The authors recommend an assessment of resectability be performed under general anesthesia for all patients with ReRuNeR OPCs deemed suitable for surgery. During assessment, the surgeon should ensure that the full mucosal extent of the tumor is visible using the robotic telescope and appropriate retractors, including a tongue stitch for traction. It is the authors' experience that a general anesthetic assessment often converts a tumor previously considered unresectable, based on clinical assessment, to amenable to resection via a TORS approach.

Special consideration should be given to the impact of trismus on access, especially if the lower extent of the tumor is not visible after robotic docking. Compounded by individual anatomy (long neck, narrow mandibular arch, and retrognathia), even mild trismus can make dissection of the anteroinferior aspects of the tumor difficult, with poor visualization and frequent instrument clashes resulting from the 3 instrument arms competing for space. If free flap reconstruction is planned (discussed later), adequate access is essential to allow for flap inset. Currently, the only available needle drivers are relatively large, at 8 mm, making suturing of the lower aspect of the flap challenging when space is limited. In the authors' experience, the most common reason for considering excision via conventional open surgery, rather than TORS, is trismus. The authors' baseline preoperative functional parameters at regarding trismus and swallow are discussed.

T STAGE AND TRANSORAL ROBOTIC SURGERY

TORS is approved as a treatment modality for early-stage oropharyngeal tumors in the primary setting and is bolstered by a considerable evidence base. Given the advantages of TORS over open surgery, however, the authors believe that, in select cases, TORS also may be suitable for tumors with higher T classifications. This is supported by data from the authors' meta-analysis,[11] in which 8.3% of the recurrent tumors identified were staged T3 or T4. In the authors' initial series, 23% of en bloc resections measured 6 cm or more, indicating that larger tumors can be removed via a TORS approach.[12]

THE TREATING TEAM AND EXPERIENCE WITH PRIMARY TRANSORAL ROBOTIC SURGERY

TORS is associated with a well-recognized learning curve. The authors caution against the use of TORS in ReRuNeR OPCs for surgeons who are early in their learning curve, especially if they have had limited experience with nonrobotic transoral surgery previously. Significant clinical judgment is needed to select appropriate cases, and the experience accrued from primary TORS is crucial to delivering a good outcome in this patient group. The postoperative course for these cancers differs from that of primary resections, and the experience the wider team gleans during the learning curve, notably in postoperative management and rehabilitation, is invaluable in counseling and caring for patients with ReRuNeR OPCs. As a guide, the authors recommend undertaking 30 primary cases, with careful assessment of postoperative outcomes and margin status, before embarking on a ReRuNeR cancer program.[13]

RELEVANT ANATOMY FOR MULTISITE OROPHARYNX RESECTIONS

Most recurrences, especially those of the tongue base, do not necessarily fall within the compartmental resection of lateralized tongue base tumor, as described by Weinstein and O'Malley.[14] If a tumor in the second subsite is superficial, then extension of the resection to the second subsite to take the tumor, a margin of mucosa, and a few millimeters of deeper tissue, should be relatively straightforward. If a tumor has substantial depth across both the tonsil and tongue base or extends deeply into the tonsillolingual sulcus, however, a greater appreciation of the deeper anatomy is warranted. In order to achieve an en bloc resection of these tumors, or tumors extending into the laryngopharynx, the surgeon must be able to identify the following structures from a transoral approach: the styloglossus muscle, the hyoid and its constrictor muscle attachments, and branches of the facial[15] and lingual arteries.[16]

Broadly, the pharyngeal constrictors are separated into 3 groups of muscles. The inferior constrictor is recognized as being divided into 2 elements, which are not relevant in transoral surgery. The subdivisions of the superior and middle constrictors are particularly important, however, when dissecting the parapharyngeal space. The superior constrictor is made up of 5 muscle slips: pterygopharyngeus, palatopharyngeus, buccopharyngeus, mylopharyngeus, and glossopharyngeus (**Fig. 1**). The window to the inverted tetrahedron of the parapharyngeal space is the pterygomandibular raphe. The raphe is the junction of the buccinator and the buccopharyngeus slip of the superior constrictor.

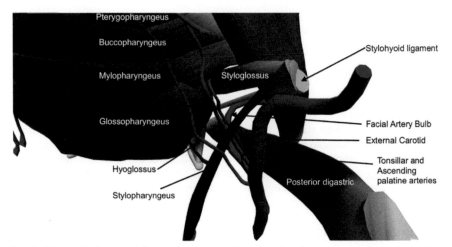

Fig. 1. Schematic from a right posterolateral view showing the various superior constrictor slips, the styloglossus muscle, and the vascular anatomy relevant to TORS in the lateral pharynx.

The styloglossus anatomy, as relevant to TORS, has been well described.[17] The styloglossus muscle merges with the glossopharyngeus, the most inferior slip of the superior constrictor. The facial and lingual branches of the external carotid are consistently lateral to the plane of the styloglossus. The 2 main branches of the facial artery, which supply the tonsils (ascending palatine and tonsillar branches) can pass either above or below the styloglossus. When passing below the styloglossus, they can either be in the space between the styloglossus and stylopharyngeus (most common variation) (see **Fig. 1**) or deep to both muscles. Dissecting lateral to styloglossus, the facial artery bulb[15] is the first major vessel to be encountered in the parapharyngeal space and often is mistaken for the lingual artery (**Fig. 2**). The bulb takes form as it arches over the posterior belly of digastric before heading into the substance of the submandibular gland (see **Fig. 1**). Encountering this vessel inevitably means a communication is created between the transoral and transcervical dissections, if performed concurrently.

If dissection continues caudally, in a plane lateral to styloglossus, then the superior thyroid artery is encountered. More medially, an early branch of the superior thyroid artery, the superior laryngeal artery, is seen as it courses through the pharyngoepiglottic fold; this vessel can be readily controlled with a clip applicator, early in the dissection of the fold, if reduced blood flow to the larynx is desired for the perioperative course.

Inferior to the glossopharyngeus, and where the styloglossus has merged with it anteriorly, the surgeon is guided by the 2 muscle slips of the middle constrictor. These are the ceratopharyngeus (attaches to the greater cornu) and chondropharyngeus (attaches to the lesser cornu) (**Fig. 3**). Their attachments to the hyoid are relevant as they pass medial to the hyoglossus. The lingual artery passes from lateral to medial proximal to where the chondropharyngeus attaches to the posterior aspect of the lesser cornu of the hyoid. After giving off the dorsal lingual branch, the artery courses toward the deep tongue musculature, entering in the plane between genioglossus and the lingual tonsils, where it is encountered during a conventional tongue base resection. Lateral to the hyoglossus muscle, almost mirroring the lingual artery from the transoral perspective, lies the hypoglossal nerve (**Fig. 4**).

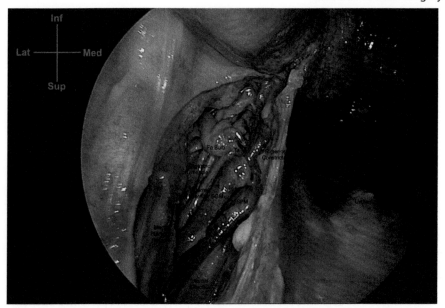

Fig. 2. A cadaver dissection of the left parapharyngeal space demonstrating the anatomy lateral to the styloglossus muscle. APa, ascending Pharyngeal artery; Fa, facial Artery; Inf, inferior; Lat, Lateral; Med, Medial; SGM, Styloglossus muscle; SPM, Stylopharyngeus muscle; Sup, Superior; TA, tonsillar Artery.

SURGICAL TECHNIQUE AND REFINEMENTS
Neck and Airway

In all cases, the ipsilateral neck should be explored to ligate the facial, lingual and ascending pharyngeal arteries; if there is concurrent metastatic neck disease, a neck dissection may need to be performed. Given the low incidence of occult metastasis, the authors do not routinely perform an elective neck dissection for recurrent cancers, except in cases of free flap reconstruction, where vascular access is required for microvascular anastomosis and limited lymph nodal clearance is needed to

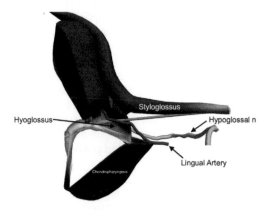

Fig. 3. Schematic showing the chondropharyngeus slip and its relation to the hyoglossus muscle and the lingual artery. N, Nerve.

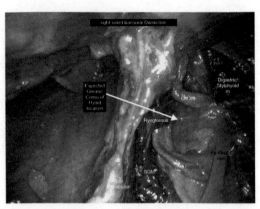

Fig. 4. A cadaver dissection of the right parapharyngeal space demonstrating the anatomy lateral and caudal to the styloglossus muscle, where the hyoglossus and the XII cranial nerve (CN) can be seen. A, Artery; M, Muscle; Facial a BULB, Facial aretry bulb; SGM, Styloglossus muscle; Sup, Superior.

accommodate the recipient vessels. The authors' preference is to perform a tracheostomy for tongue base ReRuNeR tumors because this improves transoral access and is retained for the immediate postoperative period as a safety to cover the known bleeding risk in this population (discussed later). Smaller ReRuNeR OPCs, such as tumors confined to the tonsil, may be resected with an oral endotracheal tube in situ, but this should be sutured to the contralateral oropharynx to prevent interaction with the operative field and instruments.

Retractor Choice

The Boyle-Davis retractor and the FK-WO [FK-WO TORS Laryngo-Pharyngoscope retractor (Olympus Europa, Hamburg, Germany)] retractor commonly are used for oropharyngeal resections. If both are available, the choice of retractor is influenced principally by the access required and the size of the tumor. The authors find the Boyle-Davis retractor useful for small tonsil tumors, without extension to the tongue base. In such cases, the convex profile of the Doherty blade is less problematic for instruments passing the oral cavity, and the smaller retractor gives excellent access for the first assistant at the bedside. The authors find the FK-WO retractor appropriate for a majority of other ReRuNeR OPCs undergoing TORS; its various blade attachments and adjustability allow finessed manipulation of the tongue to optimize instrument access and tumor retraction.

Tonsil Recurrence

In patients with ReRuNeR OPCs confined to the tonsillar fossa, the technique for resection is similar to the radical tonsillectomy described by Weinstein and colleagues.[18] In more advanced cases, where the tonsillar tumor extends into the tongue base, the resection can include the affected tongue musculature and floor of mouth mucosa, using the anatomic principles discussed previously.

Tongue Base Recurrence

When TORS for ReRuNeR tongue base tumors is compared with its use in the primary setting, 2 major differences emerge: (1) recurrent tumors often extend anterior to the circumvallate papillae in a submucosal plane, rendering the anterior part of the tumor is readily palpable, and (2) the tongue base tissues often are edematous and brawny as a result of the previous irradiation. These tissue changes are problematic particularly for the operating surgeon: first, it is hard to discriminate tumor from the surrounding normal tissue at the mucosal level because the visual usual haptic feedback that is helpful in primary TORS is masked; and, second, the interaction of the monopolar cautery with the noncancerous deeper tissue appears more similar to that of cancerous tissues. Both these differences are primarily responsible for the proposed technical refinements, outlined in Paleri and colleagues.[12]

The current robotic retractors and set up are neither required nor adaptable for surgery anterior to the circumvallate papillae, where direct transoral access can be obtained easily, negating the need for robotic instrumentation in this area. In such cases, a stitch is placed on the anterior aspect of the tongue, as for other TORS resections, and the tongue is pulled forward. The anterior margin of the palpable tumor is marked out with methylene blue. Using monopolar cautery and digital palpation, an anterior shelf is established to separate the base of the tongue affected by tumor from the unaffected anterior tongue (**Fig. 5**A). This shelf is extended as needed to establish and define the tumor depth, allowing, as far posteriorly as possible, for an adequate margin of normal tissue in all dimensions. With progressive anterior and medial mobilization, a surprisingly significant amount of dissection can be performed transorally with a headlight and monopolar cautery. For dissections further posteriorly, a 6-in insulated monopolar blade can be used (Conmed, Utica, New York). Laterally, these ReRuNeR tumors often extend superficially to the free margin of the tongue, and the deep margin may be formed by the posterior floor of mouth/sublingual glands. Removal of these structures may therefore be required for adequate clearance.

Once a substantial shelf is established and medial dissection as far back as possible has been performed, the FK-WO TORS retractor, with the mandible or WO blade, is placed in such a way that the blade of the retractor is anchored into the surgically created shelf; the tumor is now in the oropharyngeal lumen and the surgeon also has defined the tumor depth (**Fig. 5**B, C). This maneuver gains additional space in

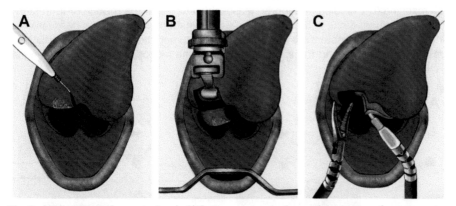

Fig. 5. (A) Creation of an anterior shelf that separates the base of the tongue from the anterior aspect of the tongue, using monopolar cautery and digital palpation (B) The FK-WO TORS retractor with the mandible blade anchored into the surgically created shelf, allowing the tumor to drop behind the blade into the oropharyngeal lumen. (C) Resection where the tongue base, vallecula, and ipsilateral epiglottis have been resected. *From* Paleri V, Fox H, Coward S, et al. Transoral robotic surgery for residual and recurrent oropharyngeal cancers: Exploratory study of surgical innovation using the IDEAL framework for early-phase surgical studies. Head Neck 2018;40(3):512-525. doi: 10.1002/hed.25032. Epub 2017 Dec 15.

the oral cavity for the robotic arms, because the mandible blade rests in the space occupied by the tongue base tumor and allows the tumor to progressively drop down into the lumen. The tumor usually is mobilized sufficiently at this point to allow the robotic arms to manipulate the tumor, aiding further dissection. In the early part of the learning curve, after incremental resection, the authors recommend that the robot be undocked repeatedly to allow the surgeon to confirm the tumor depth by direct palpation. Incremental resection, following this technique, allows progressive mobilization of the tumor, resulting in more accurate assessment of the adequacy of the resection margins.

Tonsillolingual Sulcus Recurrence

In the authors' early experience, they found deep-seated tumors in this area to be the most difficult for performing en bloc resections, given the need to resect both the tonsil and tongue base to a sufficient depth. In these instances, an appropriate margin of the tonsil is marked out, and the parapharyngeal space is entered. The surgeon must be able to define the parapharyngeal space, even when approaching it through the tonsil, because conventional access through the pterygomandibular raphe leads to an unnecessarily large resection. Once the styloglossus is identified, dissection can proceed laterally and inferiorly to it, as required, until the middle constrictor and the hyoid are identified. Appropriate tongue base cuts, as described in the section above, are performed around the tumor anteriorly, and the dissection proceeds to the required depth using the styloglossus dissection laterally as a guide. These techniques allow for an en bloc resection of these tumors (**Fig. 6**).

Intraoperative Ultrasound

Intraoperative ultrasound is useful in select instances, especially with submucosal tongue base cancers where intraoperative examination does not allow for a good assessment of the tumor extent and depth (Paleri V, Fox H, Coward S, et al. Transoral robotic surgery for residual and recurrent oropharyngeal cancers: an IDEAL phase 2a exploratory study of surgical innovation. In: Unpublished, ed., 2016).[19] The Flex Focus 800 machine (BK Medical, Peabody, Massachusetts), with the robotic drop-in ultrasound transducer 8826, is the authors' preferred instrument for tongue base lesions. After appropriate retractors are used to expose the tumor, the ultrasound transducer is grasped by the Maryland forceps and placed on the mucosal surface of the tongue

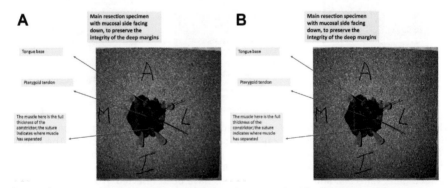

Fig. 6. The resected specimen is orientated and mounted with the deeper side facing up, taking care not to distort the convexity. (*A*) Shows the annotated mucosal side of the tumor before being orientated using pins (*B*).A, Anterior; I, Inferior; L, Lateral; M, Medial.

base. In combination with the patient's preoperative magnetic resonance imaging, the transoral ultrasound images of the tongue base are interpreted by the radiologist and TORS surgeon in combination as the tumor resection progresses.

Intraoperative Margin Assessment

It is reasonable to aim to achieve a 5-mm margin for the deep and mucosal resections where the anatomy allows. It is the authors' opinion that a greater emphasis should be placed on achieving a clear margin clinically, rather than focusing on the numerical figure attached to the resection specimen in the final pathology report. This is relevant particularly because the final reading may reduce by up to 25%, resulting from tissue necrosis induced by the energy devices commonly used in TORS, and up to 10% further when undergoing formalin fixation.[20,21]

For tonsil cancers, a 5-mm mucosal margin is achievable in most cases; but, these margins may not be possible for the deeper aspect of the mobilized specimen laterally, where the thickness of the constrictor bed measures less than 2 mm, reduced by radiation induced atrophy and formalin fixation. Smaller tongue base cancers may achieve 5-mm deep and mucosal margins if they are confined to this subsite. For tumors centered in the tonsillolingual sulcus, the deep margin may be augmented by including the constrictor and stylohyoid muscles in the resected specimen.

It is important for the surgeon to examine all aspects of the specimen once it is completely resected. The authors do not routinely slice the specimen in the operative room to assess the deep margin. Areas where the deep resection margin is felt to be close are marked with colored ink on the specimen. The specimen then is orientated and temporarily placed back into the defect, pinpointing the precise location for further resection. Frozen section examination then can be used to confirm adequate clearance. For small oropharyngeal defects, the whole tumor bed may be sampled as a single marginal biopsy if required.

Intraoperative Frozen Section

Significant input from pathology services is needed to run such a service but it can be invaluable in the management of ReRuNeR OPCs: in some cases, a definitive confirmation of malignant disease may be required before progressing with a more advanced resection, especially where chronic ulceration has affected the oropharyngeal tissues and previous attempts at more superficial biopsy have been ambiguous; in other cases, the full submucosal extent of the tumor is difficult to appreciate in the irradiated tissue and histologic confirmation of adequate resection is needed to avoid removing unaffected tissue.

Specimen Processing

Special attention should be paid to the mounting of specimens to allow for accurate margin assessment. Traditionally, specimens are orientated, pinned, and mounted with the mucosal side facing up. If this method is applied to the en bloc oropharyngeal specimen resected with TORS, then the convex shape of the deep aspect may be lost when undergoing formalin fixation while flattened against the board. Additionally, once fixed in formalin, the muscle layers on the under-surface of the tumor specimen, that were freely mobile in vivo, have become compressed and distorted, which may contribute to an underestimation of these margins. Consequently, the authors recommend that the specimen is mounted with the mucosal side facing down, to maintain the natural convexity of the deeper aspect of the resected specimen (see **Fig. 6**). Furthermore, to ensure optimal communication between surgeons and histopathologists, it is the authors' practice to photograph all resections and provide labeled diagrams to facilitate specimen orientation prior to processing.

Reconstructive Strategy

TORS oropharyngeal resections traditionally have been left to heal by secondary intention but in the salvage setting complex ablative defects often cross a variety of anatomic subsites and, as a result, may require formal reconstruction. The anatomic goals of such reconstruction include coverage of vital vascular structures and maintenance of a watertight seal. Additionally, there are functional goals, such as minimizing velopharyngeal insufficiency and improving swallow by restoring tongue volume. These aims can be achieved by the transfer of vascularized tissue either locally or more often as a microvascular free flap.[22–24]

Reconstructive algorithms have been developed to aid planning of post-TORS resection defects. de Almeida and colleagues[23] suggested 4 classes of defect: class I involves 1 subsite (tonsil, tongue base, pharynx, or soft palate) and no adverse features (internal carotid artery exposure, neck communication, or >50% of soft palate resection); class II is similar but involves more than 1 subsite; class III involves 1 subsite but has 1 or more adverse features; and class IV involves multiple subsites and adverse features. Class I and class II defects can be either left to heal by secondary intention or closed with local flaps, whereas class III and class IV defects require regional or free flap reconstruction.

Oropharyngeal surgery in the salvage setting has shifted toward minimally invasive approaches, such as TORS, which aim to avoid unnecessary tissue disruption from access procedures. The natural evolution of this progression has been the development of robotic-assisted free flap inset (RAFFI). Combining resection and reconstruction robotically is a more cost-effective and efficient use of the robotic system and avoids the need for a formal mandibulotomy. This reduces operation time and hospital stay with other potential benefits, including a more expedient return of swallow and potentially a reduced incidence of osteoradionecrosis at the osteotomy site.[25]

Selber[26] described a small series of 5 patients undergoing oropharyngeal resection and reconstruction with an intact mandible with either local or free flaps. An anterolateral thigh flap was used in 1 patient to resurface the neck and reconstruct the tongue, floor of mouth and pharyngeal defects. The inset was performed using a combination of methods: by hand through the mouth and via a pharyngectomy and robotically via TORS for the more difficult to access areas. Microneedle drivers were employed to place the sutures but the investigators did comment that some of the knots ultimately were hand-tied. Several investigators since have described their techniques for salvage oropharyngectomies using both cervical and TORS approaches, with an emphasis on a combination of hand and robotic inset of free flaps.[12,26–29]

RAFFI is technically demanding and, in common with TORS ablation in the salvage setting, should be attempted only by experienced surgeons. Surgical time can be saved by performing resection and flap raising simultaneously but this requires a careful assessment of flap dimensions. This is best achieved using a combination of preoperative imaging and on-table measurements, with the need to accept that modifications may well be necessary as the case proceeds. To conform to the complex 3-dimensional ablative cavity, thin fasciocutaneous flaps are best employed. Time efficiency is maximized using a combination of a hand and robotic approaches for inset. In general, the flap is first supported by 2 or 3 holding sutures, 1 of which is placed cervically around the hyoid bone to stabilize the most inferior aspect of the flap and help achieve a watertight seal. The robotic inset should be performed first, because this allows any excess flap to be readily excised at its superior extent under direct vision. The lack of haptic feedback makes robotic tying of knots challenging and as such alternative sutures, such as the V-Loc barbed system (Medtronic, Watford, United Kingdom) have obvious advantages during inset, but the absorption profile of V-Loc is a minimum of 90 days.

MANAGEMENT OF POSITIVE MARGINS RECOGNIZED ON FORMALIN-FIXED PARAFFIN-EMBEDDED TISSUES

Difficult decisions need to be made patients in whom a paraffin section shows cancer in the defect margin after a negative frozen section. For these patients, the margin should be considered to be positive and the authors believe that the surgeon has no option but to consider a re-resection. In many cases, it may be practically impossible to be precise about the site of the positive margin, especially in tongue base recurrences. In small tongue base ReRuNeR OPCs defects, a re-resection of the entire tumor bed may be feasible. In other instances, the sole option, the authors believe, is for open resection of the entire tumor bed and reconstruction as appropriate. In all such instances, in the authors' series (3 of the first 50 cases), no tumor was identified pathologically in the re-resected bed, but this could be a reflection of the minimal tumor volume and a sampling issue during processing.

POSTOPERATIVE CARE

The authors' policy for postoperative care is based on a patient comorbidity burden and requirement for postoperative ventilator support. If the burden is high or ventilatory support is required, such patients are sent to the critical care units; all others return to the ward.

Pain is a significant component of the postoperative phase that needs to be actively managed to assist with the rehabilitation. The authors' postoperative TORS pain management protocol includes pregabalin, 150 mg on the day of surgery, followed by 75 mg twice a day, until the pain recedes and oral intake increases. Additionally, patient-controlled analgesia is used for 24 hours to 48 hours, with morphine given as required for breakthrough pain.

REHABILITATION

It has been well documented that swallowing function remains a primary concern for patients up to 12 months after definitive organ preservation treatment of head and neck cancer (HNC).[30,31] Swallowing dysfunction has been shown to persist for many years after definitive treatment[32] and for some patients can present as a late complication, with a gradual decline occurring many years after treatment.[33] In the setting of ReRuNeR HNC, patients have the potential to present with a baseline dysphagia, related to their previous treatments, as well as new-onset dysphagia, as a symptom of their active disease. Dysphagia is associated with higher risk of pneumonia, poorer oral intake, prolonged gastrostomy use, poor nutritional status, weight loss, and significant alterations to eating patterns, social activities, and subsequently quality of life.[34] Even in the setting of minimally invasive surgery for ReRuNeR OPCs, where more favorable functional outcomes have been reported in comparison to traditional surgical techniques,[12,35] a protracted period of dysphagia rehabilitation is required.[36] Consequently, swallowing rehabilitation should be integral to the management of patients with ReRuNeR OPCs and should include prehabilitation with functional optimization before surgery. This should take place in addition to immediate postoperative therapy and followed by longer-term rehabilitation for the weeks and months after surgery. A rehabilitation model (**Fig. 7**) has been developed at the authors' center based on clinical experience and review of the existing literature in the management of dysphagia in HNC.

A multidimensional pretreatment swallowing evaluation underpins discussions regarding potential functional outcomes, as part of the informed consent process. A thorough assessment also identifies targeted prehabilitation goals, including swallowing exercises. The baseline assessment should include a range of patient-reported and clinician-reported measures, in addition to instrumental evaluation of swallowing function using videofluoroscopy and/or fiberoptic endoscopic evaluation of swallowing (FEES).[36] Baseline evaluation also informs decision making regarding nonoral feeding methods in the acute and longer term after surgery. At the authors' center, an intraoperative nasogastric tube routinely is placed; however, depending on baseline swallowing function, some patients may require gastrostomy tube placement prior to surgery. If patients do not follow an expected trajectory of recovery (see **Fig. 7**), conversion from nasogastric tube to gastrostomy takes place at 14 days after surgery.

A range of rehabilitation approaches must be used, including targeted dysphagia swallowing exercises (see **Fig. 7**). More novel methods also have been used, including expiratory muscle strength training (EMST) and intensive blocks of boot camp–style interventions.[36] The rehabilitation plan must be a patient-centered process, tailored to individual needs, with repeated outcome measures, allowing reactive changes to the plan as needed.[37]

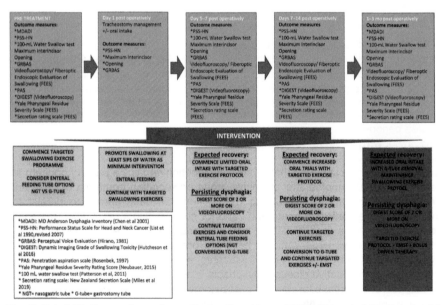

Fig. 7. Rehabilitation pathway for patients after salvage TORS. This rehabilitation model previously was presented at the Dysphagia Research Society. (*From* Brady GC, Leigh-Doyle, L, Stephen, S., Roe, J.W.G., Paleri, V. Functional Outcomes Following Transoral Robotic Surgery for Recurrent Head and Neck Cancer (HNC): A Prospectve Observational Study. In: Dysphagia, ed. Dysphagia Research Society 27th Anniversary Annual Meeting., 2019:944-1018.)

OUTCOMES

The authors' group performed a systematic review and meta-analysis of studies reporting survival data and functional outcomes for patients undergoing TORS for previously treated HNC. Of the 811 records identified, 8 were eligible for inclusion, covering 165 cases (range 1–64). There was a male preponderance, and the mean ages were approximately 60 years. Nearly all cases were squamous cell carcinoma, but HPV rates were reported inconsistently. Most cases were early-stage disease, rT0-T2 and rN0-N2b.

The pooled free flap rate was 0.9% (4 studies; range 0.0–14.3; 95% CI, 0.0–6.8; I^2 63.7%; $P = .04$).

Complications

The meta-analysis showed a pooled postoperative hemorrhage rate of 9.2% from 4 studies (range 3.3–13.3), with a pooled postoperative pharyngocutaneous fistula rate of 0.6% (4 studies, range 0.0–3.3).

Margins

All but one study reported on rates of positive resection margins, with 5 studies also reporting rates of close resection margins. The pooled positive margin rate was 18.2% (4 studies, range 6.7–33.3). The pooled close margin rate (not including positive margins) was 25.7% (3 studies, range 6.7–52.9). The criteria used for a close margin cutoff was reported by 4 studies, ranging between 2 mm and 5 mm, with only 1 study reporting the criteria used for considering a margin as positive.

Oncologic outcomes

The pooled data for oncological outcomes (**Fig. 8**) were as follows: 2-year overall survival, 73.1% (4 studies; range 64.7–75.0; 95% CI, 64.6–80.9; I^2 0.0%; $P = .9$), and 2-year disease-free survival, 75.3% (4 studies; range 60.0–92.0; 95% CI, 65.2–84.2; I^2 22.9%; $P = .3$).

Functional outcomes

Only surrogate functional outcomes were available from the systematic review. The pooled perioperative gastrostomy rate from 3 studies was 25.0% (range 16.7–35.9), with a pooled perioperative tracheostomy rate of 22.3% (3 studies; range 21.9–23.5). Some long-term results were available for functional outcomes, although the definitions of what constituted long-term outcomes were not clear in the source material. The pooled long-term gastrostomy rate was 5.0% (4 studies; range 0.0–20.0) and the pooled long-term tracheostomy rate was 1.9% (2 studies; range 0.0–10.0), indicating that a vast majority of patients were swallowing without tubes and were decannulated in the longer term.

To provide more granular data, the authors present their center results for functional outcomes. Between December 2017 and August 2019, 30 patients (4 women) underwent TORS for ReRuNeR. Previous treatments included (biochemo)radiation (n = 28) and surgery with postoperative radiotherapy (n = 2). Median age was 60 years (range 37–82 years). Patients had locally recurrent/residual disease of the oropharynx (n = 29) and hypopharynx (n = 2). TORS-assisted flap reconstruction was required in 8 patients. Tracheostomy was performed in 25 patients. Median time to decannulation was 11 days (range 4–27). Baseline and postsurgery gastrostomy use was as follows: 6 at baseline (n = 30); 15 at 3 months (n = 30); 7 at 6 months (n = 16 assessable patients); and 4 at 12 months postsurgery (n = 10 assessable patients). Median

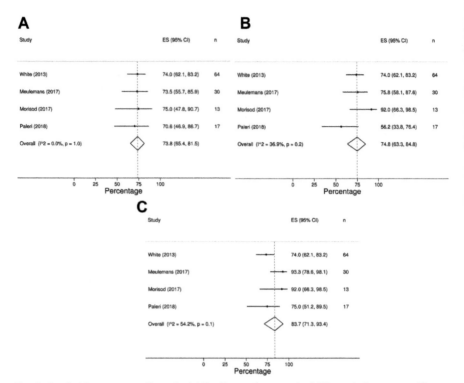

Fig. 8. Pooled 2-year overall survival (*A*), disease-free survival (*B*), and disease-specific survival (*C*) after salvage TORS for ReRuNeR cancers. (*From* Hardman J, Liu Z, Brady Get al. Transoral robotic surgery for recurrent cancers of the upper aerodigestive tract-Systematic review and meta-analysis. Head Neck 2020; 42:1089-1104.)

length of hospital stay was 14 days (range 1–30). Further objective and patient-reported outcome measures, including the MD Anderson Dysphagia Inventory (MDADI) (Chen and colleagues,[38] 2001), Performance Status Scale for Head and Neck Cancer Patients Normalcy of Diet (PSS-HN) (List and colleagues,[39] 1990), and maximum interincisor opening, are shown in **Table 1**.

FUTURE TRENDS

Revising margins after salvage TORS is a difficult prospect, so real-time assessment of margins and revision of the resection at the time of surgery are key to avoiding this predicament. Frozen sections are associated with an inevitable delay between sampling and the subsequent result, which may result in difficulty relating any positive results to precise location in the resection bed, given the complexity of the endoscopic landscape. Real-time assessment of the margins might be the way forward in this setting and several options have shown promise in this regard. Rapid evaporation ionizing mass spectrometry, where analysis of the plume from the area being cut by the electrocautery instrument, has shown promise and is one option that has been robustly validated in the laboratory setting.[40] The authors' work on snap frozen samples from 74 patients and 1051 observations offers the following diagnostic efficacy metrics: specificity, 98.47%; sensitivity, 97.78%; positive predictive value, 97.4%; and negative predictive value, 98.4%. This innovative technology will greatly increase

Table 1
Functional outcome measures from a single center cohort

	Baseline	Postoperative		
		3 Months Post	6 Months Post	12 Months Post
Mean PSS-HN Normalcy of diet score	69.3 95% CI, 62.0–76.7 n = 30	39.3 95% CI, 29.9–48.7 n = 29	51.2 95% CI, 37.6–68.4 n = 17	51.1 95% CI, 30.1–72.1 n = 9
Mean MDADI composite score	74.6 95% CI, 68–81.2 n = 24	45.6 95% CI, 3 2.7–58.5 n = 12	59.5 95% CI, 46.3–72.7 n = 11	61.8 95% CI, 34.7–88.9 n = 6
Median maximum interincisor opening (mm)	38.5 Range: 20–55 n = 26	26.5 Range: 10–43 n = 22	31 Range: 10–50 n = 9	

intraoperative confidence in the adequacy of the resection margins and is under ongoing evaluation.

Although immunotherapy approaches have shown success compared with conventional chemotherapy for unresectable nonmetastatic cancers,[41] surgery remains the sole curative option. No targeted nonsurgical therapies are available on the horizon. A recent prospective trial to assess the clinical benefit of a tailored gene set built on a next-generation sequencing platform in patients with recurrent or metastatic head and neck squamous cell carcinoma provided to clinicians to inform treatment decisions did not provide clinical benefit to the patients.[42] Promising avenues of investigation appear to be combining immunotherapy in the surgically salvageable population (ClinicalTrials.gov Identifier: NCT03565783).

DISCUSSION

TORS clearly is proving itself an acceptable treatment modality for recurrent cancers, with outcomes comparable to the results of open resections[2] and transoral laser resections.[43,44] The caveats associated with these outcomes must be interpreted carefully, however; there is a selection bias to those being offered TORS. This bias pertains mainly to 2 factors: (1) the selection of relatively smaller cancers (approximately 90%) is limited to 1 subsite vs larger tumors, and (2) smaller recurrences usually are HPV-positive cancers in patients with a better comorbidity profile compared with to HPV-negative squamous cell cancers.[45] This cohort usually has a greater respiratory reserve and tolerates larger transoral resections, which still leave them with a functional swallow. The authors hope to have greater clarity on these aspects in a forthcoming international individual patient data meta-analysis that currently is under way (IRAS 268830, RMHCCR5156).

TORS should form just one modality in the spectrum of treatments available to patients with ReRuNeR OPCs. Although transoral laser microsurgery (TLM) for ReRuNeR OPCs is not to be discounted entirely, it is the authors' experience that TLM is unsuited for anything but the smallest tonsil cancers. The ability to perform intraoperative imaging and flap inset are unique to TORS resections, expanding the patient base for transoral surgery.

As a surgeon's practice and experience evolve, it is likely that the patients deemed suitable for these procedures will expand too. The authors emphasize that prior to embarking on any TORS for ReRuNeR cancer, the members of their multidisciplinary team carefully consider all aspects of a patient's treatment, from surgical to oncological to functional perspectives, to ensure the patient may be counseled appropriately. The postoperative complication profile and the long-term rehabilitation outcomes are significantly different from those of the primary cohort and need to be understood when embarking on this service. The authors' hospital stay data may be skewed by patients from outside the region; discharge policy allows patients to return directly home (rather than to an interim closer hospital) only after the following criteria are met: the tracheostomy is decannulated; pain is well controlled; nutritional requirements are met through oral intake and/or an appropriate feeding tube; nursing support is in place for the feeding tube and any social care issues; and patient transport can be arranged to the referring area of the country. The authors' previous single-center data indicate a hospital stay of under a week when patients receive treatment at their local center and many of these logistical issues do not apply.[13]

DISCLOSURE

V. Paleri is a proctor for Intuitive Surgical Si and Xi systems.

REFERENCES

1. Culie D, Benezery K, Chamorey E, et al. Salvage surgery for recurrent oropharyngeal cancer: post-operative oncologic and functional outcomes. Acta Otolaryngol 2015;135:1323–9.
2. Jayaram SC, Muzaffar SJ, Ahmed I, et al. Efficacy, outcomes, and complication rates of different surgical and nonsurgical treatment modalities for recurrent/residual oropharyngeal carcinoma: A systematic review and meta-analysis. Head Neck 2016;38:1855–61.
3. Nichols AC, Kneuertz PJ, Deschler DG, et al. Surgical salvage of the oropharynx after failure of organ-sparing therapy. Head Neck 2011;33:516–24.
4. Patel SN, Cohen MA, Givi B, et al. Salvage surgery for locally recurrent oropharyngeal cancer. Head Neck 2016;38(Suppl 1):E658–64.
5. Hay A, Simo R, Hall G, et al. Outcomes of salvage surgery for the oropharynx and larynx: a contemporary experience in a UK Cancer Centre. Eur Arch Otorhinolaryngol 2019;276:1153–9.
6. Maruo T, Zenda S, Shinozaki T, et al. Comparison of salvage surgery for recurrent or residual head and neck squamous cell carcinoma. Jpn J Clin Oncol 2020;50:288–95.
7. Fakhry C, Zhang Q, Nguyen-Tan PF, et al. Human papillomavirus and overall survival after progression of oropharyngeal squamous cell carcinoma. J Clin Oncol 2014;32:3365–73.
8. Daly ME, Le QT, Maxim PG, et al. Intensity-modulated radiotherapy in the treatment of oropharyngeal cancer: clinical outcomes and patterns of failure. Int J Radiat Oncol Biol Phys 2010;76:1339–46.
9. Garden AS, Dong L, Morrison WH, et al. Patterns of disease recurrence following treatment of oropharyngeal cancer with intensity modulated radiation therapy. Int J Radiat Oncol Biol Phys 2013;85:941–7.
10. Goldenberg D, Begum S, Westra WH, et al. Cystic lymph node metastasis in patients with head and neck cancer: An HPV-associated phenomenon. Head Neck 2008;30:898–903.

11. Hardman J, Liu Z, Brady G, et al. Transoral robotic surgery for recurrent cancers of the upper aerodigestive tract-Systematic review and meta-analysis. Head Neck 2020;42:1089–104.

12. Paleri V, Fox H, Coward S, et al. Transoral robotic surgery for residual and recurrent oropharyngeal cancers: Exploratory study of surgical innovation using the IDEAL framework for early-phase surgical studies. Head Neck 2018;40(3): 512–25.

13. Albergotti WG, Gooding WE, Kubik MW, et al. Assessment of Surgical Learning Curves in Transoral Robotic Surgery for Squamous Cell Carcinoma of the Oropharynx. JAMA Otolaryngol Head Neck Surg 2017;143:542–8.

14. Weinstein GS, O'Malley BW Jr. Transoral robotic surgery (TORS). San Diego (CA): Plural Publishing Inc.; 2011.

15. Mohamed A, Paleri V, George A. A cadaveric study quantifying the anatomical landmarks of the facial artery and its parapharyngeal branches for safe transoral surgery. Head Neck 2019;41:3389–94.

16. Wang C, Kundaria S, Fernandez-Miranda J, et al. A description of arterial variants in the transoral approach to the parapharyngeal space. Clin Anat 2014;27: 1016–22.

17. Laccourreye O, Orosco RK, Rubin F, et al. Styloglossus muscle: a critical landmark in head and neck oncology. Eur Ann Otorhinolaryngol Head Neck Dis 2018;135:421–5.

18. Weinstein GS, O'Malley BW Jr, Snyder W, et al. Transoral robotic surgery: radical tonsillectomy. Arch Otolaryngol Head Neck Surg 2007;133:1220–6.

19. Clayburgh DR, Byrd JK, Bonfili J, et al. Intraoperative Ultrasonography During Transoral Robotic Surgery. Ann Otol Rhinol Laryngol 2016;125:37–42.

20. Johnson RE, Sigman JD, Funk GF, et al. Quantification of surgical margin shrinkage in the oral cavity. Head Neck 1997;19:281–6.

21. Mistry RC, Qureshi SS, Kumaran C. Post-resection mucosal margin shrinkage in oral cancer: quantification and significance. J Surg Oncol 2005;91:131–3.

22. Song HG, Yun IS, Lee WJ, et al. Robot-assisted free flap in head and neck reconstruction. Arch Plast Surg 2013;40:353–8.

23. de Almeida JR, Park RC, Villanueva NL, et al. Reconstructive algorithm and classification system for transoral oropharyngeal defects. Head Neck 2014;36: 934–41.

24. de Almeida JR, Park RC, Genden EM. Reconstruction of transoral robotic surgery defects: principles and techniques. J Reconstr Microsurg 2012;28:465–72.

25. Lee SY, Park YM, Byeon HK, et al. Comparison of oncologic and functional outcomes after transoral robotic lateral oropharyngectomy versus conventional surgery for T1 to T3 tonsillar cancer. Head Neck 2014;36:1138–45.

26. Selber JC. Transoral robotic reconstruction of oropharyngeal defects: a case series. Plast Reconstr Surg 2010;126:1978–87.

27. Chan JYW, Chan RCL, Chow VLY, et al. Transoral robotic total laryngopharyngectomy and free jejunal flap reconstruction for hypopharyngeal cancer. Oral Oncol 2017;72:194–6.

28. Gorphe P, Temam S, Kolb F, et al. Cervical-transoral robotic oropharyngectomy and thin anterolateral thigh free flap. Eur Ann Otorhinolaryngol Head Neck Dis 2018;135:71–4.

29. Mukhija VK, Sung CK, Desai SC, et al. Transoral robotic assisted free flap reconstruction. Otolaryngol Head Neck Surg 2009;140:124–5.

30. Wilson JA, Carding PN, Patterson JM. Dysphagia after nonsurgical head and neck cancer treatment: patients' perspectives. Otolaryngol Head Neck Surg 2011;145:767–71.
31. Roe JW, Drinnan MJ, Carding PN, et al. Patient-reported outcomes following parotid-sparing intensity-modulated radiotherapy for head and neck cancer. How important is dysphagia? Oral Oncol 2014;50:1182–7.
32. Patterson JM. Late Effects of Organ Preservation Treatment on Swallowing and Voice; Presentation, Assessment, and Screening. Front Oncol 2019;9:401.
33. Cohen EE, LaMonte SJ, Erb NL, et al. American Cancer Society Head and Neck Cancer Survivorship Care Guideline. CA Cancer J Clin 2016;66:203–39.
34. Patterson JM, Brady GC, Roe JW. Research into the prevention and rehabilitation of dysphagia in head and neck cancer: a UK perspective. Curr Opin Otolaryngol Head Neck Surg 2016;24:208–14.
35. White H, Ford S, Bush B, et al. Salvage surgery for recurrent cancers of the oropharynx: comparing TORS with standard open surgical approaches. JAMA Otolaryngol Head Neck Surg 2013;139:773–8.
36. Brady GC, Hardman JC, Paleri V, et al. Changing paradigms in the treatment of residual/recurrent head and neck cancer: implications for dysphagia management. Curr Opin Otolaryngol Head Neck Surg 2020;28(3):165–71.
37. Wade DT. What is rehabilitation? An empirical investigation leading to an evidence-based description. Clin Rehabil 2020;34(5):571–83.
38. Chen AY, Frankowski R, Bishop-Leone J, et al. The development and validation of a dysphagia-specific quality-of-life questionnaire for patients with head and neck cancer: the MD Anderson dysphagia inventory. Archives of Otolaryngology–Head & Neck Surgery 2001;127(7):870–6.
39. List MA, Ritter-Sterr C, Lansky SB, et al. performance status scale for head and neck cancer patients. Cancer 1990;66(3):564–9.
40. Dhanda J, Schache A, Robinson M, et al. iKnife Rapid Evaporative Ionisation Mass Spectrometry (REIMS) Technology In Head and Neck Surgery. A Ex Vivo Feasibility Study. Br J Oral and Maxillofac Surg 2017;55(10):e61.
41. Ferris RL, Blumenschein G Jr, Fayette J, et al. Nivolumab for Recurrent Squamous-Cell Carcinoma of the Head and Neck. N Engl J Med 2016;375:1856–67.
42. Westbrook TC, Hagemann IS, Ley J, et al. Prospective assessment of the clinical benefit of a tailored cancer gene set built on a next-generation sequencing platform in patients with recurrent or metastatic head and neck cancer. Med Oncol 2019;37:12.
43. Grant DG, Salassa JR, Hinni ML, et al. Carcinoma of the tongue base treated by transoral laser microsurgery, part two: Persistent, recurrent and second primary tumors. Laryngoscope 2006;116:2156–61.
44. Melong JC, Rigby MH, Bullock M, et al. Transoral laser microsurgery for the treatment of oropharyngeal cancer: the Dalhousie University experience. J Otolaryngol Head Neck Surg 2015;44:39.
45. Hess CB, Rash DL, Daly ME, et al. Competing causes of death and medical comorbidities among patients with human papillomavirus-positive vs human papillomavirus-negative oropharyngeal carcinoma and impact on adherence to radiotherapy. JAMA Otolaryngol Head Neck Surg 2014;140:312–6.

Complications of Transoral Robotic Surgery

Rosh K.V. Sethi, MD, MPH[a], Michelle M. Chen, MD, MHS[b], Kelly M. Malloy, MD[b],*

KEYWORDS

- TORS • Transoral robotic surgery • TORS complications

KEY POINTS

- Transoral robotic surgery (TORS) is associated with several important complications, including postoperative hemorrhage, dysphagia, and injury to surrounding structures, including nerves and mucosal surfaces.
- It is imperative that surgeons anticipate and recognize complications, and identify patients who may be at higher risk.
- Appropriate preoperative planning, and intraoperative risk mitigation strategies should be employed to ensure patient safety and to prevent unintended complications.

INTRODUCTION/BACKGROUND

Minimally invasive transoral robotic surgery (TORS) has modernized the approach to multiple head and neck disorders, including difficult-to-access oropharyngeal tumors. It has allowed surgeons to offer less morbid approaches, while also capitalizing on a technology that offers improved visualization, enhanced articular movement, and faster recovery. However, as with any new technology, there are inherent risks and complications. Many of these have become more apparent as TORS use becomes widespread. In some cases, complications related to severe bleeding can be catastrophic whereas others, such as tongue and lip injury, are minor. It is prudent to understand what complications can occur with TORS, and how to anticipate and manage them. This article summarizes major and minor complications, including discussion of prevention and management.

[a] Brigham and Women's Hospital, Division of Otolaryngology-Head and Neck Surgery, 75 Francis Street, Boston, MA 02115, USA; [b] Department of Otolaryngology–Head and Neck Surgery, University of Michigan, 1904 Taubman Center, 1400 East Medical Center Drive, Ann Arbor, MI 48109, USA
* Corresponding author.
E-mail address: kellymal@med.umich.edu
Twitter: @dockellym (K.M.M.)

Otolaryngol Clin N Am 53 (2020) 1109–1115
https://doi.org/10.1016/j.otc.2020.07.017
0030-6665/20/© 2020 Elsevier Inc. All rights reserved.
oto.theclinics.com

DISCUSSION
Postoperative Hemorrhage

Postoperative hemorrhage is the most common complication following TORS.[1,2] It may occur because of major bleeding from named arterial branches, premature scar sloughing, mucosal tears, or trauma to the surgical bed. Postoperative hemorrhage can range in severity from mild blood spotting in oral secretions to severe bleeding that, in some cases, may result in life-threatening cardiopulmonary compromise or even death. Regardless of severity, it is a feared complication that may be difficult to manage because of the location of bleeding, provider expertise, and provider comfort.

As the volume of TORS cases increase and indications for surgery continue to evolve, surgeons have been better able to understand complication rates as they pertain to postoperative bleeding. A classification system to characterize the severity of postoperative hemorrhage was developed by investigators from the Mayo Clinic in 2013 and has helped frame discussion around the subject.[3] Notably, this includes descriptors characterizing amount of bleeding and management required. Although this has not been universally adopted, it may help frame future discussion and assist with academic research nomenclature.

Overall, postoperative hemorrhage after TORS has been reported as between 1.5% and 18.5%.[1,3–13] By comparison, posttonsillectomy hemorrhage among adult tonsillectomy patients is estimated to be 4.8% nationally.[14] Many of the cited studies are single-institution based, making it difficult to assess national trends. Zenga and colleagues[16] used state-wide databases to query more than 500 TORS cases across multiple states and found that 8% of patients experienced postoperative hemorrhage. Patients typically present with bleeding between 6 and 14 days postoperatively, with most (up to 83.6%) bleeding episodes occurring within 2 weeks of surgery.[3,15,16]

Major or severe bleeding is rare and is reported to occur in between 1.7% and 16.5% of cases.[3,13,15,17] In their retrospective cohort of 906 patients, Pollei and colleagues[3] report major postoperative hemorrhage in 5.4% of cases, and severe postoperative hemorrhage in 1.8% of cases. Kubik and colleagues[15] report a major hemorrhage rate of 2.2% and severe hemorrhage rate of 3.7%. Hay and colleagues[13] report a major rate of 3.3% and severe rate of 1.6%.

Post-TORS fatality is extremely rare, with reported incidence of 0.3% to 0.7%[1,18]; however, when it does occur, it is frequently attributed to severe postoperative hemorrhage.[5] Of the 7 post-TORS deaths reported in a survey study of TORS providers, 4 were attributable to severe postoperative hemorrhage.[1]

Recent studies have attempted to identify risk factors associated with postoperative hemorrhage. In a single-institutional study by Kubik and colleagues,[15] history of radiotherapy, TORS for known primary tumor (vs unknown primary work-up), and lack of transcervical arterial ligation were significantly associated with increased risk of major/severe hemorrhage. Additional risk factors may include recurrent tumors, tumor location (eg, tonsil), comorbidities, and anticoagulation therapy.[1,3,8,17]

Variability in postoperative hemorrhage rate may be associated with surgeon volume. According to a 2013 survey study of 2015 procedures reported by 45 TORS-trained surgeons, there may be a trend toward increased risk of bleeding with fewer TORS cases performed; however, this was not statistically significant.[1] Similar findings have been reported by other groups.[19] In general, overall complication rates are lower among higher-volume surgeons (>50 cases).[1] Comprehensive understanding of anatomy relevant to TORS surgery has been touted as an educational necessity for safe and effective TORS procedures.

Achievement of adequate hemostasis in the operating room is paramount to the prevention of TORS hemorrhage. Although cautery is used in nearly all TORS procedures, it is important to identify and ligate large vessels. Ligation can be accomplished with the use of hemoclips, which have been shown to be effective and safe for vessels greater than 0.5 to 1 mm in diameter.[20]

Prophylactic transcervical arterial ligation has been shown in multiple studies to significantly mitigate severity of postoperative hemorrhage. A meta-analysis of 619 patients showed a significant risk reduction of major and severe bleeding events, although overall bleeding rate was unchanged.[21] This finding is consistent with other single-intuitional data.[15] There is currently no consensus for utility or timing of transcervical arterial ligation during TORS; however, multiple investigators advocate its use. In patients who do not undergo concurrent neck dissection, prophylactic tracheostomy for airway protection may be considered.

In most cases, patients require operative examination for control of bleeding. Prior single and multi-institutional data report operating room take-back rates as high as 71%, regardless of severity.[15] Control of postoperative hemorrhage typically does not require use of the robot. Prior studies have shown adequate control with conventional suction monopolar cautery.[6] At a minimum, most investigators advocate observing patients with sentinel bleeding for at least 1 night.[19] In the case of severe bleeding, transcervical ligation of vessels in the operating room, emergent tracheostomy, or endovascular control of bleeding may be required. However, most postoperative bleeding is managed in the operating room via a transoral approach.[1]

Dysphagia

Dysphagia is the most common functional priority of patients with oropharyngeal cancer, both during and after treatment.[22] Compared with other toxicities of treatment, dysphagia is the most strongly correlated with overall quality-of-life scores, even if it is mild.[23] A survey of 1729 oropharyngeal cancer survivors found that 15.5% showed moderate to high decisional regret with respect to their cancer treatment, and difficulty swallowing was one of the strongest drivers of decisional regret.[24] Furthermore, patient-reported dysphagia has been shown to be associated with increased risk of aspiration pneumonia.[25] Nearly all TORS patients self-report some degree of dysphagia; however, among early-stage patients, approximately 92% start oral intake by hospital discharge and 98% by 1 month postoperatively.[26] When diet outcomes are assessed over time using the Performance Status Scale, Leonhardt and colleagues[27] showed that diet scores decreased from a mean of 96.05 pretreatment to 74.44 ($P<.001$) at 6 months but then returned to baseline at around 12 months.

Another objective metric for measuring the degree of functional dysphagia is gastrostomy tube rates. Among patients with oropharyngeal cancer who are treated with nonsurgical modalities, about 62% received gastrostomy tubes.[28] Regarding prolonged gastrostomy tube dependence, 22.8% were still dependent at 6 months and 8.9% at 12 months.[28] With regard to TORs patients, 3% to 39% of all patients had a perioperative feeding tube placed; however, 0% to 9.5% of patients had chronic gastrostomy tube dependence.[1,27,29–34] However, it is hard to compare these 2 groups directly, because TORS studies tend to have a smaller proportion of patients with advanced-stage disease compared with primary chemoradiation patients. Moreover, a significant proportion of TORS patients also receive adjuvant therapy.

Several studies sought to compare functional outcomes after primary TORS compared with primary radiation therapy. Hutcheson and colleagues[35] reviewed 257 patients with oropharyngeal cancer treated with either TORS or radiation therapy and showed that 22.7% had moderate to severe dysphagia (Dynamic Imaging Grade of Swallowing Toxicity grade $\geq$2) postoperatively, but this decreased to 6.7% at 3 to 6 months posttreatment. The degree of persistent moderate to severe dysphagia was not significantly different from the radiotherapy group.[35] The ORATOR trial was the first randomized controlled trial that sought to compare radiotherapy with TORS resection and neck dissection, with the primary end point being swallowing-rated quality of life at 1 year.[36] The trial showed that the mean total MD Anderson Dysphagia Inventory (MDADI) scores at 1 year were 86.9 in the radiotherapy group compared with 80.1 in the TORS and neck dissection group ($P = .042$), but the difference did not meet the threshold for a clinical meaningful difference.[36]

Predictors of postoperative swallowing dysfunction include T stage, nodal stage, base of tongue location, and adjuvant therapy. Patients with T3 to T4 tumors, current smokers, and concurrent chemoradiation were more likely to have gastrostomy tube dependence.[28] In contrast, increasing nodal status was a predictor of poorer MDADI outcomes.[34]

NERVE INJURY

There is a low rate of nerve injury either from surgical technique or for paresis of the lingual nerve caused by pressure on the tongue from the mouth gag. A survey of 2015 procedures performed by 45 TORS-trained surgeons reported a 0.6% rate of inadvertent lingual nerve injury, 0.9% rate of temporary hypoglossal nerve injury, and 0.1% permanent hypoglossal nerve injury.[1]

MUCOSAL, CORNEAL, AND DENTAL INJURY

Although bleeding is the most common complication, additional complications may include injury to the teeth, lips, cornea, or adjacent mucosal surfaces around the site of surgery.[1] It is imperative that surgeons exercise caution when docking the robot and that their assistants monitor for unplanned collisions with surrounding structures. Few studies have cataloged these types of injury; however, some studies suggest they are rare events.[4] Early experiments designed to intentionally injure human cadavers with TORS misuse were largely reassuring and established early safety metrics for human TORS.[37] Regardless, multiple investigators advocate that adequate protection of the teeth, lips, and eyes is imperative. Cost-effective custom-molded dental guards using thermoplastic nasal splint material, and commercially available adhesive safety goggles, are among some of the recent innovations that have been introduced.[1,37,38]

MORTALITY

In the initial study of the safety of transoral lateral oropharyngectomy, Holsinger and colleagues[39] showed a 2.6% mortality in the immediate postoperative period. The mortality after TORS resections of oropharyngeal lesions has now been assessed with several national and institutional studies and noted to be low.[2] A review of 305 TORS patients treated nationally in the United States from 2010 to 2013 showed a 30-day postoperative mortality of 0.7%.[18] For deaths reported to the Food and Drug Administration, the mortality nationwide was approximately 0.3% from 2009 to 2015.[2] Aubry and colleagues[17] conducted an institutional study of 178 TORS patients treated from 2009 to 2014 and showed a 1.1% postoperative mortality.

SUMMARY

TORS is a valuable surgical tool that has permitted substantial innovation in the way clinicians evaluate and manage complex disorders in head and neck surgery.

However, with its increasingly widespread use, clinicians have also gained valuable insight into its inherent risk profile and associated complications. This article summarizes major and minor complications and discusses prevention and management therein. Continued investigation and discussion of postoperative complications is imperative as this novel surgical tool continues to be implemented in daily practice.

CLINICAL CARE POINTS

- The most common complication following TORS is postoperative hemorrhage, which is reported to occur with an incidence between 1.5% and 18.5%.
- Although dysphagia is a common functional complication, most patients are able to tolerate a regular diet and regain functional performance within 12 months after surgery.
- Overall, TORS is a safe procedure; however, mortality has been reported, usually caused by severe postoperative hemorrhage. Surgeons should exercise caution and anticipate potential complications by ensuring adequate knowledge of anatomy, considering transcervical artery ligation when indicated, and using safe surgical techniques

DISCLOSURE

The authors have nothing to disclose.

REFERENCES

1. Chia SH, Gross ND, Richmon JD. Surgeon experience and complications with Transoral Robotic Surgery (TORS). Otolaryngol Head Neck Surg 2013;149: 885–92.
2. Chen MM, Holsinger FC. Morbidity and Mortality Associated With Robotic Head and Neck Surgery: An Inquiry of the Food and Drug Administration Manufacturer and User Facility Device Experience Database. JAMA Otolaryngol Head Neck Surg 2016;142:405–6.
3. Pollei TR, Hinni ML, Moore EJ, et al. Analysis of postoperative bleeding and risk factors in transoral surgery of the oropharynx. JAMA Otolaryngol Head Neck Surg 2013;139:1212–8.
4. Weinstein GS, O'Malley BW Jr, Magnuson JS, et al. Transoral robotic surgery: a multicenter study to assess feasibility, safety, and surgical margins. Laryngoscope 2012;122:1701–7.
5. Laccourreye O, Malinvaud D, Garcia D, et al. Postoperative hemorrhage after transoral oropharyngectomy for cancer of the lateral oropharynx. Ann Otol Rhinol Laryngol 2015;124:361–7.
6. Asher SA, White HN, Kejner AE, et al. Hemorrhage after transoral robotic-assisted surgery. Otolaryngol Head Neck Surg 2013;149:112–7.
7. Lorincz BB, Mockelmann N, Busch CJ, et al. Functional outcomes, feasibility, and safety of resection of transoral robotic surgery: single-institution series of 35 consecutive cases of transoral robotic surgery for oropharyngeal squamous cell carcinoma. Head Neck 2015;37:1618–24.
8. Mandal R, Duvvuri U, Ferris RL, et al. Analysis of post-transoral robotic-assisted surgery hemorrhage: Frequency, outcomes, and prevention. Head Neck 2016; 38(Suppl 1):E776–82.

9. Moore EJ, Olsen SM, Laborde RR, et al. Long-term functional and oncologic results of transoral robotic surgery for oropharyngeal squamous cell carcinoma. Mayo Clin Proc 2012;87:219–25.

10. Park YM, Kim WS, De Virgilio A, et al. Transoral robotic surgery for hypopharyngeal squamous cell carcinoma: 3-year oncologic and functional analysis. Oral Oncol 2012;48:560–6.

11. Vergez S, Lallemant B, Ceruse P, et al. Initial multi-institutional experience with transoral robotic surgery. Otolaryngol Head Neck Surg 2012;147:475–81.

12. Hurtuk A, Agrawal A, Old M, et al. Outcomes of transoral robotic surgery: a preliminary clinical experience. Otolaryngol Head Neck Surg 2011;145:248–53.

13. Hay A, Migliacci J, Karassawa Zanoni D, et al. Haemorrhage following transoral robotic surgery. Clin Otolaryngol 2018;43:638–44.

14. Bhattacharyya N, Kepnes LJ. Revisits and postoperative hemorrhage after adult tonsillectomy. Laryngoscope 2014;124:1554–6.

15. Kubik M, Mandal R, Albergotti W, et al. Effect of transcervical arterial ligation on the severity of postoperative hemorrhage after transoral robotic surgery. Head Neck 2017;39:1510–5.

16. Zenga J, Suko J, Kallogjeri D, et al. Postoperative hemorrhage and hospital revisit after transoral robotic surgery. Laryngoscope 2017;127:2287–92.

17. Aubry K, Vergez S, de Mones E, et al. Morbidity and mortality revue of the French group of transoral robotic surgery: a multicentric study. J Robot Surg 2016; 10:63–7.

18. Su HK, Ozbek U, Likhterov I, et al. Safety of transoral surgery for oropharyngeal malignancies: An analysis of the ACS NSQIP. Laryngoscope 2016;126:2484–91.

19. Gleysteen J, Troob S, Light T, et al. The impact of prophylactic external carotid artery ligation on postoperative bleeding after transoral robotic surgery (TORS) for oropharyngeal squamous cell carcinoma. Oral Oncol 2017;70:1–6.

20. Hockstein NG, Weinstein GS, O'Malley BW Jr. Maintenance of hemostasis in transoral robotic surgery. ORL J Otorhinolaryngol Relat Spec 2005;67:220–4.

21. Bollig CA, Gilley DR, Ahmad J, et al. Prophylactic arterial ligation following transoral robotic surgery: A systematic review and meta-analysis. Head Neck 2020; 42(4):739–46.

22. Wilson JA, Carding PN, Patterson JM. Dysphagia after nonsurgical head and neck cancer treatment: patients' perspectives. Otolaryngol Head Neck Surg 2011;145:767–71.

23. Hunter KU, Schipper M, Feng FY, et al. Toxicities affecting quality of life after chemo-IMRT of oropharyngeal cancer: prospective study of patient-reported, observer-rated, and objective outcomes. Int J Radiat Oncol Biol Phys 2013;85: 935–40.

24. Goepfert RP, Fuller CD, Gunn GB, et al. Symptom burden as a driver of decisional regret in long-term oropharyngeal carcinoma survivors. Head Neck 2017;39: 2151–8.

25. Hunter KU, Lee OE, Lyden TH, et al. Aspiration pneumonia after chemo-intensity-modulated radiation therapy of oropharyngeal carcinoma and its clinical and dysphagia-related predictors. Head Neck 2014;36:120–5.

26. Albergotti WG, Jordan J, Anthony K, et al. A prospective evaluation of short-term dysphagia after transoral robotic surgery for squamous cell carcinoma of the oropharynx. Cancer 2017;123:3132–40.

27. Leonhardt FD, Quon H, Abrahao M, et al. Transoral robotic surgery for oropharyngeal carcinoma and its impact on patient-reported quality of life and function. Head Neck 2012;34:146–54.

28. Bhayani MK, Hutcheson KA, Barringer DA, et al. Gastrostomy tube placement in patients with oropharyngeal carcinoma treated with radiotherapy or chemoradiotherapy: factors affecting placement and dependence. Head Neck 2013;35: 1634–40.

29. Moore EJ, Olsen KD, Kasperbauer JL. Transoral robotic surgery for oropharyngeal squamous cell carcinoma: a prospective study of feasibility and functional outcomes. Laryngoscope 2009;119:2156–64.

30. Genden EM, Park R, Smith C, et al. The role of reconstruction for transoral robotic pharyngectomy and concomitant neck dissection. Arch Otolaryngol Head Neck Surg 2011;137:151–6.

31. More YI, Tsue TT, Girod DA, et al. Functional swallowing outcomes following transoral robotic surgery vs primary chemoradiotherapy in patients with advanced-stage oropharynx and supraglottis cancers. JAMA Otolaryngol Head Neck Surg 2013;139:43–8.

32. Van Abel KM, Moore EJ, Carlson ML, et al. Transoral robotic surgery using the thulium:YAG laser: a prospective study. Arch Otolaryngol Head Neck Surg 2012;138:158–66.

33. Iseli TA, Kulbersh BD, Iseli CE, et al. Functional outcomes after transoral robotic surgery for head and neck cancer. Otolaryngol Head Neck Surg 2009;141: 166–71.

34. Sinclair CF, McColloch NL, Carroll WR, et al. Patient-perceived and objective functional outcomes following transoral robotic surgery for early oropharyngeal carcinoma. Arch Otolaryngol Head Neck Surg 2011;137:1112–6.

35. Hutcheson KA, Warneke CL, Yao C, et al. Dysphagia after primary transoral robotic surgery with neck dissection vs nonsurgical therapy in patients with low- to intermediate-risk oropharyngeal cancer. JAMA Otolaryngol Head Neck Surg 2019;145(11):1053–63.

36. Nichols AC, Theurer J, Prisman E, et al. Radiotherapy versus transoral robotic surgery and neck dissection for oropharyngeal squamous cell carcinoma (ORATOR): an open-label, phase 2, randomised trial. Lancet Oncol 2019;20: 1349–59.

37. Hockstein NG, O'Malley BW Jr, Weinstein GS. Assessment of intraoperative safety in transoral robotic surgery. Laryngoscope 2006;116:165–8.

38. Benito D, Michel MC, Thakkar PG, et al. A cost effective custom dental guard for transoral robotic surgery. J Robot Surg 2020;14:91–4.

39. Holsinger FC, McWhorter AJ, Menard M, et al. Transoral lateral oropharyngectomy for squamous cell carcinoma of the tonsillar region: I. Technique, complications, and functional results. Arch Otolaryngol Head Neck Surg 2005;131: 583–91.

Quality of Life Implications After Transoral Robotic Surgery for Oropharyngeal Cancers

Christopher M.K.L. Yao, MD[a], Katherine A. Hutcheson, PhD[b,c],*

KEYWORDS

- Quality of life • Functional outcomes • PROMs

KEY POINTS

- Understanding the impact of transoral robotic surgery (TORS) on quality of life of patients requires consideration of functional outcomes and the emotional, psychological, and social construct placed on various symptoms.
- Patients consider swallowing to be the most important outcome after cure and survival. To fully understand a patients' swallowing outcome requires the study of their oral intake, feeding tube dependence, and physical impairment (via videofluoroscopic or endoscopic swallow study), in addition to patient-reported outcome questionnaires.
- Tumor volume, advanced T stage, and adjuvant therapy are major predictors of worse swallowing outcomes after TORS.

INTRODUCTION

As survival for human papillomavirus (HPV)-related oropharyngeal squamous cell carcinomas (HPV-OPSCC) improve, the focus in evaluating treatment strategies and clinical outcomes of patients turns toward their quality of life (QOL). QOL is a multifaceted construct that encompasses a person's physical, psychological, and social health as it relates to a particular disease.[1] It provides clinicians an insight into the patient's perception of the impact that either the disease or treatment has had on their life. Although clinicians' and patients' perception can differ markedly, widespread use of

[a] Advanced Head and Neck Surgical Oncology and Microvascular Reconstruction, Department of Head and Neck Surgery, The University of Texas at MD Anderson Cancer Center, 1515 Holcombe Boulevard, Unit 1445, Houston, TX 77030, USA; [b] Department of Head and Neck Surgery, The University of Texas at MD Anderson Cancer Center, 1515 Holcombe Boulevard, Unit 1445, Houston, TX 77030, USA; [c] Division of Radiation Oncology, The University of Texas at MD Anderson Cancer Center, 1515 Holcombe Boulevard, Unit 1445, Houston, TX 77030, USA
* Corresponding author. Division of Radiation Oncology, The University of Texas at MD Anderson Cancer Center, 1515 Holcombe Boulevard, Unit 1445, Houston, TX 77030.
E-mail address: KArnold@mdanderson.org

Otolaryngol Clin N Am 53 (2020) 1117–1129
https://doi.org/10.1016/j.otc.2020.07.018
0030-6665/20/Published by Elsevier Inc.

various QOL tools and their incorporation into clinical trials as primary or secondary outcomes assists with decision-making processes and the ability to compare anticipated treatment outcomes.

Increasingly then, it is important for clinicians to understand what is being measured, how it is measured, and how QOL data can apply to clinical situations. Indeed, applying QOL results may prove the most challenging, as there is subjectivity and lack of guidance as to how much weight QOL measures should play in clinical decision-making. This is particularly true given (1) the patient's ability to adapt over time such that patient experience in the short term (most easily and frequently measured) may become less relevant as long-term outcomes become clearer; (2) QOL measurements are weighted for survivors who are not dealing with active cancer; and (3) there is little agreed-on standard of analysis and reporting at this time.[2]

QOL is particularly important in the discussion of HPV-OPSCCs. Most of the patients do well and survive after treatment of this condition, and analyzing how each treatment modality affects a patients' perceived state of health and wellbeing is important in deciding the optimal treatment. To fully understand what outcomes are of importance after transoral robotic surgery, we need to first understand the priorities and preferences of patients with HPV-OPSCC.

WHAT ARE THE PRIORITIES FOR PATIENTS WITH OROPHARYNX CANCER?

In a recent prospective trial whereby patients completed surveys before and after treatment, patients with HPV-OPSCC were asked to rank their treatment goals. Patients ranked swallowing right after cure and survival as their top three priorities both before and after treatment.[3] Furthermore, after completion of treatment, a proportion of patients ranked moist mouth within the top 3 priorities.[3] This study brings to light the importance of swallowing outcomes in this patient population, in addition to the detrimental impact that xerostomia can have on patients, so much so that it can change their priorities as they experience new symptoms over time.

MEASURING FUNCTIONAL OUTCOMES

Intimately associated with a patient's QOL is their functional outcome. For patients with oropharyngeal cancer, the swallowing mechanism can be affected by the cancer itself or the cancer treatment. Studies of functional outcomes include various metrics such as the use of feeding tubes, the consistency of ingested food, the risk of aspiration, efficiency of swallow, as well as patient-reported swallowing outcomes.

Perioperative feeding tube use, delivered either through a nasogastric (NG) or gastrostomy (G) tube placement, varies widely (3%–100% and 18%–39%, respectively) based on institutional protocols and varying opinions on prophylactic placement.[4-7] Although the duration of perioperative NG tube placement varies from 2 to 13 days, short-term G-tube placements approach a minimum of 3 months, typically used in the adjuvant therapy period.[8] The decision of feeding tube placement should not be made lightly. G-tube placement is an invasive procedure with a small risk for serious complications and a tremendous impact on the QOL of both the patient and the caregivers due to leakage, soiling, and interference with intimacy and family life. It has even been noted to be one of the worst burdens of treatment.[9-12] Furthermore, a systematic review suggested that feeding route may in fact have unintended consequences, with a greater proportion of patients with swallowing difficulties among those receiving a prophylactic G-tube, even in the long term.[13] Long-term G-tube dependence, defined as greater than a year, ranges from 0% to 10.3% after primary surgical modality with older age, open surgical approaches, resection of more than 25% of the oral tongue, and advance T-stage found to be significant predictors of long-term G-tube dependence.[14,15] It is also worth noting that in one cohort, 10.3% of patients who received TORS followed by adjuvant therapy were G-tube dependent compared with 0.0% in those undergoing TORS alone. Other recent series have mirrored these trends, with long-term tube feeding dependence ranging from 6% to 18.8% for those with advanced stage disease requiring adjuvant treatment.[16,17] Prolonged feeding tube dependence is undoubtedly associated with adjuvant therapy, with 25% to 35% of patients percutaneous endoscopic gastrostomy (PEG)-tube dependent after chemoradiation and 10% after 2 years.[8]

However, the presence or absence of a feeding tube does not fully characterize a patient's swallowing function. In order to further characterize a patient's functional ability, it is important to understand the nature of tube use, such as how frequent patients access feeding tubes and the percentage of their nutritional intake derived from parenteral feeds. The patients' oral intake, including the time to oral intake, and consistency of food ingested provides further insight into functional status. The initiation of oral intake after surgery is closely linked with the perceived safety for swallowing both from an aspiration and from a wound contamination perspective. In addition to swallowing ability and healing, time to oral intake often reflects also the patient's overall condition, including any underlying baseline comorbidities and their pain control. That being said, most case series indicate that oral intake started as early as POD1 after TORS for early staged tumors and varied from 1 to 4 weeks postoperatively depending on the stage of the tumor.[6,18,19] More recently, in the setting of a prospective trial, 92% of patients proceeded to oral intake by discharge and 98% of patients by 1 month, with many requiring compensatory strategies to do so.[20]

Aside from the presence of feeding tube, the placement of a tracheostomy tube was also a commonly reported clinical measure in early studies. As surgeons became more experienced with TORS, placement of tracheostomy tube ranged from 0% to 3.5% at the time of surgery, with permanent tracheostomy tubes exceedingly rare (0.5%).[8,21] With the exception of the recently published ORATOR trial results,[22] contemporary series continue to report low rates of tracheostomy tube placements, occurring more commonly in the setting of complications.[23] Postoperative weight loss is another important functional indicator. A mean weight loss of 4.1% has been reported to occur primarily between POD 1 and 7.[20] Furthermore, case control data reported that surgically treated patients were less likely to experience grade 3 weight loss (per Common Terminology Criteria for Adverse Events) of greater than 5% to 10% of their body weight within 90 days of treatment than nonsurgically treated patients.[24]

Other clinical measures of swallowing include both clinician-rated functional scales such as the Performance Status Scale for Head and Neck Cancer Patients (PSS-HN) and Functional Outcomes Swallowing Score (FOSS) as well as patient-reported outcome (PRO) questionnaires such as the Eating Assessment Tool (EAT-10), MD Anderson Dysphagia Inventory (MDADI), Functional Assessment of Cancer Therapy (FACT), and the Sydney Swallow Questionnaire (SSQ).[25-29] Although there are several PRO measurement tools that capture both function and QOL outcomes, the latter 3 have been more widely used and validated for patients with head and neck cancer specifically.

The strength of the PSS-HN questionnaire is that it captures the normalcy of diet on a 0 to 100 scale, and estimates a patient's ability to tolerate various consistencies of food from liquids (10) to dry foods (60). Although it is a clinician-administered instrument, it explores the patients' comfortability with eating in public and estimates their speech understandability. When the PSS-HN tool was used for TORS patients, the normalcy of diet scores dropped from an unrestricted solid food diet preoperatively

(96.1 ± 17.0) to a range of 25 to 75 points in the 2- to 6-month time frame, before returning back to baseline around the 1-year mark.[5,7] Another clinician-rated scale, the FOSS, distinguishes patients based on the clinician-rated 5-stage scale, ranging from stage 0 = normal function and asymptomatic to stage V = nonoral feeding for all nutrition.[29] In one series, the median FOSS scores at the pre- and 1-month post-TORs interval was 1, which indicated a compensated abnormal swallow function. Patients with a normal pre-TORS FOSS stage generally returned to stage 0 at 1 month.[6]

The EAT-10 questionnaire is a 10-question likert-type PRO survey quantifying various dysphagia symptoms, and although it has primarily been used in evaluating neurologic or benign conditions that affect swallowing, it has recently been validated to correlate with unsafe swallowing in recently treated patients with head and neck cancer, and with postswallow pharyngeal residue on fiberoptic endoscopic evaluation.[30–32] The EAT-10 questionnaire was featured in 2 prospective studies of postoperative (TORS ± adjuvant therapy) patients. One study focused on the evolution of swallowing in the immediate month following surgery, finding that EAT-10 scores significantly increased between POD1 and POD7 but decreased by POD30.[20] When EAT-10 was used in a prospective cohort of patients treated with TORS ± adjuvant therapy, scores were found to significantly worsen in the postoperative period and improve but remain worse than baseline between 6 and 12 months, and for TORS-only patients, there was no difference than baseline scores after 12 months.[23] However, this contrasted with a head and neck–specific QOL eating subscale used in the same study, whereby there continued to be a difference in the TORS-only subgroup beyond 12 months, suggesting EAT-10 may not be as sensitive to changes experienced in this surgical population.

The MDADI is a self-administered 20-item questionnaire, exploring 4 domains of swallowing-related QOL, including global, emotional, functional, and physical subscales, with high scores representing better day-to-day functioning and QOL.[27] Among several studies that used the MDADI tool, composite scores over a year out from surgery ranged from 65.2 to 78.[4,18,33] Furthermore, patients with prolonged feeding tube, higher T-stage tumor, and those who had complications were found to have worse postoperative MDADI scores.[18] Finally, the FACT instrument and SSQ were recently compared with the MDADI, with the FACT-Head and neck cancer–specific questionnaire likely overlapping with the MDADI in collected information.[28]

INSTRUMENTAL SWALLOWING ASSESSMENTS

Although the inventories and questionnaires discussed earlier provide us with the perceived swallowing dysfunction, the exact cause of the dysfunction does not become revealed. More objective data from radiographic or endoscopic swallowing evaluations have not been as frequently reported after TORS. Clinically, speech language pathologists perform fiberoptic endoscopic evaluation of swallowing (FEES) and Modified Barium Swallow (MBS) to characterize oropharyngeal swallowing dysfunction.[34,35] Both studies provide complementary information. With FEES, there is direct endoscopic visualization, which allows for examination of the pharyngeal stage of swallowing including the ability to handle secretions, although the view may be lost during bolus passage as shown in **Fig. 1**.[36] FEES is attractive after TORS to visualize the wound as well as laterality of impairment and physiology such as pharyngeal constriction and velopharyngeal function during swallowing and nonswallowing tasks. The MBS allows for examination of the bolus flow in relation to the surrounding swallowing structure as shown in **Fig. 2** and may be more sensitive

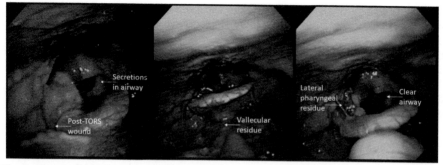

Fig. 1. Fiberoptic Endoscopic Evaluation of Swallowing (FEES). FEES 2 weeks post-TORS for T2 N1 M0 (AJCC 8th edition) HPV-associated squamous cell carcinoma of the right base of tongue with extension to the glossotonsillar fold. Endoscopy (*left image*) reveals tongue base and lateral pharyngectomy wound. After bolus trials, vallecular residue (*middle image*) and lateralized pharyngeal residue (*right image*) are evident along with clear laryngeal airway reflecting dysphagia resulting in inefficient bolus clearance but safe swallowing.

at detecting aspiration but requires the exposure to ionizing radiation.[37,38] MBS may be favored for dynamic views of oral, pharyngeal, and esophageal phases of swallowing and offers more quantitative parameters to characterize pathophysiology of dysphagia.

In order to communicate results of the MBS more universally, the Dynamic Imaging Grade of Swallowing Toxicity (DIGEST) method was developed, which translates MBS-derived assessments into a universal toxicity grade aligning to the common terminology criteria for adverse events (CTCAE) framework that is commonly used in oncology.[39] Scores reflect both the safety and efficiency of a swallow, based on the patterns and interaction of laryngeal penetration/aspiration ratings and pharyngeal residue. This method was recently used to report on a prospective collected cohort

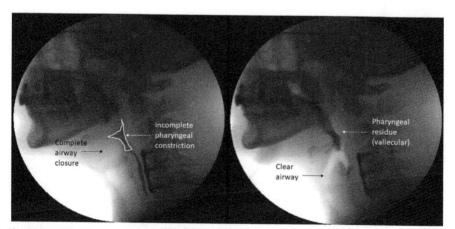

Fig. 2. Modified barium swallow (MBS) study. MBS 4 weeks post-TORS for T1 N2b M0 (AJCC 7th edition) HPV-associated squamous cell carcinoma of the right tonsil. Videofluoroscopy shows incomplete pharyngeal constriction and complete airway closure at peak swallow (*left image*) with vallecular residue and clear airway postswallow (*right image*). Mild dysphagia characterized by inefficient bolus clearance but intact airway protection.

of patients with oropharynx cancer treated with primary surgery, confirming that swallowing acutely worsened after surgery (23% prevalence of moderate to severe dysphagia on average 3 weeks post-TORS), with patients with larger tumor volume predictive of worse swallowing outcomes.[40] Swallowing function improved by 3 to 6 months after TORS, although many remained worse than baseline with up to 13.6% and 13.3% of those requiring adjuvant radiation or chemoradiation respectively, having DIGEST grades greater than or equal to 2 reflective of moderate to severe dysphagia.

QUALITY OF LIFE

Functional outcomes provide a barometer for understanding the degree to which a patient can carry an activity, without the emotional, and psychological importance that patient's may place on the activity. A patient's QOL, however, goes beyond the physical domain and includes the emotional, functional, and social domains. To assess a patient's QOL, a plethora of general and head and neck–specific questionnaires were developed, including the MD Anderson Symptom Inventory Head and Neck (MDASI-HN), University of Washington QoL (UWQOL), Functional Assessment of Cancer Therapy-Head and Neck (FACT-H&N), Head and Neck Cancer Inventory, Michigan Head and Neck Quality of Life instrument, European Organization for Research and Treatment of Cancer Core (EORTC) QLQ-C30 as well as QLQ-H&N35, SF-8, SF36 and Health Utilities Index Mark 3 (HUI3), among others.[41] Recent structured reviews outlined the most commonly used questionnaires in head and neck cancer and oropharyngeal cancers as measured by number of publications were the EORTC QLQ-C30/HN-35, UW-QOL, and the MDADI.[41,42] With the plethora of QOL instruments, the National Cancer Institute was tasked with evaluating the various instruments and their suitability for use in multicenter clinical trials. They found that most instruments can adequately assess patient's QOL, with a high degree of reliability and validity, and called for more standardization in their use for clinical trials.[43] Although going in depth with each tool is beyond the scope of this article, the authors highlight the ones that have been used specifically for evaluating patients with OPSCC.

The EORTC QLQ-C30/HN35 is one of the more detailed instruments, containing 2 modules with a 30-question cancer-specific module and an additional 35 questions specific to head and neck cancer (ie, swallowing, senses, speech, and social eating). It takes approximately 7 minutes to complete either module, and each domain is normalized to a scale between 0 to 100, with higher scores reflecting better functional scales but worse for symptom scales.[44] A change of 5 to 10 points reflects a clinically significant change.[45] In a cross-sectional survey of oropharyngeal cancer survivors, with a median of 67 months after treatment, patients treated with surgery alone had less issues with dry mouth, trouble with teeth, and other senses when compared with those treated with radiation.[46]

The UWQOL questionnaire was developed from a surgical perspective, with 15 questions, including 3 generic and 12 domain items that are aggregated into a single composite score between 0 (worse) and 100 (best).[47] A difference of 6 to 7 points indicates a clinically significant change.[48] The UWQOL has been used in 4 studies,[49–52] confirming that those treated with surgery alone had better QOL indexes particularly in the swallowing and diet domains a year out from surgery, and no patient had further deterioration of symptoms after a month. In fact, as many as 74% of surgical patients reported swallowing to be "as well as ever" compared with 32% in the nonsurgical group, although this included transoral laser microsurgery patients.[49]

The MD Anderson Symptom Inventory—Head and Neck Module (MDASI-HN), although not a QOL instrument per say, is a multisymptom survey quantifying the domain of symptom burden. MDASI-HN assesses symptom severity for 11 head and neck cancer–specific items (ie, choking, taste) in addition to 13 cancer symptoms (ie, pain, fatigue, sleep) and 6 interference symptoms (ie, work, relationship).[53] The symptom interference score is considered a QOL surrogate. This tool was recently used to characterize the symptom burden in patients with OPSCC treated surgically versus nonsurgically.[54] Initially, after surgery, patients who underwent surgery alone were significantly worse with regard to their voice, choking, and numbness scores. By 6 months, these scores were similar between the 2 groups, and instead, those who underwent radiation alone had significantly worse dry mouth, mucus, and taste disturbances. For patients treated with a single treatment modality, those who underwent surgery had better MDASI scores than those who underwent radiation at 6 months.[54] It is clear then, that when patients can be treated with surgery alone, this offers them the shortest treatment duration and shorter duration of posttreatment side effects.[55] If multimodality treatment is required, there seems to be similar symptom burden between surgical and nonsurgical cohorts, although nonsurgical cohorts continued to have worse dry mouth and taste disturbances. Use of a multisymptom instrument such as MDASI-HN can help to characterize the trade-off or distinctions in symptom profiles between treatment modalities. At this time, longer term symptom and QOL studies in the late survivorship time frame is lacking in literature, although there are suggestions that certain radiation toxicities may occur years after treatment.[56,57]

HEALTH UTILITIES

QOL measurements can be distilled to a quantified state using health utilities. Health state utilities use numbers to reflect how strongly an individual weighs a particular outcome in the face of uncertainty and are classically derived through various interview techniques such as the Time Trade Off or Standard Gamble methodology.[58,59] When these interview techniques were used to assess whether a healthy person or expert would prefer one treatment over the other, TORS alone was preferred over radiotherapy by both healthy subjects and experts.[60] Even after the addition of adjuvant radiotherapy, subjects still preferred surgery over definitive chemoradiation in paired comparisons but not when trimodality therapy was indicated. These utilities can further be used to perform cost-utility analyses to assist with treatment decision-making. A cost-utility analysis comparing TORS with nonsurgical management for early tumors was found to have a cost savings of $1,366 and an increase of 0.25 quality-adjusted life years compared with nonsurgical management.[61]

Predictors of Quality of Life and Functional Outcomes

In the management of OPSCC, TORS has provided a minimally invasive surgical approach with better functional outcomes and QOL outcomes than traditional open surgical approaches.[62] Furthermore, studies reporting the functional and QOL outcomes have all similarly demonstrated a short-term decrease of either outcome that recovers to near baseline by 6 to 12 months. However, in the treatment of OPSCCs, TORS cannot be considered alone. Upward of 70% of patients will receive either adjuvant radiation or chemoradiation.[8] With the addition of adjuvant therapy, reports have indicated a significant decrease in functional and QOL outcomes at 3 to 6 months that may not fully recover by a year's time.[40,63]

Those who do undergo TORS may receive a lower radiation dose in the adjuvant setting, compared with those treated with definitive chemoradiation. Radiation dose is known to have a logarithmic dose-toxicity scale with 3.4% increase risk of having at least grade 2 dysphagia per increase in gray to the constrictor musculature.[64–66] Indeed, even if trimodality therapy is indicated, there are reports that patients undergoing surgery have better QOL scores than those treated with definitive chemoradiation at 12 months.[4,49,67] Even after stratifying groups by T-stage and subsites, this finding remains significant, but must be interpreted cautiously, as most series are subject to selection bias. Although it is important to acknowledge this, when properly selected, TORS may be able to deliver improved outcomes compared with primary nonsurgical treatment.

Aside from adjuvant therapy, advance T-stage is also an important predictor of postoperative swallowing outcomes. Tumor volume was found to be predictive of swallowing outcomes, with tumor volume greater than 9.35 cm^3 more likely to have worse baseline swallowing dysfunction in addition to ongoing swallowing dysfunction immediately after TORS.[40] Patients with larger tumors were also more likely to have PEG placement.[8]

Despite these excellent outcomes, severe prolonged dysphagia has been reported after transoral resection of oropharynx lesions.[68] Several small case reports have suggested that bilateral glossopharyngeal nerve injury, in addition to injury to the superior pharyngeal constrictor muscles, may have contributed to prolonged swallowing dysfunction.

SUMMARY

TORS has provided an excellent surgical modality for patients with oropharynx cancer, with the potential to minimize the negative impact on functional and QOL outcomes. This is particularly apparent when compared with nonsurgical treatment modalities where studies have demonstrated patients to more readily recover from surgery than radiation or chemoradiation, and in the carefully selected patient, even in the setting of adjuvant therapy. The main predictors of poor functional and QOL outcomes are larger tumors and adjuvant treatment. Therefore, careful selection of patients, particularly those with low-intermediate disease may allow for optimal functional and QOL outcomes.

CLINICS CARE POINTS

- Patients consider swallowing to be the most important outcome after cure and survival.[3] To fully understand a patients' swallowing outcome requires the study of their oral intake, feeding tube dependence, and physical impairment (via videofluoroscopic or endoscopic swallow study), in addition to patient-PRO questionnaires.
- Patients have an acute worsening of swallowing function after TORS, which improves by 3 to 6 months.[20,40]
- Tumor volume, advanced T-stage, and adjuvant therapy are major predictors of worse swallowing outcomes after TORS.[8,40]

DISCLOSURE

C.M.K.L. Yao has nothing to disclose. Dr K.A. Hutcheson acknowledges funding support from the National Institute of Dental and Craniofacial Research, the National

Cancer Institute, the Patient-Centered Outcomes Research Institute, and the Charles and Daneen Stiefel Oropharynx Cancer Research Fund.

REFERENCES

1. Guyatt GH, Feeny DH, Patrick DL. Measuring health-related quality of life. Ann Intern Med 1993;118(8):622–9.
2. Rogers SN, Semple C, Babb M, et al. Quality of life considerations in head and neck cancer: United Kingdom National Multidisciplinary Guidelines. J Laryngol Otol 2016;130(S2):S49–52.
3. Windon MJ, Fakhry C, Faraji F, et al. Priorities of human papillomavirus-associated oropharyngeal cancer patients at diagnosis and after treatment. Oral Oncol 2019;95:11–5.
4. More YI, Tsue TT, Girod DA, et al. Functional swallowing outcomes following transoral robotic surgery vs primary chemoradiotherapy in patients with advanced-stage oropharynx and supraglottis cancers. JAMA Otolaryngol Head Neck Surg 2013;139(1):43–8.
5. Leonhardt FD, Quon H, Abrahao M, et al. Transoral robotic surgery for oropharyngeal carcinoma and its impact on patient-reported quality of life and function. Head Neck 2012;34(2):146–54.
6. Moore EJ, Olsen KD, Kasperbauer JL. Transoral robotic surgery for oropharyngeal squamous cell carcinoma: a prospective study of feasibility and functional outcomes. Laryngoscope 2009;119(11):2156–64.
7. Genden EM, Park R, Smith C, et al. The role of reconstruction for transoral robotic pharyngectomy and concomitant neck dissection. Arch Otolaryngol Head Neck Surg 2011;137(2):151–6.
8. Hutcheson KA, Holsinger FC, Kupferman ME, et al. Functional outcomes after TORS for oropharyngeal cancer: a systematic review. Eur Arch Otorhinolaryngol 2015;272(2):463–71.
9. Grant DG, Bradley PT, Pothier DD, et al. Complications following gastrostomy tube insertion in patients with head and neck cancer: a prospective multi-institution study, systematic review and meta-analysis. Clin Otolaryngol 2009;34(2):103–12.
10. Rogers SN, Thomson R, O'Toole P, et al. Patients experience with long-term percutaneous endoscopic gastrostomy feeding following primary surgery for oral and oropharyngeal cancer. Oral Oncol 2007;43(5):499–507.
11. Terrell JE, Ronis DL, Fowler KE, et al. Clinical predictors of quality of life in patients with head and neck cancer. Arch Otolaryngol Head Neck Surg 2004;130(4):401–8.
12. Mayre-Chilton KM, Talwar BP, Goff LM. Different experiences and perspectives between head and neck cancer patients and their care-givers on their daily impact of a gastrostomy tube. J Hum Nutr Diet 2011;24(5):449–59.
13. Paleri V, Patterson J. Use of gastrostomy in head and neck cancer: a systematic review to identify areas for future research. Clin Otolaryngol 2010;35(3):177–89.
14. Varma VR, Eskander A, Kang SY, et al. Predictors of gastrostomy tube dependence in surgically managed oropharyngeal squamous cell carcinoma. Laryngoscope 2019;129(2):415–21.
15. Dziegielewski PT, Teknos TN, Durmus K, et al. Transoral robotic surgery for oropharyngeal cancer: long-term quality of life and functional outcomes. JAMA Otolaryngol Head Neck Surg 2013;139(11):1099–108.

16. Canis M, Ihler F, Wolff HA, et al. Oncologic and functional results after transoral laser microsurgery of tongue base carcinoma. Eur Arch Otorhinolaryngol 2013; 270(3):1075–83.

17. Haughey BH, Hinni ML, Salassa JR, et al. Transoral laser microsurgery as primary treatment for advanced-stage oropharyngeal cancer: a United States multicenter study. Head Neck 2011;33(12):1683–94.

18. Iseli TA, Kulbersh BD, Iseli CE, et al. Functional outcomes after transoral robotic surgery for head and neck cancer. Otolaryngol Head Neck Surg 2009;141(2): 166–71.

19. Hurtuk A, Agrawal A, Old M, et al. Outcomes of transoral robotic surgery: a preliminary clinical experience. Otolaryngol Head Neck Surg 2011;145(2):248–53.

20. Albergotti WG, Jordan J, Anthony K, et al. A prospective evaluation of short-term dysphagia after transoral robotic surgery for squamous cell carcinoma of the oropharynx. Cancer 2017;123(16):3132–40.

21. Yeh DH, Tam S, Fung K, et al. Transoral robotic surgery vs. radiotherapy for management of oropharyngeal squamous cell carcinoma - A systematic review of the literature. Eur J Surg Oncol 2015;41(12):1603–14.

22. Nichols AC, Theurer J, Prisman E, et al. Radiotherapy versus transoral robotic surgery and neck dissection for oropharyngeal squamous cell carcinoma (ORATOR): an open-label, phase 2, randomised trial. Lancet Oncol 2019; 20(10):1349–59.

23. Achim V, Bolognone RK, Palmer AD, et al. Long-term Functional and Quality-of-Life Outcomes After Transoral Robotic Surgery in Patients With Oropharyngeal Cancer. JAMA Otolaryngol Head Neck Surg 2018;144(1):18–27.

24. Heah H, Goepfert RP, Hutcheson KA, et al. Decreased gastrostomy tube incidence and weight loss after transoral robotic surgery for low- to intermediate-risk oropharyngeal squamous cell carcinoma. Head Neck 2018;40(11):2507–13.

25. Belafsky PC, Mouadeb DA, Rees CJ, et al. Validity and reliability of the Eating Assessment Tool (EAT-10). Ann Otol Rhinol Laryngol 2008;117(12):919–24.

26. List MA, D'Antonio LL, Cella DF, et al. The Performance Status Scale for Head and Neck Cancer Patients and the Functional Assessment of Cancer Therapy-Head and Neck Scale. A study of utility and validity. Cancer 1996;77(11):2294–301.

27. Chen AY, Frankowski R, Bishop-Leone J, et al. The development and validation of a dysphagia-specific quality-of-life questionnaire for patients with head and neck cancer: the M. D. Anderson dysphagia inventory. Arch Otolaryngol Head Neck Surg 2001;127(7):870–6.

28. Peng LC, Hui X, Cheng Z, et al. Prospective evaluation of patient reported swallow function with the Functional Assessment of Cancer Therapy (FACT), MD Anderson Dysphagia Inventory (MDADI) and the Sydney Swallow Questionnaire (SSQ) in head and neck cancer patients. Oral Oncol 2018;84:25–30.

29. Salassa JR. A functional outcome swallowing scale for staging oropharyngeal dysphagia. Dig Dis 1999;17(4):230–4.

30. Cheney DM, Siddiqui MT, Litts JK, et al. The Ability of the 10-Item Eating Assessment Tool (EAT-10) to Predict Aspiration Risk in Persons With Dysphagia. Ann Otol Rhinol Laryngol 2015;124(5):351–4.

31. Florie M, Pilz W, Kremer B, et al. EAT-10 Scores and Fiberoptic Endoscopic Evaluation of Swallowing in Head and Neck Cancer Patients. Laryngoscope 2020. https://doi.org/10.1002/lary.28626.

32. Arrese LC, Schieve HJ, Graham JM, et al. Relationship between oral intake, patient perceived swallowing impairment, and objective videofluoroscopic

measures of swallowing in patients with head and neck cancer. Head Neck 2019; 41(4):1016–23.

33. Sinclair CF, McColloch NL, Carroll WR, et al. Patient-perceived and objective functional outcomes following transoral robotic surgery for early oropharyngeal carcinoma. Arch Otolaryngol Head Neck Surg 2011;137(11):1112–6.

34. Hiss SG, Postma GN. Fiberoptic endoscopic evaluation of swallowing. Laryngoscope 2003;113(8):1386–93.

35. Logemann JA. Role of the modified barium swallow in management of patients with dysphagia. Otolaryngol Head Neck Surg 1997;116(3):335–8.

36. Langmore SE. Evaluation of oropharyngeal dysphagia: which diagnostic tool is superior? Curr Opin Otolaryngol Head Neck Surg 2003;11(6):485–9.

37. Scharitzer M, Roesner I, Pokieser P, et al. Simultaneous Radiological and Fiber-endoscopic Evaluation of Swallowing ("SIRFES") in Patients After Surgery of Oropharyngeal/Laryngeal Cancer and Postoperative Dysphagia. Dysphagia 2019;34(6):852–61.

38. Kelly AM, Drinnan MJ, Leslie P. Assessing penetration and aspiration: how do videofluoroscopy and fiberoptic endoscopic evaluation of swallowing compare? Laryngoscope 2007;117(10):1723–7.

39. Hutcheson KA, Barrow MP, Barringer DA, et al. Dynamic Imaging Grade of Swallowing Toxicity (DIGEST): Scale development and validation. Cancer 2017; 123(1):62–70.

40. Hutcheson KA, Warneke CL, Yao C, et al. Dysphagia After Primary Transoral Robotic Surgery With Neck Dissection vs Nonsurgical Therapy in Patients With Low-to Intermediate-Risk Oropharyngeal Cancer. JAMA Otolaryngol Head Neck Surg 2019;145(11):1053–63.

41. Ojo B, Genden EM, Teng MS, et al. A systematic review of head and neck cancer quality of life assessment instruments. Oral Oncol 2012;48(10):923–37.

42. Hoxbroe Michaelsen S, Gronhoj C, Hoxbroe Michaelsen J, et al. Quality of life in survivors of oropharyngeal cancer: A systematic review and meta-analysis of 1366 patients. Eur J Cancer 2017;78:91–102.

43. Ringash J, Bernstein LJ, Cella D, et al. Outcomes toolbox for head and neck cancer research. Head Neck 2015;37(3):425–39.

44. Bjordal K, Hammerlid E, Ahlner-Elmqvist M, et al. Quality of life in head and neck cancer patients: validation of the European Organization for Research and Treatment of Cancer Quality of Life Questionnaire-H&N35. J Clin Oncol 1999;17(3): 1008–19.

45. Osoba D, Bezjak A, Brundage M, et al. Analysis and interpretation of health-related quality-of-life data from clinical trials: basic approach of The National Cancer Institute of Canada Clinical Trials Group. Eur J Cancer 2005;41(2):280–7.

46. Broglie MA, Soltermann A, Haile SR, et al. Quality of life of oropharyngeal cancer patients with respect to treatment strategy and p16-positivity. Laryngoscope 2013;123(1):164–70.

47. Weymuller EA Jr, Alsarraf R, Yueh B, et al. Analysis of the performance characteristics of the University of Washington Quality of Life instrument and its modification (UW-QOL-R). Arch Otolaryngol Head Neck Surg 2001;127(5):489–93.

48. El-Deiry MW, Futran ND, McDowell JA, et al. Influences and predictors of long-term quality of life in head and neck cancer survivors. Arch Otolaryngol Head Neck Surg 2009;135(4):380–4.

49. Chen AM, Daly ME, Luu Q, et al. Comparison of functional outcomes and quality of life between transoral surgery and definitive chemoradiotherapy for oropharyngeal cancer. Head Neck 2015;37(3):381–5.

50. Choby GW, Kim J, Ling DC, et al. Transoral robotic surgery alone for oropharyngeal cancer: quality-of-life outcomes. JAMA Otolaryngol Head Neck Surg 2015; 141(6):499–504.

51. Maxwell JH, Mehta V, Wang H, et al. Quality of life in head and neck cancer patients: impact of HPV and primary treatment modality. Laryngoscope 2014; 124(7):1592–7.

52. Park YM, Byeon HK, Chung HP, et al. Comparison study of transoral robotic surgery and radical open surgery for hypopharyngeal cancer. Acta Otolaryngol 2013;133(6):641–8.

53. Rosenthal DI, Mendoza TR, Chambers MS, et al. Measuring head and neck cancer symptom burden: the development and validation of the M. D. Anderson symptom inventory, head and neck module. Head Neck 2007;29(10):923–31.

54. Amit M, Hutcheson K, Zaveri J, et al. Patient-reported outcomes of symptom burden in patients receiving surgical or nonsurgical treatment for low-intermediate risk oropharyngeal squamous cell carcinoma: A comparative analysis of a prospective registry. Oral Oncol 2019;91:13–20.

55. Ling DC, Chapman BV, Kim J, et al. Oncologic outcomes and patient-reported quality of life in patients with oropharyngeal squamous cell carcinoma treated with definitive transoral robotic surgery versus definitive chemoradiation. Oral Oncol 2016;61:41–6.

56. Dong Y, Ridge JA, Li T, et al. Long-term toxicities in 10-year survivors of radiation treatment for head and neck cancer. Oral Oncol 2017;71:122–8.

57. Townes TG, Navuluri S, Pytynia KB, et al. Assessing patient-reported symptom burden of long-term head and neck cancer survivors at annual surveillance in survivorship clinic. Head Neck 2020;42(8):1919–27.

58. Torrance GW, Thomas WH, Sackett DL. A utility maximization model for evaluation of health care programs. Health Serv Res 1972;7(2):118–33.

59. Noel CW, Lee DJ, Kong Q, et al. Comparison of Health State Utility Measures in Patients With Head and Neck Cancer. JAMA Otolaryngol Head Neck Surg 2015; 141(8):696–703.

60. de Almeida JR, Villanueva NL, Moskowitz AJ, et al. Preferences and utilities for health states after treatment for oropharyngeal cancer: transoral robotic surgery versus definitive (chemo)radiotherapy. Head Neck 2014;36(7):923–33.

61. de Almeida JR, Moskowitz AJ, Miles BA, et al. Cost-effectiveness of transoral robotic surgery versus (chemo)radiotherapy for early T classification oropharyngeal carcinoma: A cost-utility analysis. Head Neck 2016;38(4):589–600.

62. Lee SY, Park YM, Byeon HK, et al. Comparison of oncologic and functional outcomes after transoral robotic lateral oropharyngectomy versus conventional surgery for T1 to T3 tonsillar cancer. Head Neck 2014;36(8):1138–45.

63. Sethia R, Yumusakhuylu AC, Ozbay I, et al. Quality of life outcomes of transoral robotic surgery with or without adjuvant therapy for oropharyngeal cancer. Laryngoscope 2018;128(2):403–11.

64. Tsai CJ, Jackson A, Setton J, et al. Modeling Dose Response for Late Dysphagia in Patients With Head and Neck Cancer in the Modern Era of Definitive Chemoradiation. JCO Clin Cancer Inform 2017;1:1–7.

65. MD Anderson Head and Neck Cancer Symptom Working Group, Spatial-Nonspatial Multi-Dimensional Analysis of Radiotherapy Treatment/Toxicity Team (SMART3). Chronic radiation-associated dysphagia in oropharyngeal cancer survivors: Towards age-adjusted dose constraints for deglutitive muscles. Clin Transl Radiat Oncol 2019;18:16–22.

66. Eisbruch A, Kim HM, Feng FY, et al. Chemo-IMRT of oropharyngeal cancer aiming to reduce dysphagia: swallowing organs late complication probabilities and dosimetric correlates. Int J Radiat Oncol Biol Phys 2011;81(3):e93–9.
67. Genden EM, Kotz T, Tong CC, et al. Transoral robotic resection and reconstruction for head and neck cancer. Laryngoscope 2011;121(8):1668–74.
68. Patel AB, Hinni ML, Pollei TR, et al. Severe prolonged dysphagia following transoral resection of bilateral synchronous tonsillar carcinoma. Eur Arch Otorhinolaryngol 2015;272(11):3585–91.

Cost Considerations for Robotic Surgery

James Kenneth Byrd, MD*, Rebecca Paquin, MD, DMD

KEYWORDS

- TORS • Transoral • Robotic • Surgery • ENT • Otolaryngology • Economic • Cost

KEY POINTS

- Transoral robotic surgery (TORS) is rapidly becoming a more commonly used therapeutic and diagnostic tool.
- Cost-effectiveness analysis is complex and should include evaluation of both economic impact as well as impact to the health state.
- On analysis of current data, TORS seems to be cost-effective when patient selection is appropriate.

INTRODUCTION

Robotics is growing steadily across surgical disciplines.[1–3] The demand for robotic surgery has increased significantly since its advent, creating a market worth of more than $3 billion in 2014, projected to exceed $20 billion by 2021. The da Vinci surgical robot (Intuitive Surgical, Sunnyvale, CA) is the most commercially successful robotic surgical platform to date.[4] As of 2017, an estimated 2800 of 5500 hospitals in the United States own a da Vinci robot, with an estimated 644,000 robotic surgeries performed annually nationwide.[5]

Robotic head and neck surgery has transformed the management of benign and malignant diseases of the head and neck in slightly more than a decade. Before the advent of transoral robotic surgery (TORS), oropharyngeal squamous cell carcinoma (OPSCC) was typically treated with primary open surgical approaches or with primary chemoradiation therapy (CRT), leading to cosmetic deformities, toxicities, and deleterious impacts on oropharyngeal and laryngeal function. TORS as a primary treatment modality for tongue base squamous cell carcinoma was first described in the literature in 2006; this was followed by approval of TORS for both benign and malignant diseases of the head and neck by the US Food and Drug Administration in 2009.[6,7] TORS has since developed as an option that preserves optimal patient function and

Otolaryngology – Head and Neck Surgery, Medical College of Georgia, Augusta University, 1120 15th Street BP 4132, Augusta, GA, USA
* Corresponding author.
E-mail address: ken.byrd@augusta.edu

Otolaryngol Clin N Am 53 (2020) 1131–1138
https://doi.org/10.1016/j.otc.2020.07.019
0030-6665/20/© 2020 Elsevier Inc. All rights reserved.

oto.theclinics.com

long-term quality of life.[3,8–11] Many studies show that TORS is an effective diagnostic and therapeutic oncological tool.[3,12–16] However, to gain a comprehensive understanding of outcomes, the cost implications of TORS must also be considered, because some investigators have implicated robotic technology in driving up health care costs.[17]

Aggregate surgical expenditures are expected to grow from $572 billion in 2005 (4.6% of US gross domestic product [GDP]) to $912 billion (in 2005 dollars) in the year 2025 (7.3% of US GDP). Both national surgical and overall health care expenditures are expected to grow by approximately 60% during the period 2005 to 2025. These trends have been in place since World War II, and the increase has been attributed to generously rewarded advances in medical and surgical technology, an insurance system that obscures the true cost of health care, the increasing age of the population, defensive medicine, an increasing number of available services, and so-called free-rider access to the US health care system provided to anyone who enters the system as an emergency. Per capita GDP growth in the United States is relatively flat. Based on these assumptions, by 2025, surgical health care expenditures will account for one-fourteenth of the entire US economy.[18]

Economic evaluation in health care is complex, given the number of variables affecting cost and measurement. Costs vary widely from institution to institution, among regions and countries, and based on whose perspective costs are being analyzed (payer, patient, or society). Furthermore, indirect costs such as lost time, transportation, childcare, and other factors are not well captured by looking solely at the bottom line. According to the Panel on Cost Effectiveness in Health and Medicine, a group convened by the US Public Health Service in the mid-1990s, economic evaluation of interventions and technology should analyze both health care expenditure and its impact, ideally, to the health state.[19] In general, Smith and Rudmik[20] outlined the principles and challenges of cost collection and analysis in a 2013 article in *Otolaryngology–Head and Neck Surgery*. The present article summarizes the current literature regarding cost and cost-effectiveness of robotic surgery in the head and neck.

DISCUSSION

Few articles to date have objectively analyzed the cost-effectiveness of robotic surgery in the head and neck. Some have criticized robotic surgery because of the high initial investment to purchase either of the 2 widely available systems. The initial cost of the da Vinci robot with the 4-arm system and software upgrades is approximately $1.5 million. The service contract for the robotic surgical system is approximately $150,000 per year.[5,21] However, the robot is typically a capital investment made by the hospital, shared among multiple services, and is most relevant in the setting of starting a new robotic program with limited use. The additional cost per TORS procedure using the da Vinci system is approximately $500 for disposable equipment.[22] The initial cost of da Vinci's primary competitor, the Flex robotic system (Medrobotics, Raynham MA), is estimated to be approximately $1 million. At this time, detailed cost analyses are only available for the da Vinci system.[23]

The literature generally indicates that the balance is in favor of TORS when all costs are considered. Multiple institutional series have shown that TORS is associated with a short hospital length of stay (LOS) and low morbidity and mortality.[24–28] In a 2018 literature review by Othman and McKinnon,[29] which focuses on the financial impact of TORS, the investigators found that TORS saved an average of $8355 per procedure and 1.8 hospital days compared with other surgical approaches for OPSCC. Motz and colleagues[30] showed that TORS is associated with a shorter LOS as well as lower hospital-related costs than non-TORS procedures. Hammoudi and colleagues[31] performed a comparison of TORS with open procedures and concluded that the robotic technique should result in both lower morbidity and lower treatment cost with no increase in complication rate and equivalent oncologic control. Similarly, Chung and colleagues[7] found that TORS for partial pharyngectomy and partial glossectomy for the base of tongue was associated with shorter hospital LOSs, lower charges, and lower costs than open procedures. However, the investigators did find that TORS was inferior to open surgery in cost measures for partial glossectomy of the anterior tongue. This difference indicates that the cost benefit may be limited by anatomic subsite. Dombrée and colleagues[32] compared TORS, transoral laser microsurgery (TLM), and open surgery for partial and total laryngectomies using activity-based costing, a cost-accounting system that allocates resource costs to products using a multistep allocation procedure assessed by activity consumption. Although the investigators found shorter operating times for TORS compared with TLM and open surgery, they nevertheless found an increased cost with TORS. This increased cost was still the case even when the investigators decreased the equipment depreciation and maintenance costs to zero and simulated a doubling of the annual TORS case load. They were able to attribute most of the cost associated with TORS to robot-specific activities, such as installation of the robot, sterilization of the robotic instruments, and external maintenance. These activities are different from TLM and open procedures, where the cost distribution is predominantly determined by personnel cost.[32]

As an extension of TORS for OPSCC, there has been interest in using lingual tonsillectomy to identify the primary site in cervical unknown primary (CUP). In a retrospective study that included a basic effectiveness measure, Byrd and colleagues[33,34] evaluated the incremental cost-effectiveness ratio (ICER), a measure of cost-effectiveness analysis comparing costs of 2 different procedures to localize the primary tumor in CUP, using standardized costs to compare examination under anesthesia (EUA) with tonsillectomy with sequential TORS base of tongue resection. The ICER for TORS base of tongue resection after EUA with tonsillectomy failed to localize the primary was $6208 per primary localized. Although this cannot be extrapolated to dollars per quality-adjusted life year (QALY) because of the unknown impact of limiting the radiation field, the investigators concluded that TORS lingual tonsillectomy after failed EUA with tonsillectomy is a modest expenditure.

Whether robotic surgery or nonsurgical treatment is more cost-effective is controversial. Simply considering financial data, TORS seems to be more cost-effective, provided that the number of treatment modalities is the same or lower. Moore and colleagues[35] retrospectively reviewed collections data for government and private payers treated for OPSCC at 2 academic institutions. Transoral surgery (TOS) alone as treatment of OPSCC had the lowest overall cost over a 90-day time frame compared with TOS with adjuvant radiation therapy (RT), TOS with adjuvant CRT, and primary CRT. In agreement with these findings, Tam and colleagues[36] performed a case control study comparing charges and costs for 15 stage II to IVa (AJCC seventh edition) patients with OPSCC treated with TORS versus 15 matched patients treated with CRT at a single institution over 1 year. For selected stage II to IVa OPSCC, frontline TORS was 22% less expensive than upfront CRT 4 months after the initial treatment and 14% lower 1 year after treatment. A significant number of patients were treated with cetuximab, rather than cisplatin, which contributed to the higher cost of treatment. Neither of these studies incorporated effectiveness, and Tam and colleagues[36] acknowledge that their small series may be subject to selection bias.

To accomplish cost-effectiveness analysis as recommended by the Panel on Cost Effectiveness in Health and Medicine,[19] costs are compared and utility values are incorporated to generate dollars per QALY in an ICER. Society's willingness to pay, which determines whether an intervention or technology is cost-effective, is controversial and has historically ranged from $50,000 to $100,000 per QALY in the literature, but has been suggested to be even as high as $200,000 per QALY.[37] Utility values range from 0 (death) to 1 (perfect health), representing a health state at a point in time. de Almeida and colleagues[38] published utility values generated from 50 healthy subjects and 9 experts via the Standard Gamble technique and visual analog scale in 2014. TORS-based treatments led to higher utility scores than radiation-based treatments. These values were subsequently incorporated into several cost-effectiveness analyses using decision trees and Markov models for TORS.

The 4 cost-effectiveness analyses have disparate findings based on model parameters and assumptions made. de Almeida and colleagues[39] found a cost saving of $1366 and an increase of 0.25 QALYs per case when using TORS as treatment of early T classification OPSCC compared with CRT over a 10-year time horizon. Conversely, there are 3 studies that indicate nonsurgical therapy as the more cost-effective option.[40–42] Rodin and colleagues[40] found that, under base case assumptions, TORS was associated with moderate gains in QALYs and an ICER of $82,190/QALY gained. This ICER was most sensitive to need for adjuvant therapy, cost of late toxicity, age at diagnosis, disease state utilities, and discount rate. Accounting for joint parameter uncertainty, RT had a higher probability than TORS of being the more cost-effective option (54% vs 46%). Of note, this study compared RT versus TORS alone, or with postoperative RT or CRT, but did not include definitive CRT or salvage surgery for radiation failure in the analysis. Similarly, Rudmik and colleagues[42] found that TORS is 42% likely to be cost-effective, with an ICER of $165,300 per QALY because of being approximately $5000 more costly and associated with only a gain of 0.03 QALYs. Sher and colleagues[41] analyzed T1 to T2, N2 OPSCC using regional cost data from the Chicago Medicare payment schedule and also found that CRT was the dominant strategy; this analysis was most sensitive to the likelihood of adjuvant CRT after TORS (61% in the base case) and differences in utility. In addition, the base case patient age in this study was 65 years, which could potentially limit some of the long-term benefits in quality of life for the theoretic patients who were able to avoid chemotherapy.

A consideration incorporated into the analysis by Sher and colleagues[41] is that staged neck dissection is associated with increased cost.[41] LOS, anesthesia and operative costs, and undiscounted work relative value unit compensation account for the increased direct costs. Frenkel and colleagues[43] reviewed 425 cases of adults undergoing TORS with staged versus concurrent neck dissection and found that there was no significant difference between the rate of adverse events, including inpatient complications, need for additional procedures, and readmissions, but there was a significantly shorter LOS for concurrent procedures. Clinicians must therefore weigh the increased cost associated with staged procedures versus patient benefit.

A major consideration for economic evaluation of robotic surgery is that cost-effectiveness of TORS varies greatly based on the need for adjuvant therapy.[39] Although patients who undergo primary TORS may be less likely to receive postoperative CRT than those treated with other surgical approaches, a review of the National Cancer Database (NCDB) indicates that 20% of patients treated with TOS had positive margins, thereby meeting indications for CRT.[30,44] Another NCDB study suggests that surgeons are improving in patient selection, because the percentage of patients receiving trimodality therapy decreased from 23.7% to 16.9% and was largely driven by extranodal extension.[45] Ultimately, selecting patients who are amenable to achieving negative margins and are unlikely to have extranodal extension is the most important factor in making TORS cost-effective, although predicting the latter based on imaging can be problematic.[46,47] In addition, selecting younger patients who are expected to survive longer without disease benefit makes the models more cost-effective via their higher utility values (ie, quality of life).[40]

Ultimately, prospective clinical trials may provide better evidence of the economic impact of head and neck robotic surgery. The Oropharynx: Radiotherapy vs Transoral Robotic Surgery (ORATOR) trial, a phase 2 trial comparing TORS with adjuvant therapy and CRT in 68 patients recently published its early results with 1-year follow-up; with longer follow-up, it may provide some information about the relative cost-effectiveness of the 2 strategies.[48] The Eastern Cooperative Oncology Group ECOG-E3311 phase 2 surgical trial for early stage human papilloma virus–positive OPSCC, having completed enrollment with 511 patients, will provide economic and quality-of-life data for patients treated with surgery with and without adjuvant treatment in the near future. However, as previously noted by Barber and Thompson,[49] the analysis and interpretation of cost data from clinical trials must be approached with appropriate statistical techniques, because a review of the literature indicates that inappropriate conclusions based on economic evaluation of trials are common.

SUMMARY

The use of robotic surgery in otolaryngology–head and neck surgery, as well as in other specialties, is increasing, as is the market worth of the predominant robotic surgical platforms. There seems to be a trend toward primary surgical management of OPSCC since the advent of TORS, because TORS has developed as an effective diagnostic and therapeutic tool. A full assessment of robotic surgery is not complete without an assessment of cost-effectiveness; however, evaluation of cost in health care is complex. Despite the high cost of ownership of the surgical robotic platform, TORS seems to be largely cost-effective for oropharyngeal surgery, but depends heavily on patient selection.

CLINICS CARE POINTS

- TORS seems to be equivalent to CRT in oncological outcomes for OPSCC and may provide improved functional outcomes based on retrospective studies and limited prospective data.
- The initial cost of a robotic system is a significant capital investment for the hospital, but should not weigh heavily in economic evaluation because it is a shared fixed cost among multiple services, rather than a variable cost.
- To date, TORS generally seems to be a cost-effective method of treatment of OPSCC, provided that patients are appropriately selected so that trimodality therapy is minimized.

DISCLOSURE

The authors have nothing to disclose.

REFERENCES

1. Genden EM, Kotz T, Tong CC, et al. Transoral robotic resection and reconstruction for head and neck cancer. Laryngoscope 2011;121(8):1668–74.
2. Chen MM, Roman SA, Kraus DH, et al. Transoral Robotic Surgery: A Population-Level Analysis. Otolaryngol Head Neck Surg 2014;150(6):968–75.

3. Sethia R, Yumusakhuylu AC, Ozbay I, et al. Quality of life outcomes of transoral robotic surgery with or without adjuvant therapy for oropharyngeal cancer. Laryngoscope 2018;128(2):403–11.

4. Garas G, Arora A. Robotic Head and Neck Surgery: History, Technical Evolution and the Future. ORL J Otorhinolaryngol Relat Spec 2018;80(3–4):117–24.

5. Feldstein J, Schwander B, Roberts M, et al. Cost of ownership assessment for a da Vinci robot based on US real-world data. Int J Med Robot 2019;15(5):e2023.

6. O'Malley BW Jr, Weinstein GS, Snyder W, et al. Transoral robotic surgery (TORS) for base of tongue neoplasms. Laryngoscope 2006;116(8):1465–72.

7. Chung TK, Rosenthal EL, Magnuson JS, et al. Transoral robotic surgery for oropharyngeal and tongue cancer in the United States. Laryngoscope 2015; 125(1):140–5.

8. Dziegielewski PT, Teknos TN, Durmus K, et al. Transoral robotic surgery for oropharyngeal cancer: long-term quality of life and functional outcomes. JAMA Otolaryngol Head Neck Surg 2013;139(11):1099–108.

9. Mydlarz WK, Chan JY, Richmon JD. The role of surgery for HPV-associated head and neck cancer. Oral Oncol 2015;51(4):305–13.

10. Choby GW, Kim J, Ling DC, et al. Transoral robotic surgery alone for oropharyngeal cancer: quality-of-life outcomes. JAMA Otolaryngol Head Neck Surg 2015; 141(6):499–504.

11. O'Leary P, Kjaergaard T. Transoral robotic surgery and oropharyngeal cancer: a literature review. Ear Nose Throat J 2014;93(8):E14–21.

12. Park YM, Jung CM, Cha D, et al. The long-term oncological and functional outcomes of transoral robotic surgery in patients with hypopharyngeal cancer. Oral Oncol 2017;71:138–43.

13. Weinstein GS, O'Malley BW Jr, Cohen MA, et al. Transoral robotic surgery for advanced oropharyngeal carcinoma. Arch Otolaryngol Head Neck Surg 2010; 136(11):1079–85.

14. Moore EJ, Hinni ML. Critical review: transoral laser microsurgery and robotic-assisted surgery for oropharynx cancer including human papillomavirus-related cancer. Int J Radiat Oncol Biol Phys 2013;85(5):1163–7.

15. Cohen MA, Weinstein GS, O'Malley BW Jr, et al. Transoral robotic surgery and human papillomavirus status: Oncologic results. Head Neck 2011;33(4):573–80.

16. Park YM, Lee WJ, Lee JG, et al. Transoral robotic surgery (TORS) in laryngeal and hypopharyngeal cancer. J Laparoendosc Adv Surg Tech A 2009;19(3):361–8.

17. Barbash GI, Glied SA. New technology and health care costs–the case of robot-assisted surgery. N Engl J Med 2010;363(8):701–4.

18. Munoz E, Munoz W 3rd, Wise L. National and surgical health care expenditures, 2005-2025. Ann Surg 2010;251(2):195–200.

19. Weinstein MC, Siegel JE, Gold MR, et al. Recommendations of the Panel on Cost-effectiveness in Health and Medicine. JAMA 1996;276(15):1253–8.

20. Smith KA, Rudmik L. Cost collection and analysis for health economic evaluation. Otolaryngol Head Neck Surg 2013;149(2):192–9.

21. Weinstein GS, O'Malley BW Jr, Snyder W, et al. Transoral robotic surgery: supraglottic partial laryngectomy. Ann Otol Rhinol Laryngol 2007;116(1):19–23.

22. Richmon JD, Quon H, Gourin CG. The effect of transoral robotic surgery on short-term outcomes and cost of care after oropharyngeal cancer surgery. Laryngoscope 2014;124(1):165–71.

23. Friedrich DT, Scheithauer MO, Greve J, et al. Recent advances in robot-assisted head and neck surgery. Int J Med Robot 2017;13(2).

24. Genden EM, Desai S, Sung CK. Transoral robotic surgery for the management of head and neck cancer: a preliminary experience. Head Neck 2009;31(3):283–9.
25. Hurtuk A, Agrawal A, Old M, et al. Outcomes of transoral robotic surgery: a preliminary clinical experience. Otolaryngol Head Neck Surg 2011;145(2):248–53.
26. Moore EJ, Olsen KD, Kasperbauer JL. Transoral robotic surgery for oropharyngeal squamous cell carcinoma: a prospective study of feasibility and functional outcomes. Laryngoscope 2009;119(11):2156–64.
27. Richmon JD, Agrawal N, Pattani KM. Implementation of a TORS program in an academic medical center. Laryngoscope 2011;121(11):2344–8.
28. Weinstein GS, O'Malley BW Jr, Snyder W, et al. Transoral robotic surgery: radical tonsillectomy. Arch Otolaryngol Head Neck Surg 2007;133(12):1220–6.
29. Othman S, McKinnon BJ. Financial outcomes of transoral robotic surgery: A narrative review. Am J Otolaryngol 2018;39(4):448–52.
30. Motz K, Chang HY, Quon H, et al. Association of Transoral Robotic Surgery With Short-term and Long-term Outcomes and Costs of Care in Oropharyngeal Cancer Surgery. JAMA Otolaryngol Head Neck Surg 2017;143(6):580–8.
31. Hammoudi K, Pinlong E, Kim S, et al. Transoral robotic surgery versus conventional surgery in treatment for squamous cell carcinoma of the upper aerodigestive tract. Head Neck 2015;37(9):1304–9.
32. Dombrée M, Crott R, Lawson G, et al. Cost comparison of open approach, transoral laser microsurgery and transoral robotic surgery for partial and total laryngectomies. Eur Arch Otorhinolaryngol 2014;271(10):2825–34.
33. Byrd JK, Smith KJ, de Almeida JR, et al. Transoral Robotic Surgery and the Unknown Primary: A Cost-Effectiveness Analysis. Otolaryngol Head Neck Surg 2014;150(6):976–82.
34. Byrd JK, Smith KJ, de Almeida JR, et al. Cost-effectiveness of transoral robotic surgery in the unknown primary: corrigendum and response to comments. Otolaryngol Head Neck Surg 2014;151(6):1094–5.
35. Moore EJ, Hinni ML, Olsen KD, et al. Cost considerations in the treatment of oropharyngeal squamous cell carcinoma. Otolaryngol Head Neck Surg 2012;146(6):946–51.
36. Tam K, Orosco RK, Dimitrios Colevas A, et al. Cost comparison of treatment for oropharyngeal carcinoma. Laryngoscope 2019;129(7):1604–9.
37. Neumann PJ, Cohen JT, Weinstein MC. Updating cost-effectiveness–the curious resilience of the $50,000-per-QALY threshold. N Engl J Med 2014;371(9):796–7.
38. de Almeida JR, Villanueva NL, Moskowitz AJ, et al. Preferences and utilities for health states after treatment for oropharyngeal cancer: transoral robotic surgery versus definitive (chemo)radiotherapy. Head Neck 2014;36(7):923–33.
39. de Almeida JR, Moskowitz AJ, Miles BA, et al. Cost-effectiveness of transoral robotic surgery versus (chemo)radiotherapy for early T classification oropharyngeal carcinoma: A cost-utility analysis. Head Neck 2016;38(4):589–600.
40. Rodin D, Caulley L, Burger E, et al. Cost-Effectiveness Analysis of Radiation Therapy Versus Transoral Robotic Surgery for Oropharyngeal Squamous Cell Carcinoma. Int J Radiat Oncol Biol Phys 2017;97(4):709–17.
41. Sher DJ, Fidler MJ, Tishler RB, et al. Cost-Effectiveness Analysis of Chemoradiation Therapy Versus Transoral Robotic Surgery for Human Papillomavirus-Associated, Clinical N2 Oropharyngeal Cancer. Int J Radiat Oncol Biol Phys 2016;94(3):512–22.
42. Rudmik L, An W, Livingstone D, et al. Making a case for high-volume robotic surgery centers: A cost-effectiveness analysis of transoral robotic surgery. J Surg Oncol 2015;112(2):155–63.

43. Frenkel CH, Yang J, Zhang M, et al. Compared Outcomes of Concurrent versus Staged Transoral Robotic Surgery with Neck Dissection. Otolaryngol Head Neck Surg 2017;157(5):791–7.

44. Zevallos JP, Mitra N, Swisher-McClure S. Patterns of care and perioperative outcomes in transoral endoscopic surgery for oropharyngeal squamous cell carcinoma. Head Neck 2016;38(3):402–9.

45. Zhan KY, Puram SV, Li MM, et al. National treatment trends in human papillomavirus-positive oropharyngeal squamous cell carcinoma. Cancer 2020; 126(6):1295–305.

46. McMullen CP, Garneau J, Weimar E, et al. Occult Nodal Disease and Occult Extranodal Extension in Patients With Oropharyngeal Squamous Cell Carcinoma Undergoing Primary Transoral Robotic Surgery With Neck Dissection. JAMA Otolaryngol Head Neck Surg 2019;145(8):701–7.

47. Maxwell JH, Ferris RL, Gooding W, et al. Extracapsular spread in head and neck carcinoma: Impact of site and human papillomavirus status. Cancer 2013; 119(18):3302–8.

48. Nichols AC, Yoo J, Hammond JA, et al. Early-stage squamous cell carcinoma of the oropharynx: radiotherapy vs. trans-oral robotic surgery (ORATOR)–study protocol for a randomized phase II trial. BMC Cancer 2013;13:133.

49. Barber JA, Thompson SG. Analysis and interpretation of cost data in randomised controlled trials: review of published studies. BMJ 1998;317(7167):1195–200.

Special Article Series: Otolaryngology in COVID-19

Editor

ZARA M. PATEL

OTOLARYNGOLOGIC CLINICS OF NORTH AMERICA

www.oto.theclinics.com

Consulting Editor
SUJANA S. CHANDRASEKHAR

December 2020 • Volume 53 • Number 6

Foreword

Otolaryngology During the COVID-19 Pandemic: What We Have Learned in Year One

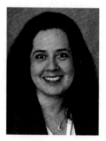

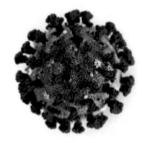

Sujana S. Chandrasekhar, MD, FACS, FAAOHNS
Consulting Editors

The year 2020 has seen disruptions in nearly every aspect of our lives, due to the global pandemic of COVID-19, caused by the virus severe acute respiratory syndrome coronavirus 2 (SARS-CoV-2). As such, we present the following 4 articles in this special series on COVID-19, guest edited by Dr Zara Patel, to detail what we have learned in this ever-changing landscape, and where we might go from here.

Coronaviruses are named for the crownlike spikes on their surface. They overwhelmingly infect animals, but at least 7 strains infect humans, including this new virus causing COVID-19. Four cause common colds. Two others rank among the deadliest of human infections: severe acute respiratory syndrome, or SARS, and Middle East respiratory syndrome, or MERS.

The original SARS outbreak first appeared in South China in 2002 but was able to be contained.[1] SARS (or SARS-CoV) was spread by respiratory droplets and person-to-person contact, and there were no cases of presymptomatic individuals transmitting disease. Between November 2002 and July 2003, a total of 8098 people worldwide became ill with probable SARS-CoV; of these, 774 died. In the United States, 8 people who had traveled to SARS-CoV transmission areas got the disease, but none died. There were no cases after July 2003, and the global outbreak was declared over. In April 2004, the Chinese Ministry of Health reported new cases, but there is no evidence of wider transmission in the community.

The current disease named COVID-19 is caused by SARS-CoV-2 virus, a related but much more contagious coronavirus, which can be spread by presymptomatic/asymptomatic individuals. The first case was identified in China at the end of 2019, which is why this disease is called **CO**rona**VI**rus**D**isease-2019. SARS-CoV-2 is very similar to known SARS-related coronaviruses in bats, especially horseshoe bats. It

Otolaryngol Clin N Am 53 (2020) xxiii–xxv
https://doi.org/10.1016/j.otc.2020.09.008
0030-6665/20/© 2020 Published by Elsevier Inc.

oto.theclinics.com

is believed that a bat virus mutated, infected an intermediate host, such as a civet or pangolin, and then mutated again, in a process called spillover, to be able to infect humans. The human form spreads via coughing, sneezing, and other contact. On March 11, 2020, COVID-19 was declared a pandemic by the World Health Organization.

Despite various degrees of lockdowns and closures worldwide, as of September 2020, there have been over 31.2 million confirmed cases of COVID-19 and 962,000 confirmed COVID-19 deaths, with cases reported in every country.[2] In the United States, there have been 6.9 million cases and 200,000 deaths. These numbers are given with the understanding that the variability in testing can skew figures and positivity rates, and the death rates do not include deaths due to failure to access health care for other reasons (for example, myocardial infarction or cerebrovascular accident) due to COVID-19 closures and fears. Over 900 health care workers in the United States have died of COVID-19.[3] Initial reports suggested that Otolaryngologists and Ophthalmologists were at higher risk of contracting this disease from their patients due to close exposure[4]; even with personal protective equipment, front-line health care workers have a 3 to 4 times increased risk of testing positive for COVID-19.[5]

The main symptoms encountered in COVID-19 are fever or chills, cough, shortness of breath or difficulty breathing, fatigue, muscle or body aches, headache, new loss of taste or smell, sore throat, congestion or runny nose, nausea or vomiting, and diarrhea. Emergency warning signs of this disease include dyspnea, chest pain or pressure, confusion, severe lethargy or stupor, and cyanosis.[6] We are finding "happy hypoxemia" in COVID-19, that is, very low blood oxygenation but no sense of dyspnea. This can lead to delays in seeking care, and its cause remains to be elucidated.[7] Many individuals have subsequently acquired pulse oximeters for use at home. While most cases of COVID-19 are self-limited and recovery is generally seen over a few days to 2 weeks, there are people with long-term issues of fatigue, cough, dyspnea, headache, joint pain, cardiopulmonary issues, blood-clotting abnormalities, cognitive and emotional issues; these people are thought to have "Long Covid," and much more remains to be learned about them.

By following the 3 W's: Wear a mask, Wash your hands, Watch your distance (maintain 6 feet from others not living in your home), some countries, states, and communities have brought their SARS-CoV-2 positivity rates down well below 1%, making reopenings possible. Unfortunately, even those successes can be undermined when people stop following that advice. In addition, as we are opening, we are using symptom and temperature screenings in physicians' offices, hospitals, schools, and so forth. COVID-19 occurring at this time has provided an opportunity to reach out via Social Media and provide teaching. I even started a YouTube channel, Dr Sujana (https://www.youtube.com/c/DrSujana) that has educational videos about COVID-19, and a livestream show called "She's On Call" (https://www.youtube.com/c/DrSujana), where we discuss COVID-19 and other health issues. Please feel free to share them with your patients.

As for educating each other, Dr Zara Patel, the Guest Editor of Special Articles: Otolaryngology in COVID-19 in this issue of *Otolaryngologic Clinics of North America*, has been at the forefront of identifying and explaining otolaryngologic manifestations of this disease and how ENT surgeons can protect ourselves and our staff members while caring for our patients. I am grateful to her for compiling the next 4 articles to encompass what we know at this point regarding this novel coronavirus disease. The authors of these articles have risen to the challenge of writing about a disease process that is evolving rapidly in real time. We hope that you find this special section useful as we all navigate our way in this global pandemic.

Sujana S. Chandrasekhar, MD, FACS, FAAOHNS
Consulting Editor, *Otolaryngologic Clinics of North America*

Past President, American Academy of Otolaryngology–Head and Neck Surgery

Secretary-Treasurer, American Otological Society

Partner, ENT & Allergy Associates LLP
18 East 48th Street, 2nd Floor
New York, NY 10017, USA

Clinical Professor, Department of Otolaryngology–Head and Neck Surgery
Zucker School of Medicine at
Hofstra-Northwell
Hempstead, NY, USA

Clinical Associate Professor, Department of Otolaryngology–Head and Neck Surgery
Icahn School of Medicine at
Mount Sinai
New York, NY, USA

E-mail address:
ssc@nyotology.com

REFERENCES

1. Available at: https://www.cdc.gov/sars/about/faq.html. Accessed September 8, 2020.
2. Available at: https://www.who.int/emergencies/diseases/novel-coronavirus-2019. Accessed September 8, 2020.
3. Available at: https://khn.org/news/exclusive-over-900-health-workers-have-died-of-covid-19-and-the-toll-is-rising/. Accessed September 8, 2020.
4. Husain IA. 2020. Available at: https://blogs.scientificamerican.com/observations/why-covid-19-is-a-special-danger-to-otolaryngologists/. April 24. Accessed September 8, 2020.
5. Nguyen LH, Drew DA, Graham MS, et al. Risk of COVID-19 among front-line health-care workers and the general community: a prospective cohort study. Lancet Public Health 2020;5(9):e475–83.
6. Available at: https://www.cdc.gov/coronavirus/2019-ncov/symptoms-testing/symptoms.html. Accessed September 8, 2020.
7. González-Duarte A, Norcliffe-Kaufmann L. Is 'happy hypoxia' in COVID-19 a disorder of autonomic interoception? A hypothesis. Clin Auton Res 2020;30(4):331–3.

Preface

Rising to the Challenge: Otolaryngologists in the COVID-19 Pandemic

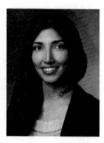

Zara M. Patel, MD
Editor

As the COVID-19 pandemic continues to wax and wane across the world and this country, it is somewhat cathartic to write this preface, at the request of our esteemed Academy Past-President and my former teacher, Dr Sujana Chandrasekhar. The realization that over 6 months have passed since the outset of this pandemic, in what feels like the blink of an eye, drives home that so many of us have had far too few chances to come up from underwater, catch our breaths, look around at the current landscape in otolaryngology, and truly appreciate the major shifts our field has undergone.

Human beings are resilient, and surgeons even more so: our shared experience of residency both demanding flexibility and adaptation while strengthening and sharpening our minds. It is likely that these qualities are what have held us together and brought us through this, despite also feeling that we have been running a never-ending race these past 6 months over ever-changing topography and with surprise obstacles around every turn.

In the United States, we owe a debt of gratitude to our international colleagues who, even while in the midst of their own most challenging time, took a moment to reach out and send a warning our way.[1] Before that time, none of us were considering the high level of virus found within the head and neck mucosal region, the widespread use of aerosol-generating procedures in our specialty, and how this may be a perfect storm for the spread of severe acute respiratory syndrome coronavirus 2 (SARS-CoV-2). With this warning in hand, otolaryngologists across the country were able to take action, supply that information to hospital administrators, obtain the appropriate high-level personal protective equipment (PPE), and shut down clinics and elective surgeries until we could safely reopen with testing protocols tailored to our higher-risk procedures and patient populations. It is a testament to our field's collective ability to rapidly

Otolaryngol Clin N Am 53 (2020) xxvii–xxviii
https://doi.org/10.1016/j.otc.2020.09.019
0030-6665/20/© 2020 Published by Elsevier Inc.

oto.theclinics.com

process information, adapt, and act to keep ourselves and our patients safe, that we have been able to reopen without any major clusters of spread of COVID-19 from our offices or operating rooms.

Most of us have been through a near complete shutdown other than surgical emergencies, a rapid ramp up of telemedicine, a fight for appropriate PPE, a myriad of testing protocols, and installment of HEPA filters or other changes to clinic rooms. Then came the reopening of clinics and operating rooms, and a return to current patient volume that is even higher than usual as we make up for lost time and patients also try to get in as soon as possible in anticipation of possible future shutdowns. With all the new information and technology we have in hand, I do not foresee another complete shutdown in our future, simply more adaptation and flexibility as the situation changes.

I am grateful to my colleagues, Dr Brandon Baird, Dr Steven Sobol, Dr Esther Vivas, and Dr Carol Yan, who I asked to write about these changes and solutions in each subspecialty in their articles for this special supplement for *Otolaryngologic Clinics of North America*. Despite the difficulty of writing on a rapidly evolving topic, they have all brought to light the most important points all of us can learn from. I am heartened by the connections formed and interaction within our community around the globe as we have come together to fight this virus and reassure each other that we will get through this. This is certainly not the end of this fight and not even the last pandemic we are all likely to face in our lifetimes. But after having this chance to reflect on the response of otolaryngologists–head and neck surgeons everywhere, I am confident that we can face and overcome any new challenge in our future, together.

Zara M. Patel, MD
Department of Otolaryngology–
Head and Neck Surgery
Stanford University School of Medicine
801 Welch Road, 2nd Floor
Palo Alto, CA 94305, USA

E-mail address:
zmpatel@stanford.edu

REFERENCE

1. Patel ZM, Fernandez-Miranda J, Hwang PH, et al. Letter: precautions for endoscopic transnasal skull base surgery during the COVID-19 pandemic. Neurosurgery 2020;87(1):E66–7. https://doi.org/10.1093/neuros/nyaa125.

Coronavirus Disease-19 and Rhinology/Facial Plastics

Morgan E. Davis, MD, Carol H. Yan, MD*

KEYWORDS

- COVID-19 • Rhinology • Facial plastic surgery • Nasal endoscopy
- Aerosol generating procedure • Viral transmission risk • Anosmia • Povidone-iodine

KEY POINTS

- The nasal and oral airway contain high viral loads, posing high risk of viral transmission even in asymptomatic individuals and possibility of false negative PCR viral tests.
- Aerosol generating procedures (AGPs) include nasal endoscopy and use of high-speed energy instruments in endoscopic nasal surgery and energy-based procedures in facial plastics; performance of AGPs require maximal PPE.
- Novel devices and techniques in the operative and clinical settings have been proposed including topical decontaminating agents, nasal tents and VENT masks, and use of HEPA filters.
- Olfactory loss is highly associated with COVID-19. For those with inflammatory sinonasal pathology or allergies, continued use of topical nasal steroids is recommended.
- Aesthetic concerns and the desire to improve self-image may increase during these high-stress times and with the use of mask-wearing and telemedicine.

INTRODUCTION

The ongoing coronavirus disease-19 (COVID-19) pandemic caused by the novel coronavirus severe acute respiratory syndrome coronavirus-2 (SARS-CoV-2) has created unprecedented challenges for our health care system and society as the number of new cases continue to increase. Here we discuss the practical and clinical implications of COVID-19 as it specifically pertains to the subspecialties of rhinology and facial plastic surgery and summarize relevant practice guidelines for clinical and surgical management as of June 2020. For the rhinologist and facial plastic surgeon, the risk of exposure to SARS-CoV-2 is high owing to close proximity and frequent manipulation of the nasal and oral cavities. A solid understanding of evidence-based recommendations to mitigate the risk of viral transmission is therefore crucial for the

Department of Surgery, Division of Otolaryngology–Head and Neck Surgery, University of California San Diego School of Medicine, 9350 Campus Point Drive, Mail Code 0970, La Jolla, CA 92037, USA
* Corresponding author.
E-mail address: c1yan@health.ucsd.edu

Otolaryngol Clin N Am 53 (2020) 1139–1151
https://doi.org/10.1016/j.otc.2020.08.002
0030-6665/20/Published by Elsevier Inc.

optimization of health preservation and patient care. Additionally, we highlight some of the recently published clinical outcomes research brought forth by COVID-19. Given the fluid nature of the current pandemic and rapidly emerging data, this article is a representation of the best evidence and information to the best of our knowledge available at the time of this literature review.

DISCUSSION

High Viral Loads Are Found in the Nasal Airway

The nasal cavity is known to be a major site of SARS-CoV-2 infection and transmission. Studies on the transmission of SARS-CoV-2 suggest the primary mechanisms of spread include inhalation of respiratory droplets or aerosols and direct contact with contaminated objects.[1–3] When comparing upper respiratory specimens, higher viral loads are detected from nasal swabs compared with that of throat swabs in symptomatic patients.[4] One theory explaining this heightened association is that susceptibility genes required for viral infection, including angiotensin-converting enzyme 2, have the highest expression in the ciliated epithelial and goblet cells of the nasal mucosa, making this anatomic region an ideal target for viral invasion and replication.[5] Viral transmission is also possible in asymptomatic patients, with some data demonstrating similar levels of viral loads among asymptomatic and symptomatic individuals, suggesting that transmission of disease is possible even early in the disease course and without clinical signs.[4] Thus, the infection route of SARS-CoV-2 poses a particular threat to the rhinologist or facial plastic surgeon whose surgical practices include diagnostic and therapeutic procedures involving the nasal airway.

Risk of False-Negative Results Owing to Nasal Pathology

The current gold standard for SARS-CoV-2 testing relies on reverse transcriptase polymerase chain reaction via nasal, nasopharyngeal, or oropharyngeal swabs. The potential for a false-negative result is not uncommon[6–8] and it has been suggested that patients with nasal pathologies, including septal deviation, nasal polyps, or masses, may be at higher risk for a false-negative result owing to inaccurate sampling.[9] Bleier and Welch[9] reported a case of a false-negative COVID-19 result during preoperative testing on a patient with chronic rhinosinusitis (CRS) with nasal polyps. As the patient underwent endoscopic sinus surgery, nasal polyps were noted obstructing the nasopharynx and a repeat intraoperative SARS-CoV-2 swab of the nasopharynx was in fact positive for COVID-19. There was inadvertent exposure for multiple health care personnel wearing only traditional surgical masks instead of higher level personal protective equipment (PPE) given the false-negative preoperative screening test result.[9] In response, DeConde and colleagues[10] have suggested performing both a nasal and oropharyngeal swab on select patients at high risk for an inadequate or inaccessible nasal or nasopharyngeal sample.

Nasal Procedures Carry a High Risk of Viral Transmission

One of the earliest reports highlighting the high risk of rhinologic procedures were 2 cases of endoscopic transsphenoidal surgery performed in Wuhan, China in January 2020 that resulted in SARS-CoV-2 transmission and illness of health care workers thought to be acquired intraoperatively.[11] Although the details and timing of the viral transmission have been debated,[12,13] the distribution of Patel and colleagues[11] letter brought attention to the uniquely high risk of viral transmission from aerosolizing nasal and endoscopic skull base procedures. Research has since been aimed at determining specific risks of aerosolization of the SARS-CoV-2 virus and categorization of true aerosol generating procedures (AGPs).

Although there is well-established evidence supporting SARS-CoV-2 transmission via droplet and direct contact, the risk of airborne transmission through AGPs (transmission of particles of <5–10 μm in size) remains controversial. One study demonstrated that aerosolized SARS-CoV-2 particles of less than 5 μm remain viable in air for at least 3 hours and on surfaces up to 72 hours depending on the surface material.[3] Simulated nasal endoscopic procedures have investigated the aerosolization risk associated with endonasal instrumentation owing to concern that potential AGPs would require enhanced safety precautions. The manipulation of nasal mucosa during endoscopy was found to distribute larger droplets up to a distance of 66 cm.[14] The use of high-speed drills and electrocautery during endonasal surgery carried the highest risk for aerosolization of virus particles, whereas cold instruments and powered suction microdebriders were lower risk.[14,15] Although diagnostic nasal endoscopy was initially thought to be non–aerosol-generating, a subsequent study by the same authors reported that both rigid and flexible nasal endoscopy can generate aerosols.[15] Perhaps, more important, they found a regular surgical mask insufficient in protecting against particle transmission generated by simulated airborne aerosol conditions in contrast to an N95 mask, which effectively contained aerosol spread.[15] Studies outside the otolaryngologic literature demonstrated similar findings of particle distribution with the use of drills and other high speed energy instruments including saws, cautery, laser, and ultrasonic technology.[14,16–18] Proposed methods to mitigate potential microscopic particle contamination include judicious use of high-powered drills with cutting burs recommended over diamond burs and use of continuous suctioning in the surgical field.[2,19] Additional research is warranted to better understand the mechanism of SARS-CoV-2 airborne transmission and further stratify risk of aerosol generation associated with different endonasal procedures and instrumentation to guide appropriate PPE use and ensure maximum safety in nonsimulated scenarios.

Oral Procedures Risk Viral Transmission

Aerosolization and risk of SARS-CoV-2 transmission during transoral facial plastic surgery procedures such as open fixation of acute facial fractures and/or removal of maxillomandibular fixation should be also considered. Although higher viral loads are typically found in the nasal cavity and nasopharynx, asymptomatic and minimally symptomatic patients have demonstrated modest levels of viral RNA in oropharyngeal samples that persists for at least 5 days.[4] As such, limited in-person evaluation was recommended for emergency department facial trauma consults and photo documentation and telehealth communication was favored.[20] Careful evaluation of specific soft tissue and hard tissue (bony) injuries can help to determine, which injuries could be treated with conservative therapy or delayed surgical management. This includes conservative treatment of mandibular and maxillary fractures and local wound care for intraoral lacerations. Hsieh and colleagues[21] proposed a facial trauma protocol for the surgical management of facial fractures which included favoring closed procedures over internal fixation when possible, use of scalpel over monopolar cautery, use of osteotome over power saw when osteotomy is required, and application of lowest speed and/or lowest power settings when such instrumentation is necessary and cannot be avoided.

General Safety Recommendations During the Coronavirus Disease-19 Era

Given the rapid spread of COVID-19 and a high degree of uncertainty of infectious transmission, prudent attention should be paid not only to the safety of the provider team and patient, but also toward environmental infection control measures during routine outpatient and surgical procedures. Although there are no universal guidelines to date, several institutions have released various versions of safety recommendations for the otolaryngologist in their clinical practices. The American Academy of Otolaryngology—Head and Neck Surgery initially recommended in March 2020 that extreme caution should be used during any transnasal or transoral procedure with use of standard universal precautions during any evaluation of these areas. These guidelines also favored limiting not only surgeries, but also routine clinic examinations (nasal endoscopy and flexible laryngoscopy), to those strictly deemed necessary.[22] Vukkadala and colleagues[23] at Stanford University proposed the following guidelines for management of otolaryngologic surgeries during the initial COVID-19 outbreak based on risk stratification and COVID status.

- All transoral and intranasal surgeries are considered high risk.
- High-risk surgeries/APGs should be performed under enhanced airborne precautions regardless of COVID status. Recommended PPE includes gloves, gown, eye protection, and a minimum of an N95 respirator.
- Patients with positive symptoms despite negative COVID test, persons with pending COVID status, and/or unknown COVID status requiring emergency surgical treatment should be treated according to enhanced airborne precautions
- For patients with confirmed COVID-19, surgery should be delayed if possible or use of powered air-purifying respirators for all OR staff is recommended if surgery involves upper airway mucosal surfaces and delay until resolution of COVID-19 infection is not possible.

Overall, with the exception of emergent conditions, surgical procedures should not proceed without preoperative confirmation of COVID-19 status.[22]

OVERVIEW OF CORONAVIRUS DISEASE-19 EFFECT ON CLINICAL PRACTICE

At the onset of the COVID-19 pandemic in March 2020, health care systems were urged to delay all elective or nonurgent surgeries in accordance with the Centers for Disease Control and Prevention (CDC) recommendations.[24] Among all surgical specialties, otolaryngology and maxillofacial surgery took a particularly hard decline in surgical activity.[25] Given the higher risk associated with upper airway exposure, Radulesco and colleagues[26] proposed the following 3 tiers of management for endonasal surgical procedures.

- Group A: patients whose surgery cannot be postponed (eg, complicated sinusitis such as cavernous sinus thrombosis, invasive fungal sinusitis, nasal foreign bodies, sinonasal cancers, life threatening epistaxis unable to be controlled by other measures) → proceed with surgery after COVID-19 testing.
- Group B: patients whose surgery can be postponed for up to 4 weeks without significant prognostic impact → surgery postponed.
- Group C: patients whose surgery can be postponed for at least 6 weeks without significant impact on prognosis or disease be controlled by other measures → surgery postponed.

As recommendations for social distancing and stay-at-home orders surfaced all over the country and worldwide, the general consensus for rhinologic and facial plastics surgical practices between late March and April was the cancellation of nonurgent in-person clinic appointments. Widespread implementation of telemedicine visits surfaced shortly thereafter. Although perhaps limited in comprehensive patient evaluation and patient–provider interaction, telemedicine can be advantageous in not only eliminating risk, but also in patient convenience, effective time management, and electronic transfer of patient files.[27]

On May 12, 2020, the CDC released a general framework outlining the gradual resumption of nonurgent hospital services and expansion of elective operative care in the United States.[24] Between late May and June, elective in-person clinic visits ensued, although the option of telemedicine visits remained. To safely carry out elective office-based practices, new clinic protocols were developed to ensure patient and health care worker safety and adherence to social distancing.[28] General considerations for safe reopenings of rhinologic and facial plastics surgical clinics included previsit patient screening and education 24 to 48 hours before scheduled appointments as well as day-of symptom screening and temperature checks. Previsit COVID-19 testing is also routinely used, when available, to screen asymptomatic carriers, especially for new patients and those who are expected to undergo AGPs.[16] One must be mindful of select patients for which COVID-19 nasal swabs are contraindicated or of low yield owing to decreased test sensitivity. This cohort includes postoperative skull base patients, patients with postoperative packing or nasal splints, and patients with unfavorable anatomy owing to severely deviated septum, obstructing nasal mass, or thick mucus and polyps.[16]

Patients necessitating high-risk in-clinic procedures should be identified early on to facilitate appropriate scheduling and ensure the availability of adequate PPE for all staff.

Full capacity clinics are difficult to implement owing to enhanced sanitation measures and appropriate downtime of rooms after AGPs. Although respiratory droplets dissipate after 30 minutes of generation, AGPs pose a greater danger for transmission owing to the production of airborne aerosol particles that can travel 23 to 27 feet and remain viable in air for up to 3 hours.[3,16] In accordance with CDC guidelines, procedure rooms without negative pressure and continual HEPA filtration and air turnover should remain vacant following any AGP before cleaning, with timing based on a room's ability for air handling and duration of time spent in room.[29]

As clinical practices continue to expand and function at higher capacities despite persistent increases in the number of COVID-19 cases, an important challenge will be finding the proper balance between resumption of sustainable and safe elective clinical and surgical care and the preservation of hospital resources in anticipation of a potential second surge of COVID-19 cases.

Safety Recommendations in the Operative Setting

Coronavirus Disease-19 testing
Current guidelines recommend perioperative COVID-19 testing to be performed within 24 to 48 hours before elective high-risk aerosol generating surgeries.[16,30]

Use of topical decontaminating agents
Given that the nasopharynx and oropharynx are key reservoirs harboring SARS-CoV-2 virus, povidone–iodine (PVP-I) rinses have been proposed as a potential oral and nasal decontaminating agent. Although there are limited data in regard to specific efficacy against COVID-19 infections, PVP-I solutions of various dilute concentrations have been reported as safe and effective in decreasing viral and bacterial colonization of other species.[31] Although studies have shown that concentrations of 2.5% and higher are associated with ciliotoxic effects on ciliated human respiratory epithelial cells, safe use has been used at concentrations of 1.25% or less.[31,32] In contrast with the nasal mucosa, the oral mucosa, which lacks cilia, has been shown to tolerate

concentrations to 5% PVP-I rinses applied intraorally for a duration of up to 6 months.[31] In regards to SARS-CoV-2, preliminary studies primarily based on viral homology with SARS-CoV-1 and anecdotal evidence suggest nasal mucosal decontamination using 0.5 to 2.0 mL of 1.25% PVP-I and oral rinses with up to 10 mL at 2.5% before scheduled surgical procedures could effectively reduce the risk of COVID-19 infection transmission to providers and health care personnel without the risk of adverse effects to the patient.[31] PVP-I solutions with concentrations as low as 0.5% have recently been shown to inactivate SARS-CoV-2 in vitro after only 15 seconds of contact,[33] which further supports the applicability of use under prophylactic perioperative surgical conditions. PVP-I should be avoided in patients who are pregnant or allergic to iodine, have thyroid disease, or are undergoing radioactive iodine treatment owing to potential systemic effects.[31,33–36]

Chlorhexidine has also been suggested as a possible solution to decrease viral load and transmission risk.[37] Studies have demonstrated that chlorhexidine alone is less effective than PVP-I and other standard disinfectants against a wide range of human viruses, not including SARS-CoV-2, in both in vitro experiments[38] and studies of disinfection of inanimate surfaces.[39] Studies investigating the efficacy of chlorhexidine specifically against the novel coronavirus do not yet exist; therefore, no recommendation has been made regarding its routine use as a disinfectant for SARS-CoV-2.

Nasal tents

The implementation of a nasal tent using a simple 160 × 200 cm clear plastic sheet to create a barrier between the patient and the provider has been proposed as a feasible and cost-effective adjunct to limit potential viral spread during high-risk nasal procedures.[40] Maharaj[40] describes using this barrier with a low-flow continuous suction circuit to filter contaminated particles as well as a setup of all necessary surgical instruments beneath the tent to avoid passage of instruments after the start of the procedure and to minimize contamination for operating room personnel. This novel technique has the potential for more widespread application if additional studies can validate its efficacy. Nevertheless, it highlights the potential for innovation in surgical protective equipment to enhance operating room safety during the current COVID-19 pandemic and future outbreaks.

Safety Recommendations in the Outpatient Setting

Use of portable high-efficiency particulate air filters

The CDC currently recommends the use of negative-pressure isolation rooms when performing AGPs or allowing adequate down time in procedure rooms after AGPs to allow clearance of SARS-CoV-2 by other means.[28,29] Negative-pressure rooms are not readily available in the outpatient setting and long wait periods in between room use is cumbersome and not conducive to efficient workflow. As a result, the use of portable air purifiers with HEPA filters have been discussed because of their theoretic ability to decontaminate airborne particles generated during in clinic AGPs.[41] The CDC supports the use of HEPA filtration systems found in powered air-purifying respirators effective against SARS-CoV-2[41,42]; however, its broader application in portable systems for clinic and procedure rooms has not been established. The implementation of portable HEPA filters intended to decontaminate airborne SARS-CoV-2 in the clinical setting should only be used as an adjunct to other already well-established measures for infection control.[41]

Use of topical lidocaine/phenylephrine

Irritative conditions that can trigger a sneeze or cough have the potential to distribute and transform larger respiratory droplets into airborne aerosols,[14–16] indicating the potential for any routine endoscopy to unexpectedly become an AGP. Ironically, the use of common anesthetic and decongestant sprays during nasal endoscopy, which are intended to increase patient comfort and decrease airway irritability, have been discouraged owing to the risk of aerosolization of viral particles with the use of nasal atomizer sprays. As alternative means of anesthesia to prevent irritation of nasal mucosa, the American Academy of Otolaryngology supports use of lidocaine- and phenylephrine-soaked pledgets.[22]

Experimental modifications in routine endoscopy

The use of nasal endoscopy plays a fundamental role in the evaluation and diagnosis of common pathologies in otolaryngology. Workman and colleagues[14,15] developed a modified valved endoscopy of the nose and throat masks using regular surgical masks and N-95 masks that they engineered to allow passage of an endoscope while maintaining a tight seal to prevent droplet and aerosol contamination. In contrast with standard endoscopy performed in unmasked conditions, the use of modified valved endoscopy of the nose and throat masks with surgical and N-95 masks prevented droplet and airborne particle distribution, respectively, during simulated AGPs.

Another proposed modification to standard endoscopy technique is the back endoscopy approach, during which the endoscopist stands behind the patient and faces the monitor to avoid standing in the direct trajectory of droplets or aerosols.[43]

Aesthetic care procedures

PPE is required for all office aesthetic treatments with surgical masks, safety glasses, gown, and gloves recommended for injectables and noninvasive body contouring. Energy-based procedures of the head and neck such as those using laser, light, and heat, may involve AGPs and thus maximal PPE including N-95 masks are recommended.[44] Smoke evacuator suction systems are necessary during these procedures. Cooling positive air pressure traditionally used for pain management during a number of laser and other energy-emitting device procedures are not recommended.

TREATMENT OF THE RHINOLOGIC PATIENT IN THE CORONAVIRUS DISEASE-19 ERA

Given the aforementioned risks of viral exposure from nasal procedures and the prior temporary cessation on elective surgical procedures, one must consider how to best manage patients with CRS in this era. The impact of systemic corticosteroids on COVID-19 infection is still being investigated[45] and not generally supported for SARS-CoV-2 pulmonary disease under guidelines from the World Health Orgnization.[46] New prescriptions of systemic corticosteroids for sinonasal symptoms is not advised.[47] However, various allergy societies including the Allergic Rhinitis and its Impact on Asthma initiative and European Academy of Allergy and Clinical Immunology Society have recommended to continue the use of intranasal corticosteroids for those with CRS or rhinitis particularly those who are at risk of worsening chronic symptoms by stopping their topical therapies.[48]

Recent studies have shown efficacy in the use of high-volume nasal steroid irrigations in patients with CRS who had not previously undergone surgery.[49,50] A double-blinded, randomized controlled trial in CRS without nasal polyposis patients without prior surgical intervention demonstrated clinically meaningful improvement in SNOT-22 scores with high-volume nasal steroid irrigations compared with steroid sprays.[49] In a retrospective study, 64.4% of all patients with CRS treated with nasal steroid irrigations did not require surgical management after treatment for at least 6 weeks.[50] These studies are preliminary but promising given the likely prolonged COVID-19 environment.

Given the high prevalence of chemosensory dysfunction and in particular, olfactory loss associated with COVID-19,[51–57] it is more important than ever to recognize smell loss and taste loss and address the impact of chemosensory loss with subjects. Otolaryngologists and rhinologists need to be aware of sudden onset hyposmia/anosmia as a predictor of SARS-CoV-2 infection, particularly in those who are otherwise asymptomatic, and gain familiarity with use of treatment options such as topical steroid rinses and olfactory training.[58–60] Of those who reported smell loss associated with COVID-19, an estimated 25% of the subjects may not regain their smell, although these data are still preliminary.[51] Thus, chemosensory dysfunction may ultimately involve a portion of a otolaryngologist's clinical practice with a potential role for validated measurements of olfactory dysfunction both during in-person visits and telehealth visits.[61]

Treatment of the Facial Plastics Patient in the Coronavirus Disease-19 Era

As elective and routine care resumes, medical aesthetic specialties including cosmetic facial plastics practices have identified a need in providing positive self-image and sense of well-being to patients following a lengthy and stressful period of quarantine.[44]

With the increased prevalence of mask wearing during the COVID-19 pandemic, there is increased attention to the upper half of one's face. Botulinum toxin treatment of the glabella complex has been suggested to decrease negative emotions and promote well-being for both the treated individual and others who come into contact with the individual.[62] One study found that more than 40% of patients without prior facial

Table 1
Proposed safety recommendations in the literature for operative and ambulatory settings

Operative Setting	Ambulatory Setting
All patients should receive COVID-19 testing within 24–48 h before surgery. With the exception of emergencies, surgeries should not proceed without confirmation of COVID-19 status.	Previsit screening questionnaires 24–48 h prior with COVID-19 testing for AGPs. Day-of symptom screening and temperature checks.
High-risk surgeries (all transoral and intranasal) should be performed under enhanced airborne precautions including gloves, gown, eye protection, and a minimum of an N95 respirator.	Maximum PPE should be worn during all potential AGPs including nasal endoscopy, injectables, noninvasive body contouring, and procedures involving lasers, light, and/or heat
Use of barriers such as nasal tents may limit potential viral spread.	Modifications in standard endoscopy technique include use of valved endoscopy of the nose and throat masks or back endoscopy approaches.
Continuous suctioning of the surgical field. Limit or avoid the use of high-powered drills with cutting burs, monopolar electrocautery, and power saws when possible.	Use of portable HEPA filters may be used as an adjunct for infection control but have not been tested specifically against SARS-CoV2.
PVP-I rinses at 1.25% and 2.5% for intranasal and intraoral use, respectively, may be safe however, in vivo efficacy against SARS-CoV2 is not well-established.	Use of topical medications on pledgets for nasal anesthesia and decongestion before nasal endoscopy is preferred over sprays, and may decrease irritative conditions resulting in aerosols.

cosmetic treatments now wished to pursue treatment after identifying concerns over their facial appearance highlighted during their initial telehealth visits.[63] These findings suggest that the increased use of video conferencing technology during the current pandemic may translate to increased number of patients pursuing nonsurgical and surgical facial cosmetic procedures, which may be challenging to achieve in a safe but timely manner.

SUMMARY

In response to the novel COVID-19, new practices have been implemented in rhinology and facial plastics, which are at high risk for viral exposure (**Table 1**). The safety of the patient and provider team are of utmost importance with the emphasis on environmental infection control measures in both practices. Safety recommendations involving procedures have included preoperative and preprocedural COVID-19 testing, enhanced PPE usage including N-95 masks for all high-risk procedures regardless of COVID status, and particular precautions while performing AGPs or using energy instruments, including high-speed drills, electrocautery, and lasers. Optional adjuncts to avoid viral transmission include prophylactic use of PVP-I rinses for nasal and oral decontamination and barrier methods such as nasal tents. The use of HEPA filters and various modifications to standard endoscopy technique to decreased risk are currently under investigation but may be promising in the future. Nonsurgical, conservative management of sinonasal and facial pathologies should be considered with the use of high-volume nasal steroid irrigations for CRS and olfactory dysfunction and increased nonoperative management of facial traumas. Olfactory dysfunction associated with COVID-19 may be seen more frequently in a rhinologic practice, and facial plastics clinics may experience an increase in patient demand for aesthetic procedures.

DISCLOSURE

None.

REFERENCES

1. Sharma A, Tiwari S, Deb MK, et al. Severe Acute Respiratory Syndrome Coronavirus -2 (SARS-CoV-2): a global pandemic and treatments strategies. Int J Antimicrob Agents 2020;106054. https://doi.org/10.1016/j.ijantimicag.2020.106054.
2. Sharma D, Rubel KE, Ye MJ, et al. Cadaveric simulation of endoscopic endonasal procedures: analysis of droplet splatter patterns during the COVID-19 pandemic. Otolaryngol Head Neck Surg 2020;163(1):145–50.
3. van Doremalen N, Bushmaker T, Morris DH, et al. Aerosol and surface stability of SARS-CoV-2 as compared with SARS-CoV-1. N Engl J Med 2020;382(16): 1564–7.
4. Zou L, Ruan F, Huang M, et al. SARS-CoV-2 viral load in upper respiratory specimens of infected patients. N Engl J Med 2020;382(12):1177–9.
5. Sungnak W, Huang N, Bécavin C, et al. SARS-CoV-2 entry factors are highly expressed in nasal epithelial cells together with innate immune genes. Nat Med 2020;26:681–7.
6. Yang Y, Yang M, Shen C, et al. Evaluating the accuracy of different respiratory specimens in the laboratory diagnosis and monitoring the viral shedding of 2019-nCoV infections. 2020. Preprint. https://doi.org/10.1101/2020.02.11. 20021493.

7. Arevalo-Rodriguez I, Buitrago-Garcia D, Simancas-Racines D, et al. False-negative results of initial RT-PCR assays for COVID-19: a systematic review. 2020. Preprint. https://doi.org/10.1101/2020.04.16.20066787.

8. Woloshin S, Patel N, Kesselheim AS. False negative tests for SARS-CoV-2 infection - Challenges and implications. N Engl J Med 2020. https://doi.org/10.1056/NEJMp2015897. 10.1056/NEJMp2015897.

9. Bleier BS, Welch KC. Pre-procedural COVID-19 screening: do rhinologic patients carry a unique risk burden for false negative results? Int Forum Allergy Rhinol 2020. https://doi.org/10.1002/alr.22645. 10.1002/alr.22645.

10. DeConde AS, Yan CH, DeConde RP. In reply: navigating personal risk in rhinologic surgery during the COVID-19 pandemic. Int Forum Allergy Rhinol 2020. https://doi.org/10.1002/alr.22649. 10.1002/alr.22649.

11. Patel ZM, Fernandez-Miranda J, Hwang PH, et al. Letter: precautions for endoscopic transnasal skull base surgery during the COVID-19 pandemic. Neurosurgery 2020;87(1):E66–7.

12. Huang X, Zhu W, Zhao H, et al. In reply: precautions for endoscopic transnasal skull base surgery during the COVID-19 pandemic. Neurosurgery 2020. https://doi.org/10.1093/neuros/nyaa145. nyaa145.

13. Patel ZM, Fernandez-Miranda J, Hwang PH, et al. In reply: precautions for endoscopic transnasal skull base surgery during the COVID-19 pandemic. Neurosurgery 2020;87(2):E162–3.

14. Workman AD, Welling DB, Carter BS, et al. Endonasal instrumentation and aerosolization risk in the era of COVID-19: simulation, literature review, and proposed mitigation strategies. Int Forum Allergy Rhinol 2020;10(7):798–805.

15. Workman AD, Jafari A, Welling DB, et al. Airborne aerosol generation during endonasal procedures in the era of COVID-19: risks and recommendations. Otolaryngol Head Neck Surg 2020. https://doi.org/10.1177/0194599820931805. 194599820931805.

16. Howard BE, Lal D. Rhinologic practice special considerations during COVID-19: visit planning, personal protective equipment, testing, and environmental controls. Otolaryngol Head Neck Surg 2020. https://doi.org/10.1177/0194599820933169. 194599820933169.

17. Nogler M, Lass-Florl C, Wimmer C, et al. Contamination during removal of cement in revision hip arthroplasty: a cadaver study using ultrasound and high-speed cutters. J Bone Joint Surg Br 2003;85:436–9.

18. Garden JM. Viral disease transmitted by laser-generated plume (aerosol). Arch Dermatol 2002;138:1303.

19. Snyderman CH, Gardner PA. Endonasal drilling may be employed safely in the COVID-19 era. Int Forum Allergy Rhinol 2020. https://doi.org/10.1002/alr.22642. 10.1002/alr.22642.

20. Edwards SP, Kasten S, Nelson C, et al. Maxillofacial trauma management during COVID-19: multidisciplinary recommendations. Facial Plast Surg Aesthet Med 2020;22(3):157–9.

21. Hsieh TY, Dedhia RD, Chiao W, et al. A guide to facial trauma triage and precautions in the COVID-19 pandemic. Facial Plast Surg Aesthet Med 2020;22(3):164–9.

22. American Academy of Otolaryngology–Head and Neck Surgery. Academy supports CMS, offers specific nasal policy. 2020. Available at: https://www.entnet.org/content/academy-supports-cms-offers-specific-nasal-policy. Accessed June 24, 2020.

23. Vukkadala N, Qian ZJ, Holsinger FC, et al. COVID-19 and the otolaryngologist: preliminary evidence-based review. Laryngoscope 2020. https://doi.org/10. 1002/lary.28672. 10.1002/lary.28672.

24. Coronavirus Disease 2019 (COVID-19). Centers for Disease Control and Prevention. 2020. Available at: https://www.cdc.gov/coronavirus/2019-ncov/hcp/ framework-non-COVID-care.html. Accessed June 20, 2020.

25. Farid Y, Schettino M, Kapila AK, et al. Decrease in surgical activity in the COVID-19 pandemic: an economic crisis. Br J Surg 2020. https://doi.org/10.1002/bjs. 11738. 10.1002/bjs.11738.

26. Radulesco T, Verillaud B, Béquignon E, et al. COVID-19 and rhinology, from the consultation room to the operating theatre. Eur Ann Otorhinolaryngol Head Neck Dis 2020. https://doi.org/10.1016/j.anorl.2020.04.013. S1879-7296(20) 30103-30104.

27. Unadkat SN, Andrews PJ, Bertossi D, et al. Recovery of elective facial plastic surgery in the post-coronavirus disease 2019 era: recommendations from the European Academy of Facial Plastic Surgery Task Force. Facial Plast Surg Aesthet Med 2020. https://doi.org/10.1089/fpsam.2020.0258. 10.1089/fpsam.2020.0258.

28. Centers for Disease Control and Prevention. Interim infection prevention and control recommendations for patients with suspected or confirmed coronavirus disease 2019 (COVID-19) in healthcare settings. 2020. Available at: https://www. cdc.gov/coronavirus/2019-ncov/hcp/infection-control-recommendations. html#take_precautions. Accessed April 28, 2020.

29. Centers for Disease Control and Prevention. Appendix B: air. Guidance for environmental infection control in health-care facilities. 2019. Available at: https:// www.cdc.gov/infectioncontrol/guidelines/environmental/appendix/air.html. Accessed June 30, 2020.

30. Taha MA, Hall CA, Rathbone RF, et al. Rhinologic procedures in the era of COVID-19: health-care provider protection protocol. Am J Rhinol Allergy 2020;34(4): 451–5.

31. Frank S, Capriotti J, Brown SM, et al. Povidone-iodine use in sinonasal and oral cavities: a review of safety in the COVID-19 era. Ear Nose Throat J 2020. https://doi.org/10.1177/0145561320932318. 145561320932318.

32. Kim JH, Rimmer J, Mrad N, et al. Betadine has a ciliotoxic effect on ciliated human respiratory cells. J Laryngol Otol 2015;129(Suppl 1):S45–50.

33. Bidra AS, Pelletier JS, Westover JB, et al. Rapid In-Vitro Inactivation of Severe Acute Respiratory Syndrome Coronavirus 2 (SARS-CoV-2) using povidone-iodine oral antiseptic rinse. J Prosthodont 2020. https://doi.org/10.1111/jopr. 13209. 10.1111/jopr.13209.

34. Foley TP Jr. The relationship between autoimmune thyroid disease and iodine intake: a review. Endokrynol Pol 1992;43(Suppl 1):53–69.

35. Furudate S, Nishimaki T, Muto T. 125I uptake competing with iodine absorption by the thyroid gland following povidone-iodine skin application. Exp Anim 1997;46: 197–202.

36. Gray PEA, Katelaris CH, Lipson D. Recurrent anaphylaxis caused by topical povidone iodine(Betadine). J Paediatr Child Health 2013;49:506–7.

37. Parhar HS, Tasche K, Brody RM, et al. Topical preparations to reduce SARS-CoV-2 aerosolization in head and neck mucosal surgery. Head Neck 2020;42(6): 1268–72.

38. Kawana R, Kitamura T, Nakagomi O, et al. Inactivation of human viruses by povidone-iodine in comparison with other antiseptics. Dermatology 1997; 195(suppl 2):29–35.

39. Kampf G, Todt D, Pfaender S, et al. Persistence of coronaviruses on inanimate surfaces and their inactivation with biocidal agents. J Hosp Infect 2020;104(3): 246–51.

40. Maharaj SH. The nasal tent: an adjuvant for performing endoscopic endonasal surgery in the Covid era and beyond. Eur Arch Otorhinolaryngol 2020;1–3. https://doi.org/10.1007/s00405-020-06149-7.

41. Christopherson D, Yao WC, Lu M, et al. High-efficiency particulate air filters in the era of COVID-19: function and efficacy. Otolaryngol Head Neck Surg 2020. 194599820941838. https://doi.org/10.1177/0194599820941838.

42. Centers for Disease Control and Prevention. Considerations for Optimizing the Supply of Powered Air-Purifying Respirators (PAPRs): for Healthcare Practitioners (HCP). 2020. Available at: https://www.cdc.gov/coronavirus/2019-ncov/hcp/ppe-strategy/powered-airpurifying-respirators-strategy.html. Accessed June 30, 2020.

43. Di Maio P, Traverso D, Iocca O, et al. Endoscopic nasopharyngoscopy and ENT specialist safety in the COVID 19 era: the back endoscopy approach to the patient. Eur Arch Otorhinolaryngol 2020;1–2. https://doi.org/10.1007/s00405-020-06093-6.

44. Dover JS, Moran ML, Figueroa JF, et al. A path to resume aesthetic care: executive summary of project AesCert guidance supplement-practical considerations for aesthetic medicine professionals supporting clinic preparedness in response to the SARS-CoV-2 outbreak. Facial Plast Surg Aesthet Med 2020;22(3):125–51.

45. Russell CD, Millar JE, Baillie JK. Clinical evidence does not support corticosteroid treatment for 2019-nCoV lung injury. Lancet 2020;395(10223):473–5.

46. Clinical management of COVID-19. Who.int. 2020. Available at: https://www.who.int/publications/i/item/clinical-management-of-severe-acute-respiratory-infection-when-novel-coronavirus-(ncov)-infection-is-suspected. Accessed June 24, 2020.

47. Herman P, Vincent C, Parietti Winkler C, et al. Consensus statement. Corticosteroid therapy in ENT in the context of the COVID-19 pandemic. Eur Ann Otorhinolaryngol Head Neck Dis 2020. https://doi.org/10.1016/j.anorl.2020.04.014. S1879-7296(20)30104-30106.

48. Bousquet J, Akdis C, Jutel M, et al. Intranasal corticosteroids in allergic rhinitis in COVID-19 infected patients: an ARIA-EAACI statement. Allergy 2020. https://doi.org/10.1111/all.14302. 10.1111/all.14302.

49. Jiramongkolchai P, Peterson A, Kallogjeri D, et al. Randomized clinical trial to evaluate mometasone lavage vs spray for patients with chronic rhinosinusitis without nasal polyps who have not undergone sinus surgery. Int Forum Allergy Rhinol 2020. https://doi.org/10.1002/alr.22586. 10.1002/alr.22586.

50. Sweis AM, Locke TB, Douglas JE, et al. Management of chronic rhinosinusitis with steroid nasal irrigations: a viable non-surgical alternative in the COVID-19 Era. Int Forum Allergy Rhinol 2020. https://doi.org/10.1002/alr.22646. 10.1002/alr.22646.

51. Yan CH, Faraji F, Prajapati DP, et al. Association of chemosensory dysfunction and COVID-19 in patients presenting with influenza-like symptoms. Int Forum Allergy Rhinol 2020. https://doi.org/10.1002/alr.22579.

52. Yan CH, Faraji F, Prajapati DP, et al. Self-reported olfactory loss associates with outpatient clinical course in COVID-19. Int Forum Allergy Rhinol 2020. https://doi.org/10.1002/alr.22592.

53. Lechien JR, Chiesa-Estomba CM, De Siati DR, et al. Olfactory and gustatory dysfunctions as a clinical presentation of mild-to-moderate forms of the coronavirus

disease (COVID-19): a multicenter European study. Eur Arch Otorhinolaryngol 2020;1–11. https://doi.org/10.1007/s00405-020-05965-1.

54. Tong JY, Wong A, Zhu D, et al. The prevalence of olfactory and gustatory dysfunction in COVID-19 patients: a systematic review and meta-analysis. Otolaryngol Head Neck Surg 2020;163(1):3–11.

55. Sayin İ, Yaşar KK, Yazici ZM. Taste and smell impairment in COVID-19: an AAO-HNS anosmia reporting tool-based comparative study. Otolaryngol Head Neck Surg 2020. https://doi.org/10.1177/0194599820931820. 194599820931820.

56. Sedaghat AR, Gengler I, Speth MM. Olfactory dysfunction: a highly prevalent symptom of COVID-19 with public health significance. Otolaryngol Head Neck Surg 2020;163(1):12–5.

57. Speth MM, Singer-Cornelius T, Oberle M, et al. Olfactory dysfunction and sinonasal symptomatology in COVID-19: prevalence, severity, timing, and associated characteristics. Otolaryngol Head Neck Surg 2020;163(1):114–20.

58. Nguyen TP, Patel ZM. Budesonide irrigation with olfactory training improves outcomes compared with olfactory training alone in patients with olfactory loss. Int Forum Allergy Rhinol 2018;8(9):977–81.

59. Yan CH, Overdevest JB, Patel ZM. Therapeutic use of steroids in non-chronic rhinosinusitis olfactory dysfunction: a systematic evidence-based review with recommendations. Int Forum Allergy Rhinol 2019;9(2):165–76.

60. Soler ZM, Patel ZM, Turner JH, et al. A primer on viral-associated olfactory loss in the era of COVID-19. Int Forum Allergy Rhinol 2020;10(7):814–20.

61. Klimek L, Hagemann J, Alali A, et al. Telemedicine allows quantitative measuring of olfactory dysfunction in COVID-19. Allergy 2020. https://doi.org/10.1111/all.14467. 10.1111/all.14467.

62. Nestor MS, Fischer D, Arnold D. "Masking" our emotions: botulinum toxin, facial expression and well-being in the age of COVID-19. J Cosmet Dermatol 2020. https://doi.org/10.1111/jocd.13569. 10.1111/jocd.13569.

63. Cristel RT, Demesh D, Dayan SH. Video conferencing impact on facial appearance: looking beyond the COVID-19 pandemic. Facial Plast Surg Aesthet Med 2020. https://doi.org/10.1089/fpsam.2020.0279. 10.1089/fpsam.2020.0279.

Coronavirus Disease-19 and Otology/Neurotology

Esther X. Vivas, MD

KEYWORDS

- Mastoidectomy • Middle ear • Skull base surgery • Neurotology • Infectious disease
- COVID-19 • SARS-CoV-2

KEY POINTS

- The use of traditional facemasks impairs communication with hard-of-hearing and deaf patients because it restricts lip reading ability. Implementing transparent windows is a strategy to help mitigate this problem.
- Preoperative screening for COVID-19 guides providers and staff in the use of adequate personal protective equipment and may potentially delay surgical intervention in positive patients, a practice driven by reports of poor perioperative prognosis.
- Respirators are used during most otologic and neurotologic procedures; the need for routine controlled air-purifying respirator and powered air-purifying respirator use is uncommon.
- Alterations to standard microscope draping to mitigate spread of pulverized bone splatter during mastoid drilling should be considered, given the unknown risk posed by aerosolized particles from the middle ear and mastoid.
- Telehealth is an option for otologic and neurotologic patients. Examples are patients with cochlear implants, tinnitus/hyperacusis management, as well as atypical migraine and some vestibular patients. Neurotologic consultations are also feasible, such as treatment planning and surveillance of vestibular schwannoma.

HISTORY

At the time of this entry, the number of worldwide Coronavirus Disease-19 (COVID-19) cases surpassed 10 million; 2.6 million claimed by the United States. Those numbers are startling, and although many countries are seeing a stabilization or even decline in cases, the United States is currently facing a surge, with no end in sight. Our hopes are heavy on the development of a safe and effective vaccine.

The field of otolaryngology has been at the forefront in creating novel ways to deliver care due to our command of the upper aerodigestive tract. Scientific endeavors were jump-started by discovery of high viral loads in the nasopharynx.[1,2] We have had to

Department of Otolaryngology–Head and Neck Surgery, Emory University School of Medicine, 550 Peachtree Street Northeast, Medical Office Tower, Suite 1135, Atlanta, GA 30308, USA
E-mail address: evivas@emory.edu

Otolaryngol Clin N Am 53 (2020) 1153–1157
https://doi.org/10.1016/j.otc.2020.08.003
0030-6665/20/© 2020 Elsevier Inc. All rights reserved.

oto.theclinics.com

alter how to examine patients, from deciphering what is adequate personal protective equipment (PPE), to the way rooms are ventilated and equipment disinfected, to how we manage patient workflow to provide proper screening and implement social distancing parameters within the clinics. We have also had to develop new preoperative and intraoperative protocols, including alterations to well-established operating room (OR) setups. The changes have been topics of much discussion and approached differently depending on the nature of the facility, each taking into account the availability of reliable COVID-19 polymerase chain reaction (PCR) testing, adequate PPE, and staff resources. Not surprisingly, these factors can be vastly different when considering, for example, a large tertiary medical center versus small independent outpatient surgical facility. The wide spectrum thus prompts protocols that reflect internal resources unique to each facility.

Although those who routinely manage the upper digestive tract endured the most drastic changes to their practice, otologists and neurotologists have not been spared. At the height of the pandemic, when much was unknown and reliable viral testing was unavailable and PPE sparse, we faced a startling stop in outpatient and surgical care. What was deemed "elective" was suspended, and only urgent and essential care provided. Many dove into telehealth visits, albeit knowing that lack of an adequate microscopic examination or audiometric and vestibular testing limited diagnosis and treatment options. As time passed, however, we faced the uncharted territory of triaging patient care. When would it be safe to offer stapedectomies? Tympanoplasties or cochlear implants? Could that draining chronic ear wait a few weeks, or a month or 2? What about vestibular schwannoma surgery or repair of cerebrospinal fluid (CSF) leaks? We flocked to online professional forums and sought guidance from national societies and international colleagues, many with weeks or months of experience behind them, all with the intent to gather a collective voice.

Patients were understandably conflicted as well, anxious at the thought of going into facilities with COVID-19–positive inpatients. Elderly individuals and those with comorbid conditions were in a precarious situation, left weighing the benefit of getting a much-awaited cochlear implant for example, with the risk of nosocomial infection. It was not until there was reliable testing for severe acute respiratory syndrome corona virus 2 (SARS-CoV-2), a steady supply of PPE, and predictable inpatient hospital resource capacity that we phased back into the OR and clinics.

During this time, we saw a surge of society consensus statements and recommendations or guidelines that were difficult to implement because of the variability in loco-regional virus burden and health care capacity between states and even counties. Ultimately, many of those statements or recommendations found themselves quickly outdated as information about the virus evolved. Given the rapid evolution of the pandemic, at the time of this entry, the published data were too scarce to implement robust evidence-based protocols. This is particularly true for the otology/neurotology practice. In the following text, I review some of the changes to the practice of otology and neurotology in the United States, in the context of the COVID-19 pandemic.

BACKGROUND

Otology and neurotology as subspecialties are unique in that we manage a wide spectrum of acuity. From elective procedures like stapedectomy, ossiculoplasty, tympanoplasty or cochlear implants, to more ominous conditions like extratemporal complications of chronic ear disease or temporal bone malignancies. On the neurotology side, we manage cerebellopontine angle (CPA) lesions, some that present as small tumors, whereas others are large enough to pose imminent brainstem compression. Similarly, with CSF leaks, some present with a chronic history of relatively asymptomatic CSF otorrhea, whereas others are acutely ill with meningitis. Some conditions clearly need to be managed urgently, because the risk of delaying care outweighs the COVID-19 exposure risk, whereas others can be delayed without affecting the overall prognosis.

There are many considerations when counseling the surgical patient, but the reality is many of the procedures we routinely provide can be postponed for weeks and even months. Although we cannot postpone a large CPA tumor with obstructive hydrocephalus or a coalescent mastoiditis with extratemporal extension, we can certainly delay an adult cochlear implant or stapedectomy. The same wide spectrum that makes the subspecialty interesting, challenges us when prioritizing care, particularly when presented with months' worth of surgical backlog, restricted OR availability, and limited hospital resources. Each practitioner, therefore, must juggle unique challenges. What may be a barrier to someone practicing in South Dakota, may not be problematic in California because of the loco-regional variability in case density and health care resources. Similar hurdles can be experienced by private practice colleagues that cannot access resources available to their academic counterparts in the same city. As a result, it would be inappropriate to provide detailed or blanket statements on how the practice has changed collectively, but change has occurred in some way for all. In addition to this, the peer-reviewed literature is nearly nonexistent as it relates to our subspecialty. With that in mind, the following discussion is largely based on exchanges with colleagues via professional forums and communications from national and international societies.

DISCUSSION

Early reports of heightened infection risk to health care workers from aerosolization of viral particles produced by high-speed drills, most notably during endonasal sinus or skull base surgery, raised the question of whether similar phenomenon was applicable to middle ear and mastoid surgery.[3] Although there have been reports of corona viruses found in middle ear specimens, there have been no data specific to SARS-CoV-2 thus far.[4,5] Given the lack of data for SARS-CoV-2, many opted for precaution and instituted alterations to the clinic and OR setup to minimize spread of aerosolized middle ear and mastoid contents. Examples of changes include the integration of filters into clinic suctions, improved ventilation in clinic rooms, and novel draping in the OR, such as the use of tentlike coverage over microscopes to capture or limit droplet splatter during mastoid drilling (**Fig. 1**). Special anesthesia protocols for intubation were procured and the use of intraoperative respirators implemented. N95 masks with or without face shields and eye protection became the most common PPE used. Other respirators were either in scarce availability or were too cumbersome to use under a microscope, most notably as experienced with controlled air-purifying respirators (CAPRs) and powered air-purifying respirators (PAPRs). Ultimately, the specifics of PPE are usually left up to the surgeon and surgical team, a decision influenced by the facility's resources, surgeon's preference, nature of surgical intervention, and the COVID status of the patient.[6] In general, it is safe to say that although N95s have been used extensively, the role of CAPR and PAPR is limited for routine otologic and neurotologic procedures, but may be necessary on patients who are positive for COVID-19.

Another change to standard operating procedures has been the implementation of preoperative COVID-19 testing for all patients undergoing surgery. The most common

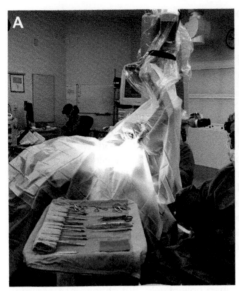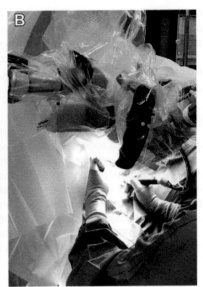

Fig. 1. (*A, B*) Microscope drape limiting splatter during mastoid drilling.

screening method is PCR testing from nasopharyngeal swab. The results help guide PPE requirements and also enable the surgeon to postpone procedures when possible for those found to be COVID-19 positive, a decision guided by published reports of poor perioperative prognosis in infected patients.[7,8]

Another change has been the implementation of face masks for all patient encounters. We have learned that consistent mask use, whether it be in the workplace or beyond, is critical in containing the spread of disease. This necessary practice has proven quite problematic by restricting ease of communication for patients who are hard of hearing because it eliminates the ability to lip read.[9] Due to the large volume of hard-of-hearing and deaf patients in an otolaryngology practice, the use of face masks with transparent windows is optimal. Although this may be a necessity for the otolaryngology or audiology provider, it is unlikely to be implemented by the rest of the medical community, as it is difficult to procure such masks.

Finally, the use of telehealth underwent significant expansion during the pandemic, particularly when shelter-in-place orders went into effect. Some institutions have been more aggressive than others with implementing these services, and although it may not be a viable option for all otologic or neurotologic patients, it has proven beneficial in specific circumstances. Examples of good telehealth candidates include cochlear implant follow-ups, tinnitus or hyperacusis counseling, and vestibular patients, such as those with established Meniere disease and lack of middle ear pathology. Telehealth neurotologic consultations for management of CPA lesions, already implemented pre-COVID by several institutions, is another example of a suitable telehealth candidate.

SUMMARY

The COVID-19 pandemic has required otologists and neurotologists to implement several changes into our practices. Due to the unforeseeable timeline in controlling the global pandemic, most of those changes are bound to be left in place for the foreseeable future. As more information on SARS-CoV-2 becomes available, we will need to continuously evaluate current practices to keep up with the changing face of this pandemic.

DISCLOSURE

The author has nothing to disclose.

REFERENCES

1. Hou YJ, Okuda K, Edwards CE, et al. SARS-CoV-2 reverse genetics reveals a variable infection gradient in the respiratory tract. Cell 2020;182(2):429–46.e14.
2. Zou L, Ruan F, Huang M, et al. SARS-CoV-2 viral load in upper respiratory specimens of infected patients. N Engl J Med 2020;382:1177–9.
3. Patel ZM, Fernandez-Miranda J, Hwang PH, et al. Letter: Precautions for endoscopic transnasal skull base surgery during the COVID-19 pandemic. Neurosurgery 2020;87(1):E66–7.
4. Pitkaranta A, Jero J, Arruda E, et al. Polymerase chain reaction-based detection of rhinovirus, respiratory syncytial virus, and coronavirus in otitis media with effusion. J Pediatr 1998;133:390–4.
5. Pitkaranta A, Virolainen A, Jero J, et al. Detection of rhinovirus, respiratory syncytial virus, and coronavirus infections in acute otitis media by reverse transcriptase polymerase chain reaction. Pediatrics 1998;102:291–5.
6. Howard BE. High-risk aerosol-generating procedures in COVID-19: respiratory protective equipment considerations. Otolaryngol Head Neck Surg 2020;163(1):98–103.
7. Aminian A, Safari S, Razeghian-Jahromi A, et al. COVID-19 outbreak and surgical practice: unexpected fatality in perioperative period. Ann Surg 2020;272:e27–9.
8. Lei S, Jiang F, Su W, et al. Clinical characteristics and outcomes of patients undergoing surgeries during the incubation period of COVID-19 infection. EClinicalMedicine 2020;21:100331.
9. Eby TL, Arteaga AA, Spankovich C. Otologic and Audiologic Considerations for COVID-19. Otolaryngol Head Neck Surg 2020;163(1):110–1.

Coronavirus Disease-19

Challenges Associated with the Treatment of Head and Neck Oncology and Laryngology Patients in the Coronavirus Disease-19 Era

Brandon J. Baird, MD[a],*, C. Kwang Sung, MD, MS[b]

KEYWORDS

- Laryngology • COVID-19 • Coronavirus • Head and neck cancer • Otolaryngology

KEY POINTS

- The landscape of ever-evolving information about COVID-19 during the pandemic has hindered the transition to normal clinical volume and efficiency.
- COVID-19 should not be a reason for delay in diagnosis or treatment with patients who have upper aerodigestive tract pathology or malignancy.
- The approach to resection, reconstruction, and surveillance for patients with head and neck cancer may need to be altered to consider severity of disease, patient comorbidity, and prevalence of regional COVID-19 infections, among other factors.
- In light of the significant number of prolonged intubations, there may be an increase in the number of patients who develop early and late sequelae of treatment of COVID-19. Tracheostomy should be performed in a safe and efficient manner when specific indications are met.

INTRODUCTION/HISTORY/DEFINITIONS/BACKGROUND

The downstream effects of COVID-19 caused by severe acute respiratory syndrome coronavirus 2 (SARS-CoV-2) have now pervaded most aspects of society and have made an indelible mark on the way that medicine, specifically otolaryngology, is being practiced. The disease represents a threat to an aging population throughout the world[1] but also has dangerous implications for providers.[2–4] Among the most at-risk group of medical providers may be those within the fields of otolaryngology[5] and ophthalmology. An otolaryngologist was among one of the first providers to succumb

Special Acknowledgment: Nishant Agrawal, MD, MS[1] for critical review.
[a] Department of Surgery, Section of Otolaryngology–Head and Neck Surgery, University of Chicago, 5841 South Maryland Avenue, MC 1035, Chicago, IL 60637, USA; [b] Division of Laryngology, Department of Otolaryngology–Head and Neck Surgery, Stanford University, 801 Welch Road, Stanford, CA 94304, USA
* Corresponding author.
E-mail address: brandonjb@uchicago.edu

Otolaryngol Clin N Am 53 (2020) 1159–1170
https://doi.org/10.1016/j.otc.2020.08.004
0030-6665/20/© 2020 Elsevier Inc. All rights reserved.

to the illness in its early days as it spread through Wuhan, China.[4] In light of the risk to patients, health care workers, and society at large, a push has been made to mitigate the risk of transmission within the field of otolaryngology–head and neck surgery.

As of September 15, there are a total of 29,723,564 COVID-19 cases reported worldwide, with a total of 939,137 deaths.[6] The United States has the highest number of cases, at 6,788,147, with the total number dead at 200,197. Given the high mortality associated with the novel virus, much of the world has enacted significant social distancing restrictions and facial covering mandates to curb the spread of the disease. The origin of the virus is not well understood, but it is thought that a bat or pangolin vector might have served as the primary reservoir.[7] The disease tends to be marked by fever (43%–98% of patients) and cough (68%–82% of patients)[1]; however, a litany of other symptoms also have been described, including gastrointestinal upset, diarrhea, shortness of breath, headache, and loss of smell/taste, among others. Severe disease is characterized by an acute respiratory distress syndrome, with a 50% to 80% mortality for patients who require mechanical ventilation.[8,9] The disease has a slight male predominance, at 58.1%. Severity of disease seems to correlate to age, because patients who are ages 1 year to 9 years have a mortality less than 0.1%, whereas those over age 80 present with a mortality approaching 15% in early studies.[1]

The nasal cavity and nasopharynx seem to harbor the highest viral load concentration[10]; thus, the nasopharynx is the preferred location for acquisition of samples for diagnostic testing. Nasal swabs, oropharyngeal swabs, bronchial alveolar lavage, saliva, and tracheal aspirates also have been suggested as possible testing sites.[11] The current preferred diagnostic assay is reverse transcription– polymerase chain reaction (RT-PCR), which has a variable sensitivity of 60% to 97%, depending on the institution and type of test.[11]

During the months of May and June, 2020, many cities, states, and countries have focused on a return to normal activity and a ramp-up of commercial activities. During this time, many otolaryngology practices have aimed at ramping up activity as well while employing telehealth, social distancing, and utilization of personal protective equipment (PPE). The American Academy of Otolaryngology - Head and Neck Surgery (AAO) recently published return to practice guidelines, detailed later.[12] As the world continues to move forward during the COVID-19 era, considerations, such as testing, including preoperative/preprocedure COVID testing; surgical triage; clinic workflow; and practice management, continue to evolve as more information becomes available. This review is intended to highlight some of the current recommendations for patient care within the laryngology and head and neck surgical oncology scope of practice.

DISCUSSION
Laryngology

As cases continue to rise, increased emphasis has been placed on protection for the provider in the clinical setting. Over the past decade, office-based management of many common laryngeal disorders has expanded significantly.[13] This includes, but is not limited to, office-based laser ablation of papilloma or dysplasia, transoral or transcervical injection laryngoplasty for vocal fold paralysis, and electromyography-guided injection of Botox for spasmodic dysphonia. Given the high number of clinic-based aerosol-generating procedures (AGPs) practiced by today's laryngologists, many providers have seen a marked reduction in their ability to treat patients and their clinical productivity. Within the category of AGPs is flexible fiberoptic laryngoscopy, one of the most widely used diagnostic tools for all otolaryngologists and speech pathologists.

A consensus statement reported by Rameau and colleagues,[14] from a virtual webinar attended by approximately 300 participants in the American laryngology community, recommended flexible laryngoscopy should be reserved for critical cases in which the findings may have an immediate impact on diagnosis or treatment. "Indications include hemoptysis, odynophagia limiting hydration and nutrition, or airway compromise—notably secondary to infectious and malignant conditions."[14] Some investigators have advocated for preclinic COVID testing prior to any AGP[4,14]; however, given the high false-negative rate of many available tests, the use of universal personal protective precautions is recommended. According to Givi and colleagues,[5] examinations should take place in negative pressure rooms if possible, with avoidance of topical lidocaine spray. A substitute to standard aerosolized anesthesia may be pledges soaked in 4% lidocaine and 0.05% oxymetazoline. The group also suggests using videolaryngoscopy whenever possible to keep the practitioner and the patient farther apart. Disposable laryngoscopes should be used whenever possible.[5] Most studies universally recommend the following PPE: N95 mask or powered air-purifying respirators (PAPRs), gloves, gown, eye shield (or goggles), and cap.[1,5,11,15,16] It also has been suggested that the patients wear a mask covering the mouth during flexible laryngoscopy to reduce aerosolization from phonatory maneuvers and in case of coughing or sneezing. At this time, transoral rigid laryngoscopy and mirror laryngoscopy are discouraged unless flexible laryngoscopy cannot be performed due to the increased risk of gagging and coughing as well as the need for patients to phonate with the mouth uncovered to allow visualization of the larynx. Additionally, universal masking is encouraged in all clinical spaces, in accordance with many state policies. Patients in the waiting rooms are encouraged to physically distance or wait in their car for a phone call prior to presenting for their appointment. Crosby and Sharma[17] also suggest offering PPE for the friends and family accompanying the patient during laryngoscopy, and certain hospitals also restrict friends and family from accompanying patients inside for the visit. Some alternatives to flexible laryngoscopy have been raised, including transcervical laryngeal ultrasound, which has a reported concordance of 70% to 95% in identifying vocal fold motion abnormalities.[18]

Another key consideration for the laryngologist in the COVID-19 era is the approach to sanitization and room turnover after AGPs. Laryngoscope turnover should include high-level disinfection, including the use of such chemical disinfectants as glutaraldehyde, chlorine dioxide, or ortho-phthalaldehyde.[14] Some investigators recommend immediate placement of the scope after use into a covered receptacle for transport from the examination room to the sterile processing areas.[17] After completion of laryngoscopy, room sanitization with an Environmental Protection Agency–registered, hospital-grade disinfectant is recommended, with a 2% to 3% hydrogen peroxide solution, 2-g/L to 5-g/L chlorine disinfectant, or 75% alcohol.[19] According to the Centers for Disease Control and Prevention (CDC) Web site, it is unknown how long the air inside a particular examination room remains infectious and likely relates to the room size, rapidity of air exchange, patient factors (like viral shedding), amount of coughing/sneezing, and length of time a patient was in the room.[20] The CDC suggests that rooms with 50 air changes per hour (ACHs) take approximately 6 minutes and 8 minutes to purify the air with 99% and 99.9% efficiency, respectively. As the number of ACHs decreases, the time between patients should be increased to allow for appropriate dissipation of theoretic infectious agents. As such, many hospitals have recommended a turnover time of 4-times the time it takes to purify the air with 99% efficiency, which may be either 20 minutes or 40 minutes, depending on the level of air turnover, or could be no additional time if any additional HEPA filtration system and negative pressure has been added. Limited data exist to support this approach for SARS-CoV-2.

Laryngology patients are quite diverse with respect to their level of acuity. Some patients require more urgent intervention, whereas others may have their care deferred.[12,21] Most guidelines advocate for a tiered approach to ramping up both clinic-based and surgical activity. AAO published guidelines for ramping up clinical activity on May 15, 2020. The AAO recommends limiting patient care to individuals with "time-sensitive-urgent and emergent medical conditions."[12] This approach is echoed in the care of head and neck cancer patients (discussed later). According to the guidelines, emergent conditions include "impending airway obstruction due to infection, neoplasm, stenosis, foreign body," which may warrant the following intervention: "flexible and rigid laryngoscopy with intervention, direct laryngoscopy/suspension laryngoscopy, bronchoscopy, and tracheostomy." Urgent conditions include "moderate or impending airway obstruction, progressive dysphonia, progressive dysphagia, glottic incompetence causing aspiration or impaired pulmonary toilet," which warrant the previously described procedures in addition to "stroboscopy, functional endoscopic evaluation of swallow, esophagoscopy with or without intervention, open airway procedures for cancer." Time-sensitive conditions include "T1 glottic carcinoma or carcinoma in situ, stable/mild dysphonia, stable dysphagia," which adds "transcervical Botox injection" to these list of procedures. Routine conditions that may be deferred for 90 days or more include "mild/moderate dysplasia, nonobstructive benign/phonotraumatic lesions of the vocal folds, glottic incompetence, glottic incompetence with mild to moderate dysphonia, gender affirmation, globus/cough without alarm signs." Comparing acuity of patients also raises an important point about the subset of patients who are typically seen for benign, phonotraumatic voice disorders. Many live vocal performance venues have shut down, concerts have been canceled or postponed, and some studies point to live singing as a potential source of massive spread.[22–24] For this reason, it might be assumed that the percentage of patients being seen for acute phonotraumatic voice disorders diminishes somewhat. Conversely, as patients continue to recover from hospitalizations related to COVID-19, it is anticipated that there may be several patients with sequelae of prolonged intubation, including posterior glottic stenosis, vocal fold granulomas, and tracheal/subglottic stenosis.

Laryngeal surgery in the era of COVID has had to undergo some significant changes in the approach to patient triage, surgical technique, and management of the airway. Preoperative evaluation of patients must weigh the risk of delaying surgery with the risk of complications related to COVID-19 infection. Lei and colleagues[25] studied a group of 34 operative patients, in whom all were COVID-19 positive within the incubation period. Mortality was 20.5% for this group, and 44.1% required ICU admission. All patients in this study underwent surgery approximately 4 days prior to demonstrating signs or symptoms of COVID-19 pneumonia. This suggests there is significant risk associated with elective surgery in seemingly asymptomatic patients who are infected with COVID-19. For this reason, many investigators have suggested preoperative COVID-19 testing,[15,26–28] although it is a subject of some debate. Some investigators advocate for a negative test within 48 hours followed by self-quarantine until the time of surgery, whereas others favor a negative test 48 hours from the time of surgery, and a point-of-care negative test on the day of surgery.[17] This not always is possible, given the limitations of the institution where the patient is undergoing surgery. As discussed previously with regard to PPE in clinic, universal precautions should be taken, including full PPE, and all patients should be presumed positive.

Airway management in the COVID-19 era has become a point of focus for quality improvement and safety groups. Endotracheal intubation is cited as one of the procedures that seems to have the highest aerosol-generating burden.[1,2,5] It is recommended that intubation be performed by the most experienced practitioner. Additionally, some investigators recommend early intubation for patients who are high risk for decompensation,[2] whereas others have advocated delaying intubation in favor of noninvasive means of ventilation. Non-invasive ventilation may include high-flow nasal cannula, which actually has minimal dispersion of exhaled air if appropriately fitted according to Meng and colleagues.[2,29] It is recommended that flexible fiberoptic intubation be avoided whenever possible.[30] Additionally, excessive bag-mask ventilation should be avoided due to the risk of dispersion of exhaled air. Furthermore, jet ventilation is considered particularly high risk and should be avoided if possible.[5]

Management of the surgical airway and the topic of tracheostomy has been well represented in the recent literature. During the SARS outbreak in 2003, open tracheostomy was the most common surgical procedure performed on infected patients.[31] Most studies seem to favor open tracheostomy over percutaneous tracheostomy[31]; however, consideration may be given for percutaneous dilatation tracheostomy in some patients if the anatomy is favorable and the practitioner has sufficient expertise with the procedure. Tay and colleagues[31] advocate for use of PAPR during tracheostomy based on the experience of 5 countries during the SARS crisis.[1] Other investigators[32] have suggested the use of an N95 mask, appropriate eye protection, gown, double gloves, and cap.[17,26] To decrease the risk of autocontamination, some investigators have recommended an infection control nurse be available to monitor donning and doffing procedures during tracheostomy.[31] Additional proposals include tracheostomy teams, which may consist of a surgeon, anesthetist, and scrub nurse, to increase efficiency and create an environment of consistent verbal and nonverbal communication (especially important given the burdens of communicating through a mask or PAPR). Portugal and colleagues[32] discuss a surgical safety checklist for performing tracheostomy in patients with COVID-19. The surgical checklist includes performing tracheostomy in the intensive care unit (ICU) whenever possible, decreasing the number of personnel in the room, and having a specific tracheostomy bundle in the ICU room to decrease the number of times providers and nurses need to break scrub to leave the room. They also recommend donning inner gloves prior to gown and outer gloves after donning gown to maintain clean inner gloves for the removal and disposal of the rest of the PPE. Two universally agreed-on maneuvers include stopping ventilation prior to entrance into the airway and holding ventilation until after the tracheostomy tube cuff has been inflated. Givi and colleagues[5] suggest that a smaller tracheotomy (6.0 cuffed) may be preferred to decrease the spread of aerosolized particles. Miles and colleagues[33] discuss the New York experience, suggesting that for intubated patients the cuff pressure should be checked every 4 hours, with a goal of 30 cm H_2O (greater pressure predisposes tracheal pressure necrosis). The group also suggests delaying the timing of tracheostomy until 21 days after onset of symptoms when feasible. Finally, some investigators have advocated for the use of specific air containment setups, including plastic draping, smoke evacuator tubing, or specifically designed negative pressure box.[15,34–36]

The field of laryngology has had to undergo significant change in the setting of the COVID 19 pandemic. As the numbers of COVID-19 patients have continued to increase during the month of June, it is clear that practice of laryngology in the post-COVID era will need to be carefully ramped up to protect patients and providers alike. Additionally, it would be expected that a continued increase in the number of recovered patients being seen for sequelae of prolonged intubation. Decisions to relax restrictions on flexible laryngoscopy and other AGPs will depend on the local incidence of COVID-19 infection, availability, and accuracy of preprocedure testing; sustainable supply of PPE; the ability to properly sanitize rooms; and, ultimately, development of an effective vaccine.

Head and Neck Surgical Oncology

Similar to laryngology, the approach to head and neck surgical oncology continues to evolve as more information becomes available during the COVID era. During the early weeks of the pandemic, the aspect of cancer care most concerning to patients and providers involved potential delays in therapy. Finley and colleagues[37] suggest that delaying cancer surgery should be done with extreme caution despite COVID-19. Additionally, delays beyond 6 weeks could significantly affect long-term outcomes and morbidity of treatment. Among patients diagnosed with severe COVID-19 requiring ICU admission, patients with cancer deteriorated faster than noncancer patients.[8] Desai and colleagues[38] discovered a higher risk of severe events in patients recently treated with chemotherapy or surgery in the past 30 days compared with noncancer COVID-19 patients. Additionally, patients with advanced-stage cancer tended to have a higher rate of severe events compared with early stage cancer. Cancer patients undergoing active treatment are predisposed to COVID-19–related complications, and critically ill patients with cancer have a higher predisposition to death.[9]

Head and neck cancer patients, especially, are considered a high-risk population for complications associated with COVID-19 infection,[8] making safe coordination of care difficult but imperative. Head and neck cancer patients are an at-risk group for several reasons. Silverman and colleagues[39] point out that head and neck cancer patients tend to present with advanced age, history of tobacco and alcohol abuse, and cardiac and pulmonary comorbidities, which are similarly found in COVID-19. Risk of respiratory sequelae in patients who have received chemotherapy and/or radiation therapy are high, with increased rates of dysphagia, aspiration, and pneumonia. Additionally, head and neck cancer patients have an increased risk of respiratory infections and aspiration pneumonitis.[39] These factors may expedite deterioration to severe adverse events in patients with COVID-19. Additionally, head and neck patients who are actively receiving chemotherapy or immunotherapy may have depressed immune function, malnutrition, and older age. For this reason, the patients need to be carefully selected and comorbidities strongly considered when constructing a treatment plan for patients with head and neck cancer.

Within the United States, mortality for patients of color (African American and Latinx) with COVID-19 is significantly higher than for white patients.[40] Unfortunately, this is a consequence of inequality within society and the health care system, rather than a biological or pathologic difference.[41] Correspondingly, these communities also tend to present with more advanced disease and have significantly worse mortality compared with their fellow white citizens. This pandemic has laid bare some of the gross inequuities within the American health care system and highlighted the need for equitable decision making for all patients with a diagnosis of head and neck cancer during the COVID-19 era.

Another consideration for the head and neck cancer patient during the COVID-19 era may include the financial burden and cost of survivorship associated with undergoing cancer treatment and financial hardship related to COVID-19's effect on the world economy and increasing levels of unemployment.[41,42] Given the significant job losses across the United States, there are preliminary data to suggest that there will be at least 1.55 million newly unemployed people who also will lose their insurance coverage in the wake of the pandemic.[43] Increased financial strain has been associated with decreased quality of life scores and subsequently mortality in head and neck cancer patients.[44–48]

Recommendations for head and neck clinic are similar to what was discussed previously for laryngology. Providers are expected to take universal precautions, regardless of a patient's COVID status. Flexible fiberoptic laryngoscopy is considered a high-risk AGP. Due to this, laryngoscopy should be reserved for instances in which it is likely to change management. One of the beneficial consequences of the COVID-19 era is the increased access of care through the widespread adoption of telehealth clinics among most hospitals.[49] Providers may use telemedicine as an initial preoperative assessment or prescreen for patients who will be seen later in clinic or prior to surgery. Although telehealth is wonderful for obtaining a detailed history, reviewing data/imaging/laboratory tests, and discussing surgical options/risks/benefits, a big drawback is the inability to perform a comprehensive head and neck physical examination.[26] Physical examination, with or without fiberoptic laryngoscopy, is important to define the extent of tumor and formulating an ablative and reconstructive plan. Fortunately, some work-arounds include anatomic and physiologic imaging for ablative planning and computed tomography angiography and virtual planning sessions for microvascular reconstruction. Telemedicine also serves a vital role in triage of post-treatment head and neck cancer patients who may not be able to be seen as frequently due to the pandemic.[5,12]

Telemedicine also serves a vital role in the coordination of care between multiple oncologic disciplines. Dharmarajan and colleagues highlighted the University of Pittsburgh approach to a virtual multidisciplinary tumor board clinic. This strategy has been adopted by multiple institutions, and works quite well to coordinate care between specialties. In their study, they found that 57.9% of virtual tumor board participants preferred virtual multidisciplinary clinic to the in-person format. Additionally, approximately 78.9% of participants indicated that they would prefer to continue the virtual multidisciplinary format once in person meeting restrictions had been lifted. Through multiple virtual meeting applications, practitioners can share imaging and laryngoscopy, which may assist with decision making for patients.

Similar to the guidelines published for laryngeal surgery, the AAO has published recommendations for ramping up clinical volume as it relates to triage for head and neck surgical oncology. Setzen note that most head and neck cases fall within the urgent category. The guidelines list emergent procedures as being tumor-obstructing airway, significant bleeding, acute or impending neurologic change, and salivary gland or deep neck abscesses. Urgent procedures (within 30 days) include all head and neck squamous cell carcinomas of the upper aerodigestive tract, benign tumors with impending complications or morbidity, anaplastic thyroid cancer, medullary thyroid cancer, bulky differentiated thyroid cancer with regional/distant metastasis, locally aggressive, or large nodules (>4 cm Bethesda 3, 4, 5, or 6), high-grade salivary malignancies, skin cancers, and parathyroid carcinomas with significant systemic effects. Time-sensitive procedures include low-risk differentiated thyroid cancer, low-grade salivary neoplasms, and slower-growing basal cell carcinomas in favorable locations. Routine procedures include benign thyroid pathology, parathyroid disease without significant systemic effects, benign salivary lesions, low-risk skin cancers, and post-treatment disease. Ranasinghe and colleagues[26] recommend a tiered approach to surgical triage, with more aggressive pathology prioritized in a similar fashion to the AAO guidelines. Similarly, the review recommends considering alternatives to long-duration microvascular reconstructive cases. It is recommended that the focus shift to simplifying reconstruction and reducing surgical duration, when it is feasible and appropriate. It also is acknowledged, however, that this approach may lead to an increase in downstream complications. Endocrine surgery is similarly tiered in a memo by Shaha,[50] which outlines a strategic approach to thyroid surgery during the pandemic. Similar to other strategies, anaplastic thyroid cancer, medullary thyroid cancer, and locally aggressive differentiated thyroid cancer, specifically with impending concern for airway obstruction, take precedent.[50] Some alternatives also are discussed, however, for instance, in patients with BRAF V600E mutations, who may have surgery delayed while being treated with appropriate targeted therapies. Additionally, de-escalation of surgical care is advocated for benign conditions like thyroid goiters that are nonobstructive and even papillary thyroid microcarcinoma (which may be followed with serial ultrasonography until resource allocation has returned to pre-COVID levels).

As institutions attempt to weigh the pros and cons of elective and essential surgery in the midst of the pandemic, some investigators have advocated for creating rating systems to allow for appropriate surgical triage during periods of limited clinical output and resource reallocation. The medically necessary, time-sensitive (MeNTS) procedures scoring system aims to "ethically and efficiently manage resource re-allocation and risk to healthcare providers" during the COVID-19 pandemic.[51] The scoring system, which uses procedural, disease, and patient factors within a 5-point Likert scale to determine the potential risk of proceeding with surgery. The cumulative MeNTS score may range between 21 and 105, with score above 64 considered within the high-risk or resource-heavy procedures, either due to patient factors (age/comorbidities) or procedure factors (head and neck surgical site, high anticipated blood loss, and ICU admission requirement). Using scoring systems like MeNTS should help hospitals triage elective and essential surgeries more appropriately and objectively in the setting of a resurgence of cases/limiting of resources.

Given the significant lack of available knowledge regarding SARS-CoV2 and its associated complications, it is difficult to characterize risk for patients undergoing ablative and reconstructive head and neck surgery. As discussed previously, in asymptomatic COVID-19 positive patients undergoing elective surgery, mortality approached 20%.[25] COVID-19 has demonstrated myriad manifestations that might interfere with the success and management of patients undergoing head and neck surgery. Tang demonstrated that coagulopathy was more common in patients with severe disease and nonsurviving COVID patients.[52] In this study, D-dimer, fibrin degradation products, prothrombin time, and partial thromboplastin time all were significantly increased in nonsurviving patients relative to those surviving COVID-19.[53] Additional studies demonstrate a prothrombotic state in certain patients, with 7 of 12 patients having deep venous thromboses on autopsy.[54] The mechanisms of this COVID-related coagulopathy are not yet well described in the literature; however, these undefined entities pose certain risk for reconstructive efforts in patients with head and neck cancer.

In lieu of significant surgical delays, radiation ± chemotherapy may be considered for certain patients. Administration of chemotherapy and fractionated radiotherapy, however, requires multiple trips to hospitals.[55] This potentially can expose patients, who already are considered high risk, to SARS-CoV2. Sharma and colleagues[55] stress the importance of making informed decisions, weighing not only the patient, comorbidities, and disease status but also the prevalence of COVID and resource availability when making decisions about preferred options for treatment.

SUMMARY

COVID-19 has forever changed the way that otolaryngologists approach laryngology and head and neck cancer care. Telemedicine has become an effective tool for the work-up of disease and interface with patients remotely. Flexible laryngoscopy should be reserved for urgent/time-sensitive cases in which it has a direct impact on management. Attempts should be made by all providers to ensure that appropriate PPE is worn and that universal precautions are taken for every patient, regardless of COVID-19 status. Given the high false-negative rate associated with nasopharyngeal RT-PCR, the role of preclinical or preoperative COVID testing has yet to be evaluated rigorously. Given the high mortality associated with elective surgery in asymptomatic COVID-19 patients, however, preoperative COVID testing is the best available option for triage of asymptomatic patients. Surgical decisions making should involve both the provider and the patient in a discussion about the necessity of surgery and other alternatives available in the context of the local COVID-19 landscape. Specific tools, like the MeNTS score, may be helpful to risk-stratify these patients and inform these decisions.

DISCLOSURE

The authors have no financial or professional conflicts of interest to disclose.

REFERENCES

1. Vukkadala N, Qian ZJ, Holsinger FC, et al. COVID-19 and the otolaryngologist: preliminary evidence-based review. Laryngoscope 2020. https://doi.org/10.1002/lary.28672.
2. Cheung JC, Ho LT, Cheng JV, et al. Staff safety during emergency airway management for COVID-19 in Hong Kong. Lancet Respir Med 2020;8(4):e19.
3. Adir Y, Segol O, Kompaniets D, et al. COVID-19: minimising risk to healthcare workers during aerosol-producing respiratory therapy using an innovative constant flow canopy. Eur Respir J 2020;55(5):2001017.
4. Vinh DB, Zhao X, Kiong KL, et al. Overview of COVID-19 testing and implications for otolaryngologists. Head Neck 2020;42(7):1629–33.
5. Givi B, Schiff BA, Chinn SB, et al. Safety Recommendations for Evaluation and Surgery of the Head and Neck During the COVID-19 Pandemic. JAMA Otolaryngol Head Neck Surg 2020. https://doi.org/10.1001/jamaoto.2020.0780.
6. Worldometer. COVID-19 CORONAVIRUS PANDEMIC. In:2020.
7. Shereen MA, Khan S, Kazmi A, et al. COVID-19 infection: Origin, transmission, and characteristics of human coronaviruses. J Adv Res 2020;24:91–8.
8. Yan F, Nguyen SA. Head and neck cancer: high-risk population for COVID-19. Head Neck 2020;42(6):1150–2.
9. Yan F, Rauscher E, Hollinger A, et al. The role of head and neck cancer advocacy organizations during the COVID-19 pandemic. Head Neck 2020;42(7):1526–32.
10. Yu F, Yan L, Wang N, et al. Quantitative Detection and Viral Load Analysis of SARS-CoV-2 in Infected Patients. Clin Infect Dis 2020;71(15):793.
11. Krajewska Wojciechowska J, Krajewski W, Zub K, et al. Review of practical recommendations for otolaryngologists and head and neck surgeons during the COVID-19 pandemic. Auris Nasus Larynx 2020. https://doi.org/10.1016/j.anl.2020.05.022.

12. Setzen G. Guidance for return to practice for otolaryngology-head and neck surgery part two. In: Setzen G, Anne S, Brown EG III, et al, editors. American Academy of Otolaryngology Head and Neck Surgery; 2020.

13. Tibbetts KM, Simpson CB. Office-Based 532-Nanometer Pulsed Potassium-Titanyl-Phosphate Laser Procedures in Laryngology. Otolaryngol Clin North Am 2019;52(3):537–57.

14. Rameau A, Young VN, Amin MR, et al. Flexible Laryngoscopy and COVID-19. Otolaryngol Head Neck Surg 2020;162(6):813–5.

15. Reddy PD, Nguyen SA, Deschler D. Bronchoscopy, laryngoscopy, and esophagoscopy during the COVID-19 pandemic. Head Neck 2020;42(7):1634–7.

16. UK E. Guidance for ENT during the COVID-19 pandemic. In: ENT UK at The Royal College of Surgeons of England 35-43 Lincoln's Inn Fields London WC2A 3PE Tel: 020 7404 8373 | Email: entuk@entuk.org | Web. 2020. Available at: www.entuk.org. Accessed June 10, 2020.

17. Crosby DL, Sharma A. Evidence-based guidelines for management of head and neck mucosal malignancies during the COVID-19 Pandemic. Otolaryngol Head Neck Surg 2020;163(1):16–24.

18. Noel JE, Orloff LA, Sung K. Laryngeal Evaluation during the COVID-19 pandemic: transcervical laryngeal ultrasonography. Otolaryngol Head Neck Surg 2020;163(1):51–3.

19. Chen P, Xiong XH, Chen Y, et al. Perioperative management strategy of severe traumatic brain injury during the outbreak of COVID-19. Chin J Traumatol 2020;23(4):202–6.

20. Control CfD. Interim Infection Prevention and Control Recommendations for Healthcare Personnel During the Coronavirus Disease-19 (COVID-19) Pandemic. In:2020.

21. Hogikyan ND, Shuman AG. Otolaryngologists and the doctor-patient relationship during a pandemic. Otolaryngol Head Neck Surg 2020;163(1):63–4.

22. Asadi S, Wexler AS, Cappa CD, et al. Aerosol emission and superemission during human speech increase with voice loudness. Sci Rep 2019;9(1):2348.

23. Marshall A. When will it be safe to sing together again? In:2020.

24. Waldstein D. Coronavirus Ravaged a Choir. But Isolation Helped Contain It. In:2020.

25. Lei S, Jiang F, Su W, et al. Clinical characteristics and outcomes of patients undergoing surgeries during the incubation period of COVID-19 infection. EClinicalMedicine 2020;21:100331.

26. Ranasinghe V, Mady LJ, Kim S, et al. Major head and neck reconstruction during the COVID-19 pandemic: The University of Pittsburgh approach. Head Neck 2020;42(6):1243–7.

27. Yuen E, Fote G, Horwich P, et al. Head and neck cancer care in the COVID-19 pandemic: A brief update. Oral Oncol 2020;105:104738.

28. Ota I, Asada Y. The impact of preoperative screening system on head and neck cancer surgery during the COVID-19 pandemic: Recommendations from the nationwide survey in Japan. Auris Nasus Larynx 2020. https://doi.org/10.1016/j.anl.2020.05.006.

29. Meng L, Qiu H, Wan L, et al. Intubation and Ventilation amid the COVID-19 Outbreak: Wuhan's Experience. Anesthesiology 2020;132(6):1317–32.

30. Bowman R, Crosby DL, Sharma A. Surge after the surge: Anticipating the increased volume and needs of patients with head and neck cancer after the peak in COVID-19. Head Neck 2020;42(7):1420–2.

31. Tay JK, Lim WS, Loh WS, et al. Sustaining Otolaryngology Services for the Long Haul during the COVID-19 Pandemic: Experience from a Tertiary Health System. Otolaryngol Head Neck Surg 2020;163(1):47–50.
32. Portugal LG, Adams DR, Baroody FM, et al. A surgical safety checklist for performing tracheotomy in patients with coronavirus disease 19. Otolaryngol Head Neck Surg 2020;163(1):42–6.
33. Miles BA, Schiff B, Ganly I, et al. Tracheostomy during SARS-CoV-2 pandemic: Recommendations from the New York Head and Neck Society. Head Neck 2020;42(6):1282–90.
34. Pollaers K, Herbert H, Vijayasekaran S. Pediatric Microlaryngoscopy and Bronchoscopy in the COVID-19 Era. JAMA Otolaryngol Head Neck Surg 2020; 146(7):1–5.
35. Canelli R, Connor CW, Gonzalez M, et al. Barrier Enclosure during Endotracheal Intubation. N Engl J Med 2020;382(20):1957–8.
36. Bertroche JT, Pipkorn P, Zolkind P, et al. Negative-pressure aerosol cover for COVID-19 Tracheostomy. JAMA Otolaryngol Head Neck Surg 2020;146(7): 672–4.
37. Finley C, Prashad A, Camuso N, et al. Lifesaving cancer surgeries need to be managed appropriately during the COVID-19 pandemic. Can J Surg 2020; 63(2):S1.
38. Desai A, Sachdeva S, Parekh T, et al. COVID-19 and cancer: lessons from a pooled meta-analysis. JCO Glob Oncol 2020;6:557–9.
39. Silverman DA, Lin C, Tamaki A, et al. Respiratory and pulmonary complications in head and neck cancer patients: Evidence-based review for the COVID-19 era. Head Neck 2020;42(6):1218–26.
40. Krouse HJ. COVID-19 and the Widening Gap in Health Inequity. Otolaryngol Head Neck Surg 2020;163(1):65–6.
41. Patel ZM, Li J, Chen AY, et al. Determinants of racial differences in survival for sinonasal cancer. Laryngoscope 2016;126(9):2022–8.
42. Gaubatz ME, Bukatko AR, Simpson MC, et al. Racial and socioeconomic disparities associated with 90- day mortality among patients with head and neck cancer in the United States. Oral Oncol 2019;89:95–101.
43. Baddour K, Kudrick LD, Neopaney A, et al. Potential impact of the COVID-19 pandemic on financial toxicity in cancer survivors. Head Neck 2020;42(6): 1332–8.
44. Woolhandler S, Himmelstein DU. Intersecting U.S. Epidemics: COVID-19 and Lack of Health Insurance. Ann Intern Med 2020;173(1):63–4.
45. Carrera PM, Kantarjian HM, Blinder VS. The financial burden and distress of patients with cancer: Understanding and stepping-up action on the financial toxicity of cancer treatment. CA Cancer J Clin 2018;68(2):153–65.
46. Fenn KM, Evans SB, McCorkle R, et al. Impact of financial burden of cancer on survivors' quality of life. J Oncol Pract 2014;10(5):332–8.
47. Kale HP, Carroll NV. Self-reported financial burden of cancer care and its effect on physical and mental health-related quality of life among US cancer survivors. Cancer 2016;122(8):283–9.
48. Ramsey SD, Bansal A, Fedorenko CR, et al. Financial Insolvency as a Risk Factor for Early Mortality Among Patients With Cancer. J Clin Oncol 2016;34(9):980–6.
49. Prasad A, Brewster R, Newman JG, et al. Optimizing your telemedicine visit during the COVID-19 pandemic: Practice guidelines for patients with head and neck cancer. Head Neck 2020;42(6):1317–21.

50. Shaha AR. Thyroid surgery during COVID-19 pandemic: Principles and philosophies. Head Neck 2020;42(6):1322–4.
51. Prachand VN, Milner R, Angelos P, et al. Medically necessary, time-sensitive procedures: scoring system to ethically and efficiently manage resource scarcity and provider risk during the COVID-19 pandemic. J Am Coll Surg 2020;231(2): 281–8.
52. Tang N, Li D, Wang X, et al. Abnormal coagulation parameters are associated with poor prognosis in patients with novel coronavirus pneumonia. J Thromb Haemost 2020;18(4):844–7.
53. Zhang Y, He L, Chen H, et al. Manifestations of blood coagulation and its relation to clinical outcomes in severe COVID-19 patients: Retrospective analysis. Int J Lab Hematol 2020. https://doi.org/10.1111/ijlh.13273.
54. Wichmann D, Sperhake JP, Lütgehetmann M, et al. Autopsy Findings and Venous Thromboembolism in Patients With COVID-19. Ann Intern Med 2020;173(4): 268–77.
55. Sharma A, Crosby DL. Special considerations for elderly patients with head and neck cancer during the COVID-19 pandemic. Head Neck 2020;42(6):1147–9.

Pediatric Otolaryngology in the COVID-19 Era

Steven E. Sobol, MD, MSc, FRCS(C)[a],*, Diego Preciado, MD, PhD[b], Scott M. Rickert, MD[c]

KEYWORDS

- COVID-19 • Pediatric otolaryngology • Pediatric ear • Nose and throat

KEY POINTS

- Families are afraid to leave their quarantined spaces and frequently delay needed care.
- Many system-based initiatives instituted in hospitals across the country have helped to mitigate risks and improve the patient experience.
- Otolaryngology has a unique set of conditions that make providers particularly vulnerable to upper respiratory pathogens.
- Managing children has several unique features, which potentially increase COVID exposure risk to the provider, including a high frequency of upper respiratory tract infections, asymptomatic carriage, and poor patient compliance with routine examination.
- Pediatric otolaryngology practices have been disproportionately affected by the financial fallout from COVID owing the specialty's elective nature and delays in receiving government financial relief made available to Medicare but not Medicaid providers.

INTRODUCTION

Although the majority of attention to the health care impact of coronavirus disease-19 (COVID-19) has focused on adult first responders and critical care providers, the pandemic has had a profound effect on the entire health care industry, including the pediatric otolaryngology community. As a result of resource limitations and social distancing measures, the day-to-day practice of pediatric otolaryngology has been abruptly altered, requiring rapid adaption to secure the health and financial viability of providers and their practices. The result of these adaptations has included the development of telemedicine, elaborate protective protocols to allow for limited

[a] Division of Otolaryngology, Department of Otorhinolaryngology–Head and Neck Surgery, Children's Hospital of Philadelphia, University of Pennsylvania, Perelman School of Medicine, 3401 Civic Center Boulevard, Philadelphia, PA 19104, USA; [b] Pediatric Otolaryngology, Children's National Health System, George Washington University School of Medicine, 111 Michigan Avenue Northwest, Washington, DC 20010, USA; [c] Division of Pediatric Otolaryngology, Department of Otolaryngology, Pediatrics, and Plastic Surgery, Hassenfeld Children's Hospital at NYU Langone, NYU Langone Health, 240 East 38th Street, New York, NY 10016, USA
* Corresponding author.
E-mail address: sobols@email.chop.edu

Otolaryngol Clin N Am 53 (2020) 1171–1174
https://doi.org/10.1016/j.otc.2020.08.005
0030-6665/20/© 2020 Elsevier Inc. All rights reserved.

oto.theclinics.com

exposure to potential aerosol-generating procedures (AGP) or manipulations, and a national discussion regarding how to resume "normal" practice following the peak of the pandemic. The objective of this article is to highlight the unique ramifications of COVID-19 on pediatric otolaryngology, with a focus on the immediate and potential long-term shifts in practice.

CARE FOR THE PATIENT

As the prevalence of COVID-19 increases throughout the United States, care for the patient in need becomes increasingly complex. Families are afraid to leave their quarantined spaces and frequently delay needed care. This practice may not only delay medical and surgical care, but also may cause a delay in developmental milestones. In the age of remote learning, apt medical care is an important component of keeping a child mentally and physically well. A child with unresolved chronic otitis media may have further speech delay. A child with chronic infections may be undertreated and not be able to perform at their best. Therefore, it is important that providers simultaneously help to protect patients from contracting COVID-19 and render essential pediatric otolaryngology expertise to those patients in need of it.

Many system-based initiatives instituted in hospitals across the country have helped to mitigate risks and improve the patient experience. Because each system is unique, the approaches have been unique to the individual system. The general concept of a better and safer patient experience is to screen patients before a visit to identify their medical needs as well as to screen patients for their and other patients' safety.

Telemedicine can act as an adjunct to in-person visits and helps to initiate medical care and carefully plan a further treatment plan. Once telemedicine has been initiated, the decision to continue remotely or follow-up with in-person visitation can be determined at that time because examinations are limited in the remote setting.

If in-person visitation is needed, screening procedures aim to decrease the risks to patients and practitioners for those coming to the office or operating room. Nearly all pediatric otolaryngology practices screen symptomatology and temperature routinely. Many screen and objectively test (via polymerase chain reaction) before office-based AGP procedures or any operative surgical procedure to ensure a COVID-negative patient (within the error of the test). Any screening or objective test that is found to be positive typically warrants rescheduling, unless it is considered an emergency and unavoidable. This process allows for the office and the operating room to mitigate risks and protect both patients and practitioners.

Other endeavors, such as decreasing clinic volumes, social distancing in the waiting rooms, and allowing time for air circulation to adequately clear the examination rooms of potential contamination, help to keep the office setting safer to cross-contamination.

CARE FOR THE PRACTITIONER AND THE HEALTH CARE TEAM

By its very nature, otolaryngology has a unique set of conditions that make providers particularly vulnerable to upper respiratory pathogens. After all, we are "ear, nose, and throat" specialists and we spend our entire work day literally in the faces of our patients. There is now an abundance of information suggesting that AGPs are a risk factor for exposure to a high viral burden, thus putting otolaryngologists at a high risk of contracting the infection. The unique risk of close patient contact and AGPs has resulted in the necessity to take immediate steps to mitigate risk to providers. In the pediatric otolaryngology community, this has meant the rapid adoption of telemedicine for evaluating patients and the development of elaborate protocols to mitigate risk of exposure with AGPs.

There are several unique features of pediatric otolaryngology practice that have made these changes particularly challenging. First, children are inherently more susceptible to viral upper respiratory tract infections and their sequelae. Whereas it is easy to set criteria to avoid seeing adult patients with respiratory tract infection symptoms, this is impractical for children because it is often the reason why they need to be seen. It would be impractical to obtain COVID testing for all patients with a runny nose who need to be examined in the office and, even if that were possible, we know that COVID testing has a false-negative rate of at least 3% to 5% in the best case circumstances.[1,2] In addition, current scientific evidence suggests that children may be asymptomatic carriers of COVID, which would indicate that prescreening for illness would not help to mitigate any potential risk to providers.

An additional unique feature of pediatric otolaryngology practice is that children are often not willing participants in the examination process. This factor creates an additional risk to providers because even a basic oral cavity or nasal examination can turn into an AGP in a screaming, gagging, coughing, or spitting child. To make matters more complex, the examination process most often requires close contact with not only the child, but also their caregiver, creating an additional exposure risk to the provider.

As stated elsewhere in this article, the risks of COVID exposure have resulted in the rapid adoption of telemedicine and safety protocols when physical contact with the patient becomes necessary. Although telemedicine has for the most part become a great immediate solution for patient access,[3] it is significantly limited by the same challenges that practitioners face with an in-person office visit; the child is often not a willing participant and if they refuse to open their mouth, there is only so much that can be evaluated virtually. In addition, much of pediatric otolaryngology practice is focused on otologic complaints and at this point there is no uniformly available replacement for the in person otologic examination. Although this process is evolving, most institutions have developed protocols that incorporate screening with or without COVID testing, social distancing measures, and cleaning protocols to minimize the risk of exposure to health care providers. A more in-depth discussion of these measures is beyond the scope of this article and is discussed elsewhere.[4,5]

It is becoming apparent that what we at first anticipated to be short-term adaptations to practice are likely to be with us for the foreseeable future. Therefore, it is very likely that the practice of pediatric otolaryngology will permanently become a hybrid of virtual and in-person visits, even beyond the acute crisis. The hybrid model does offer several advantages to both the patient and the practitioner in this time of unease. Its widespread use helps families to obtain initial medical care and treatment despite trepidation. It allows a patient–doctor relationship to develop despite distance. It helps the practitioner to triage those with more serious issues and to streamline their care. Currently, its disadvantages are that it is time consuming and limited in its ability to elicit a quality examination of the patient. On a positive note, as we develop technologies to overcome the examination limitations of telemedicine, this may become an attractive alternative for many patients (and providers) because it will significantly decrease the time commitment and cost related to the visit.

CARE FOR THE PRACTICE

The entire world has seen an economic contraction and the otolaryngology community has not been immune to this fact. Much of what we do is quality of life management, rather than immediately necessary life preservation. This factor is even more apparent in general pediatric otolaryngology practice, where complex, life-threatening, and/or cancer diagnoses represent only a minority of cases and where the bread-and-butter management is largely geared to improve patient comfort (ear infections), hearing (ear fluid), or sleep (adenotonsillar hypertrophy). During the acute phase of the COVID pandemic, both office-based visits and elective surgical practice abruptly ceased, essentially arresting the financial pipeline of otolaryngology practices primarily treating children. Even as we reintegrate into the clinics and the operating room, volumes will be significantly lower for the foreseeable future for a variety of reasons, including enhanced safety protocols, parental fear of taking their child to the doctor and lost family income and/or insurance.

In addition to a significantly decreased revenue, pediatric surgical practices in the United States have largely been left behind their adult counterparts in receiving government financial relief made available to Medicare but not Medicaid providers. To make matters worse, the majority of pediatric otolaryngologists practice in hospital-based settings and have, thus, been unable to obtain the small business loans available to others specialists who practice in a private practice setting. The net result of these financial constraints have led to significantly reduced personal incomes for physicians, the necessitation of reducing cost by arresting new hires and/or furloughing employees, and the reduction of expenses related to nonessential activities (meetings, dues, etc).

In summary, although the post-COVID framework of pediatric otolaryngology practice is unknown, it is highly likely that the new reality will incorporate telemedicine, enhanced safety protocols, new indications for direct patient contact, and reduced patient volumes. Finally, the economic fallout from COVID may result in a sustained contraction of general pediatric otolaryngology practice nationwide.

DISCLOSURE

The authors have nothing to disclose.

REFERENCES

1. Parikh SR, Bly RA, Bonilla-Velez J, et al. Pediatric otolaryngology divisional and institutional preparatory response at Seattle Children's Hospital after COVID-19 regional exposure. Otolaryngol Head Neck Surg 2020;162(6):800–3.
2. Vinh DB, Zhao X, Kiong KL, et al. An Overview of COVID-19 testing and implications for otolaryngologists. Head Neck 2020;42(7):1629–33.
3. Ning AY, Cabrera CI, D'Anza B. Telemedicine in otolaryngology: a systematic review of image quality, diagnostic concordance, and patient and provider satisfaction. Ann Otol Rhinol Laryngol 2020. https://doi.org/10.1177/0003489420939590. 3489420939590.
4. Mukerji SS, Liu YC, Musso MF. Pediatric otolaryngology workflow changes in a community hospital setting to decrease exposure to novel coronavirus [published online ahead of print, 2020 Jun 5]. Int J Pediatr Otorhinolaryngol 2020;136:110169.
5. Francom CR, Javia LR, Wolter NE, et al. Pediatric laryngoscopy and bronchoscopy during the COVID-19 pandemic: a four-center collaborative protocol to improve safety with perioperative management strategies and creation of a surgical tent with disposable drapes. Int J Pediatr Otorhinolaryngol 2020;134:110059.

Moving?

Make sure your subscription moves with you!

To notify us of your new address, find your **Clinics Account Number** (located on your mailing label above your name), and contact customer service at:

Email: journalscustomerservice-usa@elsevier.com

800-654-2452 (subscribers in the U.S. & Canada)
314-447-8871 (subscribers outside of the U.S. & Canada)

Fax number: 314-447-8029

Elsevier Health Sciences Division
Subscription Customer Service
3251 Riverport Lane
Maryland Heights, MO 63043

Printed and bound by CPI Group (UK) Ltd, Croydon, CR0 4YY

03/10/2024

01040404-0010